THE IRON DISORDERS INSTITUTE
GUIDE TO
HEMOCHROMATOSIS

SECOND EDITION

SCIENTIFIC ADVISORS:

Robert T. Means Jr., MD · P. D. Phatak, MD · E. D. Weinberg, PhD

Herbert Bonkovsky, MD · Ralph G. DePalma, MD

CHERYL GARRISON, Editor · Cofounder, Iron Disorders Institute

CUMBERLAND HOUSE™
AN IMPRINT OF SOURCEBOOKS, INC.®
WWW.SOURCEBOOKS.COM

Published by Cumberland House, an imprint of Sourcebooks, Inc.
P.O. Box 4410, Naperville, Illinois 60567-4410
(630) 961-3900
Fax: (630) 961-2168
www.sourcebooks.com

Library of Congress Cataloging-in-Publication Data

The Iron Disorders Institute guide to hemochromatosis / [edited by] Cheryl Garrison. — 2nd ed.
        p. cm.
    Includes bibliographical references and index.
    1. Hemochromatosis—Popular works. I. Garrison, Cheryl D. II. Iron Disorders Institute. III. Title: Guide to hemochromatosis.

    RC632.H4I76 2009
    616.1'52—dc22

                                    2009030761

Printed and bound in the United States of America.
                    VP 10 9 8 7 6 5 4 3 2

Contents

Foreword. vii
Acknowledgments. xi
Introduction: Hemochromatosis, A Common,
Under-diagnosed Iron Disorder .xiv

Part One: Iron—A Little Bit Goes a Long Way
1. Hemochromatosis: Not Just an
   Old Man's Disease. 3
2. Iron in Your Body 7
3. Our One-Sided View of Iron 16

Part Two: Detecting and Diagnosing Hemochromatosis
4. Symptoms and Clues. 20
5. Tests That Lead to Diagnosis. 27
6. Biopsies, Quantitative Phlebotomies, and Scans . . . 41
7. Benefits of Screening for Hemochromatosis. 47
8. The HFE Gene 51
9. Role of a Genetic Counselor 55
10. Who Is a Candidate for Genetic Testing?. 58

Part Three: Hemochromatosis and Body Systems
11. Liver, Spleen, Gallbladder, and Pancreas 64
12. Joints and Bones 77
13. Heart and Arteries 85
14. Brain and Spinal Cord 92
15. Hormone-Producing Organs: The
    Endocrine System 96
16. Skin, Nails, Hearing, and Vision. 103
17. Lungs 108
18. Immune System 113

Part Four: Challenges

19. Frustrations of Getting the Diagnosis—Part 1 118
20. Frustrations of Getting the Diagnosis—Part 2 120
21. Women Don't Get Hemochromatosis, Do They?. . 128
22. Heterozygotes and the Other Homozygote...... 140
23. Emotions Crowd Out Reason. 142
24. The Wrong Diagnosis 145
25. Multiple Symptoms That Can Prompt Diagnosis . . 148
26. You Must Be a Drinker. 153
27. Lost Opportunity: Elevated Serum Iron 155
28. Ignoring the Doctor 158
29. Ignoring Diagnosed Family Members 161
30. One Woman's Legacy 163

Part Five: Hemochromatosis: How It Was, How It Is, How It Must Be

31. How It Was 168
32. The Way It Is Now 189
33. How It Must Be 194

Part Six: Taking Care of Yourself

34. Finding a Doctor and Treatment Center 198
35. Treatment Routine: Phlebotomy and
    Blood Donation. 202
36. Specialized Treatment. 212
37. Diet, Supplements, and Behavior. 220
38. Being Prepared for Emergencies 237

Part Seven: Support

39. About the Iron Disorders Institute 242
40. Support across the United States
    and around the World 251
41. Role of U.S. Government Health Agencies 258

Appendix A: QUICK Checklist for Physicians 267
Appendix B: QUICK Checklist for Patients 269
Glossary 270
Bibliography 308
Index. 341
Contacts 349

DISCLAIMER

Content in this publication is not intended to be a substitute for professional medical advice, nor is it intended to replace the services of a medical professional or impair the relationship between patients and healthcare providers or caregivers. Content in this publication should be used as information only and be discussed with a medical professional, who is the only one qualified to diagnose and treat your condition. The Iron Disorders Institute, all contributors, and the publisher of this book are not responsible for the content on websites listed in the resources, nor do we endorse products promoted on such sites. We advise you to always seek the advice of a qualified health provider before making any changes to your diet or supplementation, or before starting any new treatment. Any application of the information or recommendations in this book is made at the reader's discretion.

Foreword

Until the discovery of the HFE gene and its mutations, hereditary hemochromatosis (HHC) was not a commonly diagnosed condition. However, we now know that HHC is the leading cause of iron-overload disease and the most common hereditary disease that affects Caucasians of northern European ancestry. The common form of HHC is due to a mutation at a single point in the HFE gene. Two of these mutations (known as an autosomal recessive condition) must usually be present in a person in order for that person to develop heavy iron overload. Such people have lifelong excessive intestinal absorption of iron, which leads to deposition of the metal in the liver, heart, pancreas, and other organs. Excess iron can be toxic and even fatal. Timely diagnosis of HHC and treatment with phlebotomy can prevent organ damage. Physicians can perform a simple blood test to determine whether a patient is at risk for iron overload. This test is the serum transferrin iron-saturation percentage (TS percentage). If TS percentage is elevated above 55 percent, a repeated fasting test should be run. If the fasting TS percentage is greater than 45 percent, the physician and patient should suspect iron overload and proceed with additional tests such as serum ferritin and HFE-gene mutational analysis.

Two mutations in the HFE gene have been linked to the hemochromatosis phenotype: the major mutation is called C282Y, and the minor mutation, called H63D, is less strongly associated with HHC. Iron overload occurs chiefly in people who have two copies of the C282Y mutation (homozygous, or

C282Y +/+) and less often in those who have one copy of each compound, heterozygous for both C282Y and H63D (C282Y +/– or H63D –/+). Tests for both are now widely and commercially available; the tests have helped to establish definitive diagnoses, particularly in patients and their families with the classic form of HHC.

In the United States, about 80 to 85 percent of patients with iron overload have the mutations in the HFE gene associated with HHC. However, many people who are homozygous for the major mutation (C282Y +/+), especially women, do not express the iron-overload phenotype. Then, too, there are other types of HHC (e.g., those occurring in black Africans or Melanesians) in which causative mutations occur in other still-unidentified genes.

Before discovery of the HFE gene and identification of the major mutations that cause HHC, physicians relied on liver biopsy for diagnosis because the liver is the principal organ responsible for the storage and detoxification of iron. It is also the first and foremost organ damaged by heavy iron overload. Indeed, the gold standard for the diagnosis of iron overload is still liver biopsy, to determine the hepatic iron index. The hepatic iron index is defined as the hepatic iron concentration, expressed as micromoles of iron per gram of dry liver, divided by the age of the patient in years. Values greater than 1.9 indicate HHC. Liver biopsy, however, is invasive and may, though rarely, be associated with complications. Furthermore, there may be considerable variability in measured hepatic iron concentrations in small liver samples from patients with cirrhosis. Genetic testing has revolutionized diagnosis of HHC because doctors can now make firm diagnoses in most patients without liver biopsies. Biopsies continue to be important to assess the presence and severity of hepatic fibrosis (scar tissue). However, among C282Y +/+ patients who have normal liver enzymes in the serum (AST, ALT) and normal livers on physical examination, when serum ferritin levels are less than 1,000 ng/mL, we now know that cirrhosis is unlikely.

We also have made progress in developing noninvasive methods for estimating hepatic iron concentrations. A dedicated device for measuring magnetic susceptibilities, the superconducting quantum interference device, is accurate for the estimation of hepatic iron concentrations but is not widely available. Although computed tomography (CT) scanning demonstrates an increase in the attenuation of the liver in hepatic iron overload, it is relatively insensitive to mild degrees of increased hepatic iron, especially if there is associated fatty change in the liver. Special magnetic resonance imaging (MRI) is a more promising noninvasive modality for estimating hepatic iron concentration. An increase in hepatic iron concentration decreases the signal intensity and makes the liver appear dark on typical MR images. Some centers now use a test called FerriScan, which uses special MRI algorithms to provide an accurate estimate of hepatic iron concentrations.

Breakthrough diagnostic approaches such as HFE DNA analysis and specialized MRI are revolutionizing the way we can help people with conditions of excessive tissue iron. We are still on the threshold of understanding the many details and intricacies of iron metabolism. We need additional studies of the duodenum (the main site of iron absorption), liver, pancreas, heart, joints, and brain (especially the pituitary gland) and of how iron-mediated damage contributes to chronic diseases such as atherosclerosis, cancer, chronic viral hepatitis, and other liver diseases. More studies on diet are needed to help us better understand the bioavailability and absorption of iron and which dietary measures decrease iron absorption and which do not.

Joint efforts by the scientific and medical communities, governmental health resources (the Centers for Disease Control and Prevention, the National Institutes of Health, and others), private industry, and national voluntary health agencies (such as the Iron Disorders Institute) can improve patient and physician education and research funding for such studies. Additional research and its translation into clinical care are the cornerstones of further progress.

This book is designed particularly for patients with iron overload and their families. It provides up-to-date practical information and is developed with laypeople in mind. The people at the Iron Disorders Institute deserve our thanks for the many hours of work that brought this book to fruition. For them, it is truly a labor of love.

Herbert L. Bonkovsky, MD
Chair, Iron Disorders Institute Medical
and Scientific Advisory Board
Vice President for Research, Carolinas HealthCare System
Professor, University of Connecticut and
University of North Carolina

Acknowledgments

The Iron Disorders Institute (IDI) Guide to Hemochromatosis is a reality because of the people mentioned here.

As I think back over the events that made this book happen, four people in particular come to mind: my father-in-law, Webb Garrison Sr.; Gene Weinberg, professor of microbiology at Indiana University and chair of publications for the Iron Disorders Institute (IDI) Medical and Scientific Advisory Board; my husband, Webb Garrison Jr.; and my son, David. Without their encouragement, patience, kindness, and generosity of time, this book would not exist.

Chris Kieffer, one of IDI's founding directors, and her husband, Harry, are two people who especially should be noted for their countless hours of time and talent. A particular contribution is the statement about hemochromatosis that Chris obtained from the former U.S. surgeon general David Satcher, MD. His was the first-ever public statement made about the disease. Dr. Shel Reyes, the U.S. Centers for Disease Control and Prevention, officially announced Dr. Satcher's statement at the Iron Disorders Institute IRONUSA 2002 Patient Conference in Greenville, South Carolina.

So many kind and generous people gave voluntarily of their time and talents to make the first and second editions of this book possible. They are Ron Pitkin, Paul Mikos, Lisa Taylor, Sara Kase, Regan Blinder, and the rest of the team at Cumberland House and Sourcebooks; Fran Weinberg; Kay and Mickey Owen; Donna Duncan; Dolores and Bob Forman; Laura,

Dick, and Matthew Main; Missy Kendall; Mary Jane Thomson; Bonnie Ritter; Sandy and Jeff Bowers; Julie Stegall; Ron DeKett; Ellie Leuthie; Jen Opperman; John McGruder; Barbara Taylor; Cliff Stitcher; Dr. Shel Reyes; Dr. William Dietz; Dr. Stephen Nightingale; and Dr. David Sundwall. Thanks also go to the Iron Disorders Institute Medical and Scientific Advisory Board: Herbert Bonkovsky, MD, chair; P. D. Phatak, MD, vice chair; Ann Aust, PhD, Utah State University; Bruce R. Bacon, MD, Saint Louis University; George Bartzokis, MD, University of California, Los Angeles; John Beard, PhD, Pennsylvania State University; Arthur L. Caplan, PhD, University of Pennsylvania; James Connor, PhD, Pennsylvania State University; James Cook, MD, University of Kansas Medical Center; Joanne Jordan, MD, MPH; Thurston Arthritis Research Center, University of North Carolina at Chapel Hill; Kris Kowdley, MD, Virginia Mason Medical Center, Seattle; John Longshore, PhD, Carolina Medical Center, Charlotte, North Carolina; Patrick MacPhail, MD, University of the Witwatersrand, South Africa; Arch Mainous III, PhD, Medical University of South Carolina; Gordon D. McLaren, MD, University of California, Irvine, and VA Long Beach Healthcare System; Robert Means, MD, University of Kentucky; David Meyers, MD, Kansas University College of Medicine; Mark Princell, MD, Spartanburg Healthcare System; Barry Skikne, MD, University of Kansas Medical Center; Gene Weinberg, PhD, Indiana University; Lewis Wesselius, MD, Mayo Clinic, Scottsdale, Arizona; Mark Wurster, MD, Ohio State University; Leo R. Zacharski, MD, Norris Cotton Cancer Center at Dartmouth-Hitchcock Medical Center. I especially thank Susan Leitman, MD, Warren G. Magnuson Clinical Center, National Institutes of Health. Other contributors include Vincent Felitti, MD; Ernest Beutler, MD; Naomi Howard; Sharon McDonnell, PhD; Francis Collins, MD; Elizabeth Thomson, MD; Priscilla Short, MD; Phyllis Sholinsky, MD; H. Ralph Schumacher, MD; Joe McCord, PhD; Barbara Bowman, PhD; Frank Vinicor, MD, PhD; Louis Heck, MD; Daniel Bailey, MD; Tug Nix; Chris Stitcher; Rosalie Yee; Bobby Montgomery; Johnny Taylor; Tom Mowell; Betty Thomas; David Remer; David Kitzman; Larry Archibald; Ruth Oakes; Vera Tanner; Mardi Brick; Carol Ann Gale; Caroline

Alexander; Rick Kauffman; Peggy Clark; Lee Woods; Stephanie Clary; Peggy Queen; Sherry Stewart; and Amy McConnell.

I deeply appreciate the hundreds of people who provided their personal stories, which gave this book its personal touch. These stories will no doubt ring familiar with someone out there who needs help.

Cheryl Garrison
Executive Director, Iron Disorders Institute

Introduction: Hemochromatosis, A Common, Under-diagnosed Iron Disorder

Hemochromatosis is the most common disease that most people do not know about. Mention of hemochromatosis generates odd looks, winces, or total disregard. The word *hemochromatosis* does not roll easily off the tongue. Describing the condition to a person unfamiliar with this devastating disease requires patience—that is, if you can get someone to listen to you. Patients with hemochromatosis quickly build up a knowledge base that they are eager, almost frantic, to share. This intimidates some or labels the person trying to convey information about a serious disease as a hypochondriac. Given that hemochromatosis can be easily diagnosed and treated, this is a serious concern.

Hemochromatosis is easy to diagnose, if you know how. It is easy to treat, if you know how, and it is relatively easy to manage, if you know how. So why is hemochromatosis such a mystery? Why is it not a household word? These are questions asked frequently by patients who wait years for a complete diagnosis that often occurs after seeing multiple physicians. Prior to the diagnosis, symptomatic patients may be labeled as hypochondriacs and shunned by family and friends, who avoid contact with whom they believe to be chronic complainers or "hemo-fanatics."

During a time of unprecedented access to Internet information, sometimes too much of it, physicians may be guarded or skeptical of a person showing up for an appointment with papers, books, articles, and a litany of diverse and seemingly unrelated symptoms. The healthcare provider might ask, "How can one person have so much going on at the same time and not be a bit unbalanced?" The evidence suggests that this is not uncommon. In a 1996 CDC survey of hemochromatosis patients, 12 percent were diagnosed as psychiatric, 17 percent were prescribed iron pills, and another 18 percent reported that they had taken iron pills (likely for a complaint of fatigue). Patients saw an average of three physicians and waited an average of nine years before a diagnosis was established.

Which brings us back to our original questions: if this disease is so common, why is it not a household word? If is so easy to diagnose, treat, and manage, why are patients still waiting for a diagnosis, being told diet doesn't matter and that iron supplements are harmless? Why are they not being treated by calibrated bleeding to reduce toxic iron overload, and why are some even dying because of missed diagnosis?

No simple answer to these questions exists, but the root cause of this difficulty is singular: failure to think about and then diagnose this disease. Barriers to sensitizing the medical community and skeptical family members remain a challenge even in this modern age of genetics and information access. One of the questions is, "Should we call it a disease or a disorder?" Patients prefer *disorder* or *condition*, but an unaware public might better respond to the word *disease*. Another barrier is that the groups needed to arouse awareness are nonmedical. For many diseases, drugs, procedures, and diagnostic aids are advertised and discussed at medical conferences and within clinical practice settings.

Symptoms such as abdominal pain, which can be associated with liver disease such as cirrhosis; frequent urination and unquenchable thirst, which are symptoms of diabetes; and heart attack, especially at an early age, are among the late effects of hemochromatosis. Chronic fatigue and joint pain are among the earliest complaints by patients, but these symptoms can be due to causes other than hemochromatosis and may therefore be overlooked if not considered in a differential diagnosis.

There is no drug for its treatment. Therapy for HHC is bloodletting, popularly regarded as a barbaric relic of the past. The concept of phlebotomy for disease triggers images of crude surgeries done by barbers or leeches strategically placed. As reviewed by DePalma, Hayes, and Zacharski in the 2007 *Journal of the American College of Surgeons*, Egyptians (1000 BC) used bloodletting to rid the body of "impurities and excess fluid." Bloodletting gained popularity by Greek and Roman practitioners, endured through the Middle Ages, and became the standard of practice for barber surgeons. According to Celsus (25 BCE to AD 50), "To let blood by incising a vein is no novelty: what is novel is that there should be scarcely any malady in which blood should not be let."

The red and white barber pole became a surgical symbol, related to a white cloth tourniquet and the flow of blood. Bloodletting arrived in America on the Mayflower and gained widespread advocacy during the eighteenth and nineteenth centuries. Lawsuits and heated arguments were won and lost, but bloodletting prevailed. On December 14, 1799, General George Washington lay dying after the onset of an acute illness treated by vigorous bloodletting. General Washington, who had a severe infection, insisted on being bled. His attending physician had removed one fairly substantial volume of blood, but Washington felt no improvement and ordered a larger needle and additional blood removed. It is reported that nearly two quarts were drawn; thirty-six hours later, General Washington died. William Osler, the author of *The Principles and Practice of Medicine* (1892) said about bloodletting, "During the first five decades of this century the profession bled too much, but during the last five decades we have certainly bled too little. Pneumonia is one of the diseases in which a timely bleed may save life." Osler continues, "Bleeding to be of service must be done early...in a full blooded man with high fever, the abstraction of 20 to 30 ounces (600–900 mL) is in every way beneficial." The 1935 edition of Osler's text, edited by McCrae, continued to advocate bleeding!

It would be many more decades before science realized the inappropriateness of bloodletting for patients with high fevers. However, even with advances in knowledge, for patients with hereditary hemochromatosis, therapeutic blood letting (phlebotomy) is still performed inconsistently and inappropriately. Many patients have also required liver transplantation.

Better answers and more action are needed. In 1998,

the Centers for Disease Control and Prevention and the Iron Disorders Institute partnered for hemochromatosis education and the training of healthcare providers. In 1999 the Secretary of Health and Human Services Blood Safety and Availability Advisory Panel declared hemochromatosis blood safe for use; IDI participated to bring about this significant change in policy. In 2000, Susan B. Leitman, MD, led a team of scientists including Janet N. Browning, Yu Ying Yau, Glorice Mason, Harvey G. Klein, Cantilena Conry-Cathy, and Charles D. Bolan to write a protocol for hemochromatosis. This was accepted and funded by the National Heart, Lung, and Blood Institute. In January 2001 the Warren G. Magnuson Clinical Center received its FDA variance, and included a provision for Double Red Cell Apheresis. Patients were referred to the center, and those who met the eligibility criteria were enrolled. The initial study group was 130 patients; 96 percent were Caucasian, 3 percent were African American, and 2 percent were Asian. All were homozygous for C282Y or H63D mutation. Of these 130 donors, 76 percent met allogeneic criteria.

During this time, The IDI Hemochromatosis Reference Guide was distributed to thousands of medical professionals by mail, personal visit, the Internet, and health system Intranets. This chart is among the most widely accepted hemochromatosis reference pieces used by healthcare professionals because of its medically reviewed content and illustrations.

As a result of a decade of policy changes, increased awareness, evidence, and expert diagnosis and treatment guidelines, the situation has slowly improved. Patients have become better informed and medical professionals continue to receive reference materials based on sound scientific evidence and expert opinion.

Ralph G. DePalma, MD, FACS
National Director of Surgery and Transplantation,
Department of Veterans Affairs, Washington, DC
Professor of Surgery, Uniformed University of
the Health Sciences, Bethesda, Maryland
Author: *Practicing and other Stories—A Memoir*
(Xilibris Corporation, 2005)

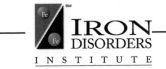

PART ONE

Iron—A Little Bit Goes a Long Way

1

Hemochromatosis: Not Just an Old Man's Disease

"Hemochromatosis, a disorder of iron metabolism, has been described as one of modern medicine's biggest oversights."

—*Dr. Randy Lauffer,* Iron and Your Heart

By the time John was thirty, he was impotent, depressed, exhausted, and experiencing severe chest pain. Before his fortieth birthday, he developed excruciating upper-right-quadrant abdominal pain, which added to his list of symptoms, now constant companions for John. He had seen five different private practice physicians and been to the emergency room on twenty different occasions. Of the countless doctors John encountered, most reached the same conclusion: he was a hypochondriac and needed psychiatric help. One physician, however, noted that John had mildly elevated liver enzymes and wrote "Hemochromatosis?" on John's chart, but he never mentioned the word or the test results. At the age of forty, John found himself undergoing shock treatment for severe depression. Now addicted to Xanax and inconsolably sad, he added to his expanding list of symptoms coppery-red skin and severe heart palpitations. John would not learn that he had hemochromatosis for another two years, at which time he would have advanced liver disease, permanent chronic fatigue, weakness, and extreme sensitivity to cold.

John is one of the numerous victims of undetected hemochromatosis. Once diagnosed, John thought back to his years in high school and recognized that delayed maturation and chest pain during his early twenties were part of the disease pattern for him. His disability and disease are due to years of unchecked iron accumulation, which was absolutely preventable, if only his physician had been knowledgeable about iron and the disorder called hemochromatosis.

What Is Hemochromatosis?

Hemochromatosis is an inherited condition of faulty iron metabolism. Individuals who have this metabolic disorder can absorb as much as four times more iron from their diets than can people with normal iron metabolism. The excess iron cannot be excreted; therefore, over three to five decades, iron accumulates to toxic levels (known as iron overload) in vital organs such as the liver, heart, joints, pancreas, bone marrow, and the hormone-producing organs of the pituitary, thyroid, and gonads. The unnatural iron burden in these organs leads to impaired function and eventually to diseases, such as heart attack or heart failure, liver cirrhosis or liver cancer, osteoarthritis, osteoporosis, hypothyroidism, hypogonadism, infertility, impotence, or depression. Without treatment, hemochromatosis will result in organ failure and death by heart attack, liver cancer, or multi-organ failure. Hemochromatosis is sometimes not diagnosed until autopsy.

The word *hemochromatosis*, used by most people in the United States, is also spelled *haemochromatosis*, which is used more abroad. The word is pronounced "HEE-mah-CROW-mah-TOE-sus." Some people, including several doctors, occasionally mispronounce the word as "HEE-mah-TOEMAH-crow-sus." Abbreviations for hemochromatosis include HH, for hereditary hemochromatosis; HC, for hemochromatosis; GH, for genetic hemochromatosis; and HHC, for hereditary hemochromatosis classic (also called hemochromatosis type 1).

Hemochromatosis is sometimes used interchangeably with *iron overload*, but there are distinctions. Some people state that hemochromatosis is a condition caused by iron overload, which is more in keeping with the origin of the word. Others state that hemochromatosis is a disorder that results in iron overload. This latter definition emerged after the hemochromatosis gene discovery and with the term *hereditary hemochromatosis*. Not everyone with HHC develops iron overload, and not everyone with iron overload has hereditary hemochromatosis.

Most people who are at risk for HHC are adult white men and adult white women who do not have a monthly period. The classic form occurs rarely in children, although cases have been reported. Type 1 classic hemochromatosis can be detected with a DNA test. Excess iron (or iron overload) can be determined by liver biopsy or with three blood tests: fasting serum iron, total iron-binding capacity (TIBC), and serum ferritin (SF). Blood removal—such as blood donation or therapeutic phlebotomy—is the therapy. With early detection, therapy, and proper management of iron levels, a person with HHC can expect to live a normal life span. Undetected and untreated, iron overload is fatal.

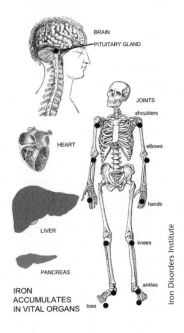

Recognition of hemochromatosis can be traced back to the late nineteenth century. In 1889 the German scientist H. von Recklinghausen noted a relationship between tissue injury, as in cirrhosis, and increased tissue iron. He termed this phenomenon *haemochromatosis*; *haem-* for "blood," *-chroma* for "bronze-colored skin," and *-osis* for "condition." A few years earlier in France, Dr. Armand Trousseau had noted a relationship between skin color and diabetes. Because of the bronze coloring of the skin, which seemed to accompany many of his diabetic patients, he named the condition "bronze diabetes." Many older clinicians and scientists still use *hemochromatosis* and *bronze diabetes* interchangeably.

In the early 1920s, Dr. A. S. Strachan, of Scotland, observed iron overload in Bantu-speaking people of Africa. Strachan believed that these individuals were becoming iron loaded because they consumed a traditional, home-brewed beer that was prepared in large iron pots. He speculated that filings from the pots were mixing with the beer and causing iron overload in those who drank large quantities of the beverage. Later termed *African siderosis* and classified as an important type of iron overload in sub-Saharan Africans, no genetic connection to the HFE gene could be made in this group. In the United States, however, there are cases of African Americans who are HFE heterozygote (i.e., inherited one copy of a gene mutation) and homozygote (i.e., inherited two copies of a gene mutation) because of the genetic admixture that occurred after Africans arrived in the Americas as slaves. The ancestors of many African Americans with these genotypes were born in the southern states of Alabama, Mississippi, Georgia, and South Carolina.

Finally, in 1927 the British physician J. H. Sheldon suggested that an inherited metabolic disorder causes iron deposition. He conducted an exhaustive review of opinion, compiling all the information he could obtain on the subject of hemochromatosis. In 1935 Sheldon published his consolidated effort in an Oxford University Press book titled simply *Haemochromatosis*. In this monograph, Sheldon wrote, "The most reasonable explanation of haemochromatosis is that it should be classed as an inborn error of metabolism, which has an overwhelming incidence in males, and which at times actually has a familial incidence." In 1996 Sheldon's observation was confirmed with the discovery of HFE, the principal gene for HHC.

2

Iron in Your Body

If you had to describe iron to someone, how would you do it? You might say that iron is the second most common mineral on Earth and the stuff used to make magnets, barbells, nails, the rust stains in your bathtub, bridges, tall buildings, and even Granny's skillet. Or would you add that iron is a pill you can take to correct iron-deficiency anemia? All of these descriptions are correct. However, you may not know that iron is a metal so essential that, without it, most life on this planet would cease to exist. Plants would wither and die; animals and human beings would suffocate.

Plants require iron to make chlorophyll. Plants, animals, and human beings require iron to make DNA, which encodes all life. Animals and humans also need iron to make hemoglobin, which delivers oxygen to the body, and we need iron to make myoglobin in muscles. Myoglobin is a protein like hemoglobin, except that it is an oxygen-storage protein contained in muscles of the body. We call on the oxygen stored in myoglobin when we use our muscles to walk, run, climb, or move in any way.

In contrast, iron can be so deadly that only 450 milligrams can poison a small child. Too much iron absorbed from diet, injections, or repeated blood transfusions can accumulate to levels that rust the vital organs and cause them to fail. Remember that streak of iron in the bathtub? That's rust, or iron oxide; the same thing can be present in your liver, joints, pancreas, heart, brain, lungs, and skin if too much iron gets into your system.

So what is this magical but potentially lethal metal? Where does it come from, and how do we get it? Iron is a metallic element found in plants, animals, soil, meteorites, and rocks, including ones found on the surface of the moon. Here on Earth, plants absorb iron through their root systems, animals eat those plants, and humans consume those plants and animals.

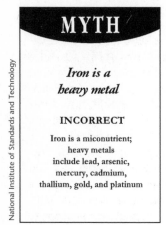

MYTH

Iron is a heavy metal

INCORRECT

Iron is a miconutrient; heavy metals include lead, arsenic, mercury, cadmium, thallium, gold, and platinum

Most of us can get sufficient amounts of iron from daily diets that include a moderate amount of meat. However, humans can get iron in other ways that might be harmful. We can inhale it in first- or secondhand tobacco smoke, take excessive amounts of supplemental iron, or receive iron by injection or in blood transfusions. We can also drink too much alcohol, which enhances iron absorption and impairs the body's ability to produce sufficient antioxidants.

Some Forms of Iron Must Be Changed to Be Absorbed
Iron in Granny's skillet is elemental iron. This form of iron cannot be absorbed by the body; the iron must be oxidized, or changed, by being united with oxygen. Bound with oxygen, elemental iron becomes ferric oxide, or common rust. The body cannot absorb iron in this form either. The body must change iron into ferrous iron, which occurs when ferric oxide is exposed to an acidic environment. This change is accomplished in the stomach, where ferric oxide mixes with adequate hydrochloric acid (HCl, or stomach acid).

Iron Is Ready to Be Absorbed, Bound, and Transported
Iron moves out of the stomach into the duodenum, the portion of the small intestine where the majority of absorption takes place. The body is able to absorb ferrous iron in the duodenum. With the exception of a small amount of absorption that may take place later in the digestive system, all other iron continues on to be excreted. Absorbed iron is grabbed by fingerlike

8

projections called villi, which line the surface of the intestinal wall. Villi can pull iron into cells that then pass the metal into the bloodstream, where it is met by the transport protein molecule transferrin. Each molecule of transferrin can bind with and carry two atoms of iron.

Iron Transport and Use

Scientists have been studying iron transport since the early 1940s. Two New York scientists, A. L. Schade and L. Caroline, noted an anti-infective agent in human plasma. They called it siderophilin, and that name was later changed to transferrin. The term *siderophilin* also applies to lactoferrin. Transferrin and lactoferrin form a unique class of proteins. Transferrin is the best-known transporter protein for iron, though other candidate transport proteins are on the scientific horizon.

Lactoferrin is found in human secretions, such as tears, perspiration, vaginal fluid, and mother's milk. It binds with iron, but lactoferrin is not considered a transporter of iron; instead, the role of lactoferrin is mainly defense related. Lactoferrin can withhold iron from invading microorganisms. However, *Helicobacter pylori*, a bacterial cause of gastric ulcers, actually seeks out lactoferrin-bound iron contained in the lining of the stomach. Lactoferrin-bound iron gives *H. pylori* its initial nourishment, enabling the microorganism to bore through the stomach wall, where it then obtains iron directly from hemoglobin.

Normally, transferrin is about 25 to 35 percent saturated with the metal, but trouble can develop when too much iron is there for transferrin to carry. Transferrin molecules that are heavily saturated lose the ability to bind iron tightly. Uncontrolled iron (or iron that is unbound or contained) is highly destructive and dangerous. Unbound iron can trigger free-radical activity, which can cause cell death and destroy DNA. Free iron can also provide nourishment for pathogens.

When working normally, one molecule of transferrin binds to two molecules of iron and transports the iron to various places in the body, such as the liver and bone marrow, so that normal metabolism, DNA synthesis, and red-blood-cell production can take place. Research has discovered that transferrin does not work completely alone in the transport of iron. Ceruloplasmin, a protein that binds with copper, is also involved in iron transport. Iron needs adequate amounts of copper to reach some of its intended destinations, such as the brain.

The protein transporters called divalent metal transport ions (DMT1) were observed in mice and rats to have an iron-binding and iron-transport ability. However, DMT1 activity seems to occur at a different phase of iron's journey. Some scientists theorize that there is more than one pathway through which iron is transported. Speculation is that, because there are different types of iron, there is more than one pathway available for transport. In any event, absorbed iron that is not needed for metabolism, production of DNA, or hemoglobin synthesis is placed in ferritin within cells.

Contained for Future Use or to Protect Us

Ferritin is a protein that nearly every cell of the body produces. It is a huge molecule: one ferritin molecule alone can hold up to 4,500 atoms of iron. Ferritin serves as a containment device for iron when it is in ample quantity or when there can be some potential harm to one's health. Elevated serum ferritin is an indicator that disease or disease-causing microorganisms are present.

Like transferrin, ferritin can also become unstable and ineffective. Ferritin is like a big sink; when the sink gets full, the body can change ferritin and its iron into a precipitate called hemosiderin.

Hemosiderin can accumulate in cells of the heart, liver, lungs, pancreas, joint synovia, and anterior pituitary, thereby restricting the ability of these organs to function. For example, when beta cells (insulin-producing cells of the pancreas) are loaded with hemosiderin, the cells become unable to produce or store adequate amounts of the hormone insulin, which results in diabetes mellitus.

Scientists can obtain small amounts of tissue with a needle biopsy, stain it, and see hemosiderin in cells. For hemosiderin to be removed, it must be placed back into ferritin, which then can release the metal to form hemoglobin, which then can be removed by phlebotomy.

Clearly, excessive accumulation of iron endangers health, but iron can be harmful to a person's health in other ways as well.

Oxidative Stress or Free-Radical Activity

Iron can reduce or change oxygen in two ways. First, as a chemical component of heme in hemoglobin, iron is able to carry oxygen throughout the body. Behaving in this way, iron is a lifesaver. However, free or unbound iron can produce free radicals that can damage cells.

Free radicals are atoms or a group of atoms that have at least one unpaired electron and are normal by-products of human metabolism as oxygen is utilized. More stable and less reactive chemical structures as a rule have all of their electrons paired to one another. Free radicals are on the hunt for an additional electron and are highly reactive with other chemicals in the body.

Programmed from their creation to find their missing parts, free radicals steal electrons from anywhere in the body to make up for the missing partner. The free radicals can steal from any cell in any organ, including the heart, pancreas, brain, liver, joints, and so on. They can also change the structure of DNA. Once DNA is changed or mutated, it is passed on in the mutated form to all future generations. The free radical doesn't care about preserving a human cell or DNA; it only wants its missing part. Ravaged atoms within the cell then also are missing a part, which creates a chain reaction of unleashed free-radical activity, oxidation, and oxidative stress at increasing speed.

Examples of oxidation include rotting foods and rust you might see on a car or lawn furniture. Often oxidation sets off chain reactions—as in the case of the oxidation of fats—with one radical causing the destruction of hundreds or thousands of previously normal molecules. Iron-triggered free-radical activity can contribute to liver disease, pancreatic burnout (type 2 diabetes), joint disease, heart disease, neurological problems, osteoporosis, sarcopenia, and accelerated aging, to name a few of the consequences of oxidative stress on the body.

Antioxidants protect the body from free-radical damage. An antioxidant donates or gives up the sought-after electron to a free radical and renders it harmless. Our bodies both manufacture antioxidants and obtain them from the fresh fruits and vegetables in our diets. When our diets lack fresh fruits and vegetables or are high in fats and sugars, we can have an overabundance of free-radical activity.

Taking antioxidants, however, is not enough for those with elevated iron levels. Removing excess iron from the body is the only way to lower the risk of disease for such individuals. Excess levels of iron can be removed through therapeutic phlebotomy, regular blood donation, or in rare cases iron-chelation therapy.

Unabsorbed Iron

In normal iron metabolism, unabsorbed iron, or about 90 percent of iron ingested through diet, is taken up by specific cells called enterocytes in the intestinal tract. These cells become engorged with iron, die, drop off, and are excreted in feces. The portion of iron that is absorbed is in the form of heme from consumed meat, nonheme from the plants we eat, and inorganic or chelated iron from supplements and food additives.

How Much Iron Is in the Body?

Men have about 4 grams of iron in their body, women have about 3.5 grams, and children usually have 3 grams or less. The 3 to 4 grams are distributed throughout the body in hemoglobin, tissue, muscles, bone marrow, blood proteins, enzymes, ferritin, hemosiderin, and transport in plasma.

IRON DISTRIBUTION	males 4 grams females 3.5 grams children 3 grams
hemoglobin	70%
myoglobin and enzymes	15%
ferritin	14%
transit in serum	1%

U.S. Centers for Disease Control and Prevention

The greatest portion of iron in a normal human being is in hemoglobin. Except in cases of great blood loss, pregnancy, or growth spurts, for which larger amounts of iron are required, our bodies only need about 1 to 1.5 milligrams of iron per day to replace what is lost. Normal daily excretion of iron through urine, vaginal fluid, sweat, feces, and tears totals about 1 to 1.5

milligrams, or the equivalent of what most of us require per day to function normally. Tiny amounts of iron can also be lost because of blood loss when medicines such as aspirin are used regularly.

Our natural iron-regulatory mechanisms are elaborate, but when they are functioning normally, the mechanisms ensure proper iron balance. These systems step up absorption when the need is great, lower absorption when iron levels are adequate, and protect us by withholding iron from harmful invaders, such as bacteria or cancer cells.

The average daily diet of an American vegetarian contains about 6 to 10 milligrams of iron. American nonvegetarian daily diets, which contain meat with most meals, are reported to contain up to 23.5 milligrams of iron. Iron is not easily absorbed unless one has a metabolic disorder associated with iron loading like hemochromatosis.

Daily Intakes of Iron

The RDA for iron and all other nutrients is established by the Food and Nutrition Board of the National Academies. You may also see references to Dietary Reference Intakes (DRI), Estimated Average Requirement (EAR), Adequate Intake (AI) level, and Tolerable Upper Intake Level (UL). The RDA represents a daily nutrient intake goal for healthy individuals that should prevent deficiency disease in 97 percent of the healthy population.

Tolerable upper intake level (UL) represents a ceiling—the largest amount of a nutrient that healthy individuals can take each day without being placed at increased risk of adverse health effects or any kind of adverse reaction (negative side effect). **The UL for iron is 45 milligrams per day**, based on findings of adverse gastrointestinal effects, such as constipation and nausea

U.S. Centers for Desease Control and Prevention RDA-IRON 1989	
Age in Years	1989 RDA (mg/day)
FEMALES AND MALES	
<1	6-10
1-5	10
FEMALES ONLY	
6-11	10
12-49	15
50->70	10
MALES ONLY	
6-11	10
12-19	12
20->70	10

U.S. Centers for Disease Control and Prevention

13

that can occur when consuming iron supplements, especially when taken on an empty stomach.

Some nutrients that are not easily absorbed, such as iron, receive higher recommended dietary allowances (RDAs) (now referred to as dietary reference intake [DRI]) from the U.S. Department of Agriculture (USDA) in an attempt to ensure that people ingest adequate amounts of the essential nutrient within the course of a day. Attempts to meet daily requirements by ingesting quantities of iron that exceed daily need are, for many people, a waste of time and money. Humans have a natural regulatory mechanism that controls the amount of iron absorbed according to individual needs. Under normal metabolic circumstances, when we take in large amounts of supplemental iron the regulatory mechanism signals the body to absorb less of the metal. Continuing to take large doses of unneeded iron simply causes stomach and intestinal discomfort without added benefit.

Drs. Fariba Roughead and Janet Hunt, of the USDA's Grand Forks Human Nutrition Research Center, demonstrated this mechanism at work in people with normal iron metabolism. In a randomized, placebo-controlled trial, heme and nonheme iron absorption by healthy men and women were measured from a test meal containing a hamburger, potatoes, and milkshake. The absorption measurements were made before and after a period of twelve weeks, when the fifty-seven participants were given 50 milligrams of supplemental iron or placebo daily while they consumed their usual diets.

Serum ferritin and fecal ferritin were measured during supplementation and for six months after supplementation was discontinued. Volunteers who took iron supplements, even those with initial ferritin of less than 21 ng/mL, adapted to absorb less nonheme iron but not less heme iron from meat.

Daily iron supplements caused the volunteers to absorb 36 percent less nonheme iron and 25 percent less total iron from food, and to have higher iron stores than those in the placebo group. The higher ferritin levels persisted for six months post-supplementation, except in individuals who had low iron stores at the beginning of the study. Because iron stores were greater after iron supplementation, the study demonstrated

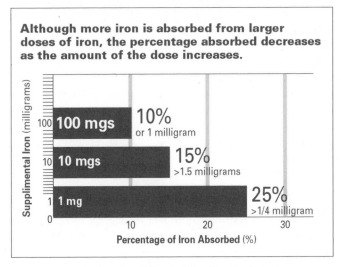

Although more iron is absorbed from larger doses of iron, the percentage absorbed decreases as the amount of the dose increases.

100 mgs — 10% or 1 milligram

10 mgs — 15% >1.5 milligrams

1 mg — 25% >1/4 milligram

Supplemental Iron (milligrams)

Percentage of Iron Absorbed (%)

Z. K. Roughead and J. R. Hunt, "Adaptation in Iron Absorption: Iron Supplementation Reduces Nonheme-Iron but Not Heme-Iron Absorption from Food." *American Journal of Clinical Nutrition* 72 (2000): 982–89.

that adaptation in absorption did not completely prevent differences in body iron stores.

The adaptation to reduce iron absorption even in volunteers with low iron stores may indicate the presence of a localized control system to prevent excessive iron exposure of intestinal cells. The study is consistent with two systems at work, one that regulates how much iron we must absorb for normal function and the iron-withholding defense system, which protects us from nurturing harmful pathogens with excesses of iron that we don't need.

For individuals with HHC, the classic type of hemochromatosis, this system is faulty; the body continues to absorb rather than limit iron absorption.

People with high body iron are at risk for contracting a number of chronic and acute diseases—and people with high body iron can actually set off metal detectors! "What sets off airport metal detectors is the metal itself. Iron is after all, a metal," said Gene Weinberg, PhD, professor of microbiology at Indiana University, and member of the Iron Disorders Institute Medical and Scientific Advisory Board.

3

Our One-Sided View of Iron

J. B. Williams Company, one of the smaller drug companies of the 1950s, needed a gimmick to sell one of its products, a multivitamin called Geritol. Instead of selling it for what it was, a nutritional supplement for iron deficiency, the company decided to sell it as a quick-fix remedy for fatigue, a known symptom of iron-deficiency anemia. Even though the medical community knew that fatigue could be a symptom of any number of conditions, a large portion of the public did not. By using the prefix *Geri-*, for "geriatric," the company was pushing iron to one of the groups of people who need it least.

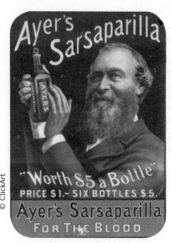

Although ads selling Geritol as a remedy for fatigue ran for only six years and were banned in 1969 by the Federal Trade Commission, Americans were hooked. The Geritol success sensitized the nation to iron deficiency. Even for people who continue to believe that iron causes fatigue, the incessant commercials had an effect. "Tired blood" and "My wife, I think I'll keep her" are phrases still familiar to millions of Americans some forty years later.

With repeated claims such as "Geritol contains twice the iron as a pound of calf's liver!" and "Tired blood is iron-poor blood," it was only a matter of time before the medical community was influenced. Many physicians were prompted to write prescriptions for iron at a patient's first mention of fatigue. Although iron supplementation may be necessary in confirmed cases of iron-deficiency anemia, it is not appropriate for those with iron-loading disorders such as hemochromatosis, even though the No. 1 complaint of people with such disorders is often fatigue.

Of 2,851 people with hemochromatosis who responded to a 1996 HHC patient survey, 17 percent had been prescribed iron supplements by their doctor, and another 18 percent reported that they had taken iron supplements for their health.
—*1996 HHC Patient Survey, Centers for Disease Control and Prevention*

Iron-deficiency anemia remains a worldwide health concern, but undiagnosed iron overload is also a major concern. The supplemental iron contained in fortified foods is potentially harming millions of Americans. Seventy-five million American are carriers of iron-loading genes, and some of those carriers also absorb too much iron. The labeling of food products to indicate iron content will help those who already know that they have abnormal iron metabolism. But what about the millions who are unaware that they are at risk of developing an iron-loading condition?

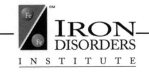

PART TWO

Detecting and Diagnosing
Hemochromatosis

4

Symptoms and Clues

There are more than 1,300 known metabolic disorders; hemochromatosis is one of them. Many of these disorders share similar symptoms with other conditions, which makes metabolic disorders among the most baffling and difficult to diagnose. A metabolic disorder exists because of defects in the body's production of energy. This energy-production process is a complex series of events that involves specific enzymes, genes, blood proteins, hormones, vitamins, electrolytes, water, and minerals—such as iron, copper, zinc, and calcium. Further, normal metabolism requires than an individual is able to use these components, which involves absorption, transport, and synthesis. One abnormality, one missing enzyme, or one defect anywhere in the process can disrupt normal metabolism.

Some scientists believe that, because HHC is an inherited condition, the error of iron metabolism occurs in more than one process and in more than one organ system. Every cell of the body contains DNA. When a gene is mutated, or flawed, its message is flawed throughout the entire human system. Therefore, the wrong message can reach anywhere within the iron regulatory and utilization process, thereby creating several different symptoms and combinations of test results.

Sick patients go to the doctor to get well. It's that simple. Getting the proper diagnosis, however, is not so simple. The process of diagnosis is complex, filled with twists and turns. A physician can see a patient with multiple symptoms of hemochromatosis, such as chronic fatigue and joint pain, heart arrhythmia, abdominal pain, depression, and loss of libido, and then take a number of different directions in diagnosis. It is highly unlikely that hemochromatosis is the first condition that occurs to a physician.

> According to Vincent Felitti, MD, former director of Kaiser Permanente's Preventive Medicine Department in San Diego, where more than two hundred thousand individuals have been screened for HHC, "Statistically, a family practice physician will likely see one case of homozygous hemochromatosis every two weeks."

Preexisting Disease Conditions May Offer Subtle Clues

Sometimes unplanned events, such as abnormal test results, can lead to proper diagnosis of HHC. Elevated liver enzymes or elevated serum iron can prompt a physician to suspect hemochromatosis and confirm diagnosis with further testing. When a patient mentions having a history of arthritis, diabetes, heart trouble or arrhythmia, liver problems, or previous experience with evaluated liver enzymes, especially mildly elevated liver enzymes, these can be clues to suspect hemochromatosis. Other conditions where hemochromatosis might be suspect include "amenorrhea, anterior pituitary failure, type 1 and 2 diabetes, impotence and loss of libido, inappropriate increase in skin pigmentation, infertility, liver cancer, and porphyria cutanea tarda (PCT)" (Pietrangelo, 2000).

In addition to your own health history, your primary care physician should collect information about your family's health history. This will provide additional clues for determining your risk of developing certain diseases. The Office of the Surgeon General has a family health history tool called My Family Health Portrait, which is available at the U.S. Department of Health and Human Services' website (www.hhs.gov/familyhistory/).

In 1996 the Centers for Disease Control and Prevention (CDC) conducted a survey of 2,851 hemochromatosis patients. Of respondents, 67 percent reported that they had been diagnosed first with arthritis, liver or gallbladder disease, stomach disorders, hormonal deficiencies, psychiatric problems, or diabetes before being properly diagnosed with hemochroma-tosis; 75 percent of respondents had chronic fatigue and joint pain. Further, 554 respondents had been diagnosed because the diagnosis of a family member led them to get tested. Of all respondents, 58 percent reported having symptoms, 30 percent had no symptoms, and 12 percent could not recall whether they had symptoms. Respondents experienced symp-toms for an average of nine and a half years, and usually had to consult more than three physicians before receiving a proper diagnosis of HHC.

Symptoms Reported by Patients

Many physicians will not make a connection between hemo-chromatosis and patients' complaints of joint pain or chronic fatigue, which are among the symptoms that people with hemochromatosis experience most frequently. Joint pain in the first two knuckles (called iron fist) is fairly specific to HHC. Other early signs of hemochromatosis are weakness, arthralgias, hepatomegaly, and elevated liver enzymes.

"Liver disease such as cirrhosis and liver cancer top the list of the main causes of death among those with hemochromatosis."
—A. Pietrangelo, "EASL International Consensus, Conference on Haemochromatosis," Journal of Hepatology, 2000

However, it is an eye-opening experience the first time that a physician successfully diagnoses and treats his or her first case of HHC. The physician will become receptive to the possibil-ity of hemochromatosis in anyone who complains of chronic fatigue, joint pain, or other vague symptoms.

"Symptoms don't help doctors recognize zebras when they're looking for horses."
—Mark Princell, MD, member of the Iron Disorders Institute Medical and Scientific Advisory Board

---

The Iron Disorders Institute has maintained a database of information about iron disorders such as HHC since early 1997. Information about symptoms, how diagnosis was reached, how individuals became educated about their disorder, and their response to treatment are among the types of data collected.

The following list includes among the most common and typically reported symptoms by individuals with hemochromatosis, in alphabetical order:

- Abdominal pain (associated with liver trouble)
- Changes in skin color (e.g., bronzing or reddening, jaundiced (yellowish) or ashen gray or olive green coloring, redness in the creases of the palms of the hands, dark circles under the eyes)
- Chest pain (associated with heart trouble)
- Chronic fatigue
- Depression
- Elevated cholesterol
- Impotence, amenorrhea (premature cessation of menstrual cycle)
- Infertility
- Irregular heartbeat (arrhythmia) (associated with heart trouble)
- Joint pain
- Loss of body hair, including baldness
- Loss of libido (sex drive)
- Slow maturation (delayed physical development)
- Sterility
- Weight gain (associated with type 2 diabetes and hypothyroidism)
- Weight loss (associated with diabetes)

Symptoms vary from person to person. Sometimes symptoms may seem to be unrelated, until a pattern begins to point to hemochromatosis. Then again, patients with hemochromatosis often feel that any symptom is a sign of hemochromatosis. Individuals with hemochromatosis have reported the following list of symptoms to IDI:

- Attention deficit disorder (ADD)
- Attention deficit/hyperactivity disorder (ADHD)
- Blisters on the back of the hands
- Confusion
- Elevated hemoglobin or hematocrit
- Elevated liver enzymes (most strikingly, these were slightly elevated)
- Emotional outbursts
- Excessive thirst and urination
- Fibromyalgia
- Frequent fever blisters
- Frequent infections
- Headache (including migraine)
- High blood pressure
- Irritable bowel syndrome
- Itchiness
- Loss of short-term memory
- Moodiness
- Rashes
- Restless legs syndrome
- Seizures
- Sleep disturbances, including sleep apnea
- Social withdrawal
- Visual disturbances

All of the symptoms reported were obtained from individuals diagnosed with hemochromatosis. However, it is important to note that not all of these symptoms are common to hemochromatosis. Some of the symptoms are associated with conditions that can occur in cases of iron-deficiency anemia, kidney problems, red-blood-cell production problems, bone marrow failure, or maldistribution of brain iron.

Over time, symptoms and signs began to be recognized as iron related. Depending on which vital organ's function has been impaired by excessive iron levels, symptoms can be quite varied. Why symptoms manifest differently among individuals is still unknown.

Prevalence of Selected Signs or Symptoms and Response to Treatment in 2,851 Patients with Hemochromatosis Treated with Phlebotomy			
Symptom	Reported Sign or Symptom, Number (%)	Improved with Therapy, Number (%)	Worse Despite Therapy, Number (%)
Extreme fatigue	1,296 (45.5)	705 (54.4)	223 (17.2)
Joint pain	1,241 (43.5)	115 (9.2)	422 (34.0)
Impotence (or loss of libido)	735 (25.8)	93 (12.7)	204 (27.8)
Skin bronzing	733 (25.7)	431 (58.8)	30 (4.1)
Heart fluttering	679 (23.8)	42 (6.2)	69 (10.1)
Depression	592 (20.8)	242 (40.8)	61 (10.3)
Abdominal pain	578 (20.3)	129 (22.3)	69 (11.9)

S. M. McDonnell, B. L. Preston, S. A. Jewell, J. C. Barton, C. Q. Edwards, P. Adams, and R. Yip, "A Survey of 2,851 Patients with Hemochromatosis: Symptoms and Response to Treatment." *American Journal of Medicine*, 106 (1999): 619–24.

Frequency of Conditions Reported in the General U.S. Population and U.S. Participants in the Hemochomatosis (HHC) Survey, by Age*				
	WOMEN NUMBER (%)		MEN NUMBER (%)	
Condition	General Population	HHC Survey	General Population	HHC Survey
Arthritis				
17-39 years	1,921 (5.9)	10 (10.3)	1,680 (5.2)	15 (8.9)
40-59 years	5,070 (23.4)	147 (34.9)	3,120 (14.7)	194 (22.2)
60-84 years	9,154 (51.1)	212 (42.8)	4,725 (33.8)	203 (31.5)
Diabetes mellitus				
17-39 years	538 (1.6)	3 (3.1)	457 (1.4)	2 (1.2)
40-59 years	950 (4.4)	31 (7.4)	1,087 (1.5)	65 (7.5)
60-84 years	2,437 (13.6)	31 (6.3)	1,991 (12.1)	62 (9.6)
Liver disease or gallbladder disease				
17-39 years	1,887 (7.2)	5 (5.2)	700 (2.7)	16 (9.5)
40-59 Years	2,674 (16.9)	84 (20.0)	1,106 (7.3)	154 (17.7)
60-84 Years	2,135 (25.6)	115 (23.2)	932 (12.2)	113 (17.5)
Extreme fatigue				
17-39 Years	14,235(43.4)	48 (49.5)	9,647 (29.9)	61 (36.0)

* General population data for liver disease or gallbladder disease from NHANES 11 (1976-1980, reference 19); other general population data from NHANES 111 (1988-1994, reference 20). Arthritis, diabetes, and liver or gallbladder disease based on response to the question: "Have you ever been diagnosed by a physician with fatigue." Based on self-reported severe fatigue. Data include only white subjects, ages 17 to 84. These data not available in NHANES for older subjects.

Social Implications
Expressed in Percent Reporting (%)

Type of Change	Severe HHC* (n=1,255)	Without Severe HHC* (n=1,596)
Divorce or breakup with significant other	6.5	2.0
Troubles with spouse or significant other	7.7	14
Marriage or relationship stronger	13.4	4.8
Family members in denial of my disease	12.3	3.8
Family members in denial of own risk	25.2	12.7
Family members supportive	44.5	38.1
Job loss	19.6	2.8
Reduced ability to do daily tasks	33.4	7.3
Loss of health insurance	8.7	5.8
Loss of life insurance	7.7	6.4
Other	5.6	3.3
No real change	28.7	60.0

* **HHC** = Hemochromatosis

5

Tests That Lead to Diagnosis

Blood Tests

Hereditary hemochromatosis classic can be confirmed with genetic testing. Iron overload, which can accompany HHC and several other conditions, can be confirmed with blood testing, biopsy, or specialized imaging. The presence of a genetic mutation does not always result in abnormal iron metabolism; therefore, determining the iron levels in one's body is the most critical first step. Establishing a benchmark for iron levels can result in early intervention, which reduces the risk of life-threatening disease or premature death.

Genetic Testing

Genetic testing examines DNA for mutations in genes that define a particular disease. This type of test examines DNA from a blood, saliva, or tissue sample for certain mutations. Genetic information does not provide information about iron levels, but it does expose the potential risk of developing iron disorders. Chapters 8–10 provide greater detail about genetics.

Lab Tests

Lab tests are biochemical tests that examine and determine levels of specific elements such as iron or components of blood, urine, or tissue. Results can help to diagnose, to determine treatment, and to provide prognosis. Lab ranges are not universally consistent, though, and ranges for all categories vary depending on the sample population examined by a given laboratory. Therefore, hemochromatosis patients are encouraged to compare lab outcomes with the reference ranges recommended by the Iron Disorders Institute.

Determining Reference Ranges

The reference range of a lab test is determined by testing a large number of healthy people within a variety of groups defined by age, sex, or other variables (such as pregnant women) and observing what appears to be "normal" for each group for a specific test. The results are then averaged and a range of normal values is established.

For example, hemoglobin and hematocrit both decline as a natural part of the aging process. Or blood loss through menstruation may cause lower hemoglobin and hematocrit levels in premenopausal women. These are examples of tests with reference ranges keyed to both age and sex.

Out-of-Range Test Results

According to the laws of probability, every one out of twenty determinations (or 5 percent) will fall outside the established reference range; thus, a single test value may not be significant. Generally, the test value is only slightly greater or less than the reference range. To put this in perspective, if a doctor runs twenty different tests on you, there's a good chance that one result will fall out of a reference range, despite the fact that you are in good health.

Of course, the result may indicate a problem. The first thing your doctor is likely to do is rerun the test. Perhaps something went awry with the sample being measured that day, such as the blood specimen was not refrigerated, or the serum either was not separated from the red cells or was exposed to heat.

Factors Affecting Test Values

Numerous additional factors can affect lab test results: caffeine, tobacco, alcohol, and vitamin C; your diet (vegetarian versus nonvegetarian); and stress or anxiety. Laboratories generally report your test results accompanied by a reference range for your age and sex. Your physician then will interpret the results on the basis of his or her personal knowledge of your particulars, including any medications you are taking, alternative treatments, diet, level of physical activity, alcohol consumption, or pregnancy.

Blood Testing for Iron Overload

Iron levels can be determined with a relatively inexpensive blood test, or lab test, called an iron panel. Iron panels are sometimes also referred to as iron studies, iron indices, or iron profiles. Specific tests include fasting serum iron (SI), total iron-binding capacity (TIBC), and serum ferritin (SF). Equally important is a test for hemoglobin/hematocrit (Hgb/Hct), which is a component of the complete blood count (CBC) blood test. Other tests that are less common but that can be helpful in diagnosing iron overload are unsaturated iron-binding capacity (UIBC) and serum transferrin receptor (sTfR).

Your doctor may require additional blood tests to determine the effects, if any, of excess iron on your body's systems. These include tests for levels of liver enzymes (liver function tests LFT), thyroid-stimulating hormone (TSH), glucose (FBS, OGTT, or GTT), glycated hemoglobin (HbA1C), amylase, testosterone, cortisol, and alpha-fetoprotein (AFP). These and other tests are explained in greater detail in the chapters that address specific body functions (chapters 11–18).

Iron Panel FAQs

As mentioned in the previous chapter, the Iron Disorders Institute maintains a database of information about iron disorders such as HHC. That database includes questions asked by many HHC patients and their families. In the past, patients have asked the following questions about iron panel blood tests.

What is an iron panel?

Iron panels can also be referred to as iron studies, iron indices, or iron profiles. The iron panel is a group of blood tests that provide levels of iron in key functions of transport and storage. Generally, an iron panel consists of the serum ferritin (SF), fasting serum iron (SI), and total iron-binding capacity (TIBC) blood tests. Transferrin saturation (TS) percentage is also an important component of iron measurement. The TS percentage is computed from the results of the SI and TIBC tests. Unsaturated iron-binding capacity (UIBC) is an alternative blood test to the TIBC. Both UIBC and SI can be used to compute TS percentage. Hemoglobin or hematocrit are also part of an iron panel. Some laboratories and physicians prefer the serum transferrin receptor (sTfR) test. This test is used more often in research settings; however, the advantage of sTfR is that it is not affected by inflammation and is therefore helpful in distinguishing between iron-deficiency anemia and anemia of inflammatory response.

What is the purpose of an iron panel?
An iron panel is a series of blood tests that measure the amount of iron in your tissues along with your body's ability to use iron. In general, your physician uses these tests to determine whether your body has a problem using iron.

Why is it important to measure iron?
Iron is important for your body to function normally. Hemoglobin in red blood cells uses iron to bind with and transport oxygen to all parts of your body. Too little iron or too much iron in the body can have serious health consequences.

Where is iron located in the body?
About 85 percent of the iron in the body is found in hemoglobin (in red blood cells) and myoglobin (in skeletal muscle). Approximately 14 percent of the iron in the body is stored (as ferritin or hemosiderin) in the liver, bone marrow, and spleen. A small percentage of the body's iron is in transport between various parts of the body or is a component of proteins in cells throughout the body.

What is transferrin?
Transferrin is a protein with the ability to bind two molecules of iron; it then transports iron to all tissues, vital organs, and bone marrow, or into containment in ferritin.

What is serum ferritin?
Serum ferritin (SF), or ferritin, is a complex protein formed by cells throughout the body. Serum ferritin is huge: each molecule

has the ability to hold 4,500 atoms of iron. The amount of SF found in blood serum is directly related to iron storage in the body. Serum ferritin serves as a containment or storage device for iron that is not needed at the moment. In ferritin, iron is stored for future use in making new red blood cells or is contained to protect against free iron that can lead to free-radical activity and tissue destruction. When ferritin molecules become full, iron is changed into hemosiderin. Serum ferritin is a good indicator of iron overload, but it has some drawbacks because it is an acute phase reactant, which means that it is affected by any kind of inflammation. Ferritin levels can become elevated as a result of certain medications, such as hormone replacement therapy or nicotine products, or in the presence of chronic disease and infection, such as viral hepatitis and alcoholic liver disease. The combination of elevated SF with an elevated TS percentage is fairly predictive of iron loading in a patient with HHC.

What is hemosiderin?
Hemosiderin can accumulate in cells of the heart, liver, lungs, pancreas, and other organs, and affect their ability to function properly. For example, when the beta cells of the pancreas are loaded with hemosiderin, they become unable to produce or store adequate amounts of the hormone insulin, which results in diabetes. Dr. Gene Weinberg refers to hemosiderin as "gunk," sort of like the residue you see at the bottom of a cup of cocoa.

What is serum iron?
Serum iron (SI) is a measure of circulating iron that is bound to transferrin, and it reflects total body iron. Serum iron measurements can be affected by menstrual cycle, time of day, diet, hepatitis, and from taking some oral contraceptives that contain iron. Therefore, it is important to refrain from eating before having an SI test; this means that, except for water or prescribed medications, you can take nothing by mouth after midnight before your blood work. Not fasting can result in an inaccurate measurement of TS percentage.

What do serum iron values indicate?
On its own, serum iron (SI) is a snapshot of your iron levels and is not very helpful for defining a chronic iron deficiency or

other iron problems. However, when the test value is examined in comparison with other iron tests, it can help provide information leading to a proper (complete) diagnosis.

What is total iron-binding capacity?
Total iron-binding capacity (TIBC) is a measurement of all the proteins available for binding free iron in the body.

What does the TIBC measurement indicate?
When TIBC is elevated, it may indicate iron-deficiency anemia, which means that there are lots of proteins available to bind with iron. When TIBC is low, it may indicate iron overload, which means that there are few proteins available to bind with iron.

> Think of TIBC as a bus. When TIBC is elevated, there are plenty of seats left on the bus for iron; when TIBC is low, there are fewer seats available on the bus for iron.

What is transferrin saturation percentage?
Transferrin saturation (TS) percentage indicates the percentage of transferrin that is saturated with iron, demonstrating how much iron is in transport and how much capacity is left to bind iron and move it to appropriate sites, such as ferritin. The TS percentage can be calculated by dividing the serum iron (SI) level by the total iron-binding capacity (TIBC), multiplying by 100, and rounding to the nearest tenth of a decimal place. The normal range of TS percentage is 25 to 35 percent.

Calculating the TS Percentage
(SI/TIBC) × 100 = TS percentage
For example:
If your SI is 96 µg/dL and your TIBC is 242 µg/dL, then your computation would appear as follows:
Step 1: 96/242 = .3966
Step 2: .3966 × 100 = 39.66%
Step 3: 39.66% is rounded to 39.7%

What is unsaturated iron-binding capacity?

Unsaturated iron-binding capacity (UIBC) is the difference between levels of TIBC and serum iron. In other words, the sum of SI and UIBC is equal to TIBC. Sometimes UIBC is referred to as extra iron-binding capacity or nonbound transferrin iron (NTBI). Levels of UIBC are lower than normal in iron overload and greater than normal in iron-deficiency anemia. Free or unbound iron can trigger free-radical activity, causing cell damage or cell death, and can destroy DNA.

$$(TIBC - SI) = UIBC$$

Can UIBC test results help determine TS percentage?

Yes. The TS percentage can be calculated by adding the unsaturated iron-binding capacity (UIBC) value to the serum iron (SI) value to derive total iron-binding capacity (TIBC), dividing SI by the resulting TIBC, multiplying the new results by 100, and rounding to the nearest tenth of a decimal place.

$[SI/(SI + UIBC)] \times 100 = TS$ percentage

For example:

If your SI is 96 µg/dL and your UIBC is 146 µg/dL, then your computation would appear as follows:

Step 1: $96 + 146 = 242$

Step 2: $96/242 = .3966$

Step 3: $.3966 \times 100 = 39.66\%$

Step 4: 39.66% is rounded to 39.7%

Should I keep a record of my blood tests?

Yes! Keeping a record of your blood tests is especially important if you move frequently or when traveling, as your medical records may not be immediately available. A spiral notebook, electronic spreadsheet, and the Personal Health Profile offered by IDI are several techniques that you can use to record your treatments. You can also download the Iron Panel Blood Test Data spreadsheet from IDI's website. One advantage of using a spreadsheet is that you can create a graph, which can then be used to convey your medical information pictorially.

Serum ferritin is one test that varies by age and gender as depicted in the ferritin chart below. For hemochromatosis patients, the IDI recommends maintaining a serum ferritin range of 25–75ng/mL.

Important Ferritin Reference Ranges ferritin	Adult Males	Adult Females
Normal Range	up to 300ng/mL	up to 200ng/mL
In treatment*	below 100ng/mL	below 100ng/mL
Ideal maintenance	25-75ng/mL	25-75ng/mL
Adolescents, Juveniles, Infants & Newborns of normal height and weight for their age and gender		
Male ages 10-19 23-70ng/mL	Infants 7-12 months 60-80ng/mL	
Female ages 10-19 6-40ng/mL	Newborn 1-6 months 6-410ng/mL	
Children ages 6-9 10-55ng/mL	Newborn 1-30 days 6-400ng/mL	
Children ages 1-5 6-24ng/mL		

*In treatment applies only to patients with hereditary hemochromatosis undergoing therapeutic phlebotomy

Iron Panel as a Diagnostic Tool

As illustrated on the HHC diagnostic algorithm chart that doctors use as a step-by-step procedure, the finding of a TS percentage greater than 45 percent with an accompanying elevated serum ferritin of greater than 200 ng/mL suggests early iron loading and should be addressed with volunteer blood donation and iron-level tracking with follow-up lab tests.

The Complete Blood Count FAQs

As in the case of the iron panel, many patients have asked the following questions about the complete blood count (CBC) test.

A specific result within the reference range for a CBC blood test does not ensure health, just as a result outside the reference range may not indicate disease.

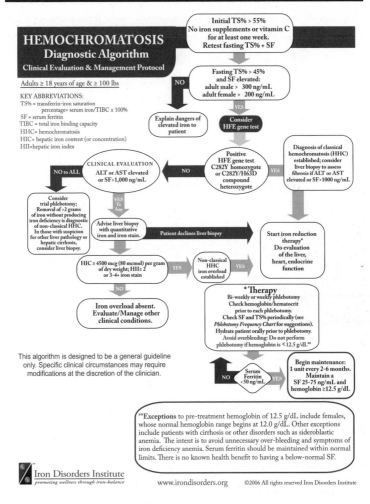

HEMOCHROMATOSIS
Diagnostic Algorithm
Clinical Evaluation & Management Protocol

Adults ≥ 18 years of age & ≥ 100 lbs

KEY ABBREVIATIONS:
TS% = transferrin-iron saturation
percentage= serum iron/TIBC x 100%
SF = serum ferritin
TIBC = total iron binding capacity
HHC= hemochromatosis
HIC= hepatic iron content (or concentration)
HII=hepatic iron index

Initial TS% > 55%
No iron supplements or vitamin C
for at least one week.
Retest fasting TS% + SF

Fasting TS% > 45%
and SF elevated:
adult male > 300 ng/mL
adult female > 200 ng/mL

NO — Explain dangers of elevated iron to patient

YES — Consider HFE gene test

Positive HFE gene test C282Y homozygote or C282Y/H63D compound heterozygote

Diagnosis of classical hemochromatosis (HHC) established; consider liver biopsy to assess fibrosis if ALT or AST elevated or SF >1000 ng/mL

CLINICAL EVALUATION ALT or AST elevated or SF >1,000 ng/mL

NO to ALL

Consider trial phlebotomy; Removal of >2 grams of iron without producing iron deficiency is diagnostic of non-classical HHC. In those with suspicion for other liver pathology or hepatic cirrhosis, consider liver biopsy.

YES To Any

Advise liver biopsy with quantitative iron and iron stain.

Patient declines liver biopsy

Start iron reduction therapy* Do evaluation of the liver, heart, endocrine function

HIC ≥ 4500 mcg (80 mcmol) per gram of dry weight; HII≥ 2 or 3-4+ iron stain

YES — Non-classical HHC iron overload established — YES

NO

Iron overload absent. Evaluate/Manage other clinical conditions.

***Therapy**
Bi-weekly or weekly phlebotomy
Check hemoglobin/hematocrit prior to each phlebotomy.
Check SF and TS% periodically (see *Phlebotomy Frequency Chart* for suggestions).
Hydrate patient orally prior to phlebotomy.
Avoid overbleeding: Do not perform phlebotomy if hemoglobin is <12.5 g/dL**

This algorithm is designed to be a general guideline only. Specific clinical circumstances may require modifications at the discretion of the clinician.

NO — Serum Ferritin <50 ng/mL — YES

Begin maintenance:
1 unit every 2-6 months.
Maintain a
SF 25-75 ng/mL and hemoglobin ≥12.5 g/dL

Exceptions to pre-treatment hemoglobin of 12.5 g/dL include females, whose normal hemoglobin range begins at 12.0 g/dL. Other exceptions include patients with cirrhosis or other disorders such as sideroblastic anemia. The intent is to avoid unnecessary over-bleeding and symptoms of iron deficiency anemia. Serum ferritin should be maintained within normal limits. There is no known health benefit to having a below-normal SF.

What is a CBC blood test?

The complete blood count (CBC) is one of the most common blood tests used. It analyzes the three major types of cells in blood: red blood cells, white blood cells, and platelets. The CBC counts these cells, measures hemoglobin (the oxygen-carrying molecule in red blood cells), estimates the volume of red blood cells, and sorts the white blood cells into five subtypes (which is referred to as the CBC differential).

What do the acronyms on CBC blood test results mean?

CBC Blood Test Components	
Acronym	**Definition**
WBC	White Blood Cells
RBC	Reb Blood Cells
Hgb	Hemoglobin
Hct	Hematocrit
MCV	Mean Corpuscular Volume
MCH	Mean Corpuscular Hemoglobin
MCHC	Mean Corpuscular Hemoglobin Concentration
RDW	Red Cell Distribution Width
PLT	Platelets
MPV	Mean Platelet Volume

What is the purpose of white blood cells?

White blood cells (WBCs), sometimes referred to as leukocytes, are produced by the immune system to help defend the body against infection. They are formed in the bone marrow and enter the blood to migrate to key organs, such as the spleen or lymph nodes. These cells are bigger than red blood cells, and there are far fewer white blood cells in the bloodstream. A high white-blood-cell count likely indicates that an infection is present somewhere in the body, whereas a low count might indicate that an infection or disease has slowed the ability of the bone marrow to produce new white blood cells.

Typically 1 cubic milliliter of blood contains about ten thousand white blood cells. There are several different types of white blood cells, which are identified in a CBC with differential blood test.

What is the purpose of red blood cells?

Red blood cells (RBCs), often referred to as erythrocytes, are responsible for delivering oxygen throughout the body. There are between 3.6 million and 6.1 million red blood cells in a single milliliter of blood. A low red-blood-cell count can indicate anemia.

What is hemoglobin?

Hemoglobin (Hgb) is an iron-containing oxygen-transport protein found inside red blood cells that gives blood its red color. Oxygen bound to hemoglobin travels through the bloodstream. The amount of hemoglobin in the blood is an indicator of the amount of oxygen the blood can carry throughout the body. Without the life-preserving capabilities of hemoglobin to deliver oxygen to cells, a person would suffocate and die.

In patients with HHC, the hemoglobin level should always be measured before a therapeutic phlebotomy or blood donation to ensure that the individual can tolerate the blood loss. A low hemoglobin count is a good indicator of anemia, though dehydration can temporarily increase hemoglobin levels.

For the majority of HHC patients, the Iron Disorders Institute recommends a pretreatment hemoglobin level of 12.5 g/dL to avoid overbleeding and unnecessary iron-deficiency anemia. There are exceptions to this recommendation, such as some women or patients with liver disease. Physicians determine these exceptions. It is noteworthy that hemoglobin does not confirm iron overload. Often hemoglobin levels are normal in HHC patients. Elevated hemoglobin levels are generally due to smoking, the need for fluids, or a condition called polycythemia. A low hemoglobin count can indicate anemia of inflammatory response or iron-deficiency anemia.

What is hematocrit?

Hematocrit (Hct) is the amount of your blood that is occupied by red blood cells. A low hematocrit percentage is a good indicator of anemia. The value is expressed as a percentage of cells in blood. For example, a hematocrit value of 42 percent means that there are 42 milliliters of red blood cells in 100 milliliters of blood.

What is mean corpuscular volume?

Mean corpuscular volume (MCV) measures the size of red blood cells. Larger red blood cells may indicate anemia caused by deficiency in vitamin B6 or folic acid; smaller red blood cells may indicate anemia caused by iron deficiency. Some drugs can increase mean corpuscular volume without necessarily causing anemia. Also, mean corpuscular volume can be used to determine when an HHC patient has achieved normal iron status.

What is mean corpuscular hemoglobin?

Mean corpuscular hemoglobin (MCH) measures the amount of hemoglobin in red blood cells. Both hemoglobin and hematocrit are used to calculate this number. Low levels indicate anemia.

What is red-blood-cell distribution width?

Red blood cells can come in different sizes. The red-blood-cell distribution width (RDW) looks at the range of these sizes in a blood sample. If anemia is suspected from other blood counts, RDW test results are often used together with mean corpuscular volume to figure out possible causes of the anemia.

What are platelets?

Platelets are tiny cells produced by the bone marrow to help blood clot in the event of a cut or scrape. A high number of platelets might be found in people with cancer, a blood disease, or rheumatoid arthritis. A decreased platelet count is called thrombocytopenia. There are a number of possible causes of thrombocytopenia, including a disorder of the immune system that causes antibodies produced by the spleen to kill platelets (idiopathic thrombocytopenia purpura [ITP]). This condition can be problematic and often warrants immediate medical care.

What is mean platelet volume?

Mean platelet volume (MPV) measures the average volume (size) of platelets. A higher-than-normal mean platelet volume has been shown to be associated with a greater risk of heart attacks and stroke.

What do the CBC Differential Values represent?

The CBC differential is a breakdown of the different types of white blood cells. There are actually two main types of white blood cells: phagocytes and lymphocytes. Phagocytes attack germs directly and are powerful defenses against certain infections. Lymphocytes, which include T cells, play a large role in fighting chronic infections.

The five subtypes of white blood cells are displayed both as a percentage of white blood cells and as an absolute number of cells. Each subtype acronym is followed by a percentage sign (%) and a pound sign (#), which represent the percentage and absolute number of cells, respectively. Multiplying the percentage of the cell type by the total number of white blood cells provides the absolute number of cells. The number of white blood cells is equal to the sum of the absolute value of the subtype cells. The sum of the percentages of these cells should always equal 100 percent.

CBC Differential Test Names

Acronym	Definition
NEU	Neutrophils *(Sometimes labeled GR or Grans.)*
LYM	Lymphocytes
MONO	Monocytes
EOS	Eosinophils
BASO	Basophils

What is the purpose of the different white blood cells?
Neutrophils (also known as segs, Polymorphonuclear Neutrophils [PMNs], or grans[GRs]) surround, engulf, and destroy invading microbes, and they normally account for anywhere between 38 percent and 80 percent of the white-blood-cell count. A low neutrophil count can put you at a greater risk of sickness from a bacterial infection.

Lymphocytes produce antibodies, which are specific proteins that attack and help destroy specific germs, but most lymphocytes circulating in the blood either attack invaders (called cytotoxic lymphocytes) or coordinate the attack of antibodies. Lymphocytes include T cells, B cells, and natural killer cells, and normally account for between 15 percent and 49 percent of the total white-blood-cell count. Viral infections can either increase or decrease the total percentage of lymphocytes.

Monocytes, or mononuclear phagocytes, are the largest white blood cells in the bloodstream; they remove dead cells and microbes from the blood. A low monocyte count can put you at a greater risk of getting sick from an infection, particularly those caused by bacteria.

Eosonophils, a type of phagocyte that produces the anti-inflammatory protein histamine, are usually elevated in people with allergies or parasitic infections.

Basophil cells are responsible for controlling inflammation and tissue damage in the body, such as liver inflammation due to hepatitis.

What do my CBC test results mean?

Test results are reported numerically and are interpreted according to the test's reference range, which may vary by the patient's age and sex, as well as the instrumentation or kit used to perform the test. High or low results are normally reported with an *H* or *L* next to the test result value. A specific result within the reference (normal) range for a CBC blood test does not ensure health, just as a result outside the reference range may not indicate disease. The Iron Disorders Institute recommends that you consult your physician to discuss your test results as a part of a complete medical examination.

6
Biopsies, Quantitative Phlebotomies, and Scans

Before the 1996 discovery of the HFE gene and before evidence of the association of certain iron levels and disease, the liver biopsy was the gold standard for diagnosing hemochromatosis. In cases when patients declined liver biopsy, physicians used quantitative phlebotomy as a means of diagnosis. Specialized scanning techniques are becoming more widely available to patients as a means of detecting and measuring iron in various organs. These alternatives are described later in this chapter.

Presently, the recommendation is against the routine use of liver biopsy to diagnose classic hereditary hemochromatosis (HHC). Instead, screening blood tests (serum iron, TIBC, ferritin) and HFE genetic testing are preferred. However, liver biopsy still has an important role, especially in persons with abnormal liver tests (such as elevated serum aminotransferases, abnormally large or firm livers on physical examination, or abnormal liver imaging studies [ultrasound, CT, or MRI scans]), with focal abnormalities that may be tumors, or with markedly elevated serum ferritin levels (greater than 1,000ng/mL). Liver biopsies with quantitative liver iron concentrations are also important to make (or exclude) as diagnosis of non-classical (non-HFE linked) hemochromatosis.

Liver Biopsy
Liver biopsy is no longer considered the gold standard for diagnosing HHC, but it is still the most certain way to determine the severity of liver disease and to establish for certain a diagnosis of liver cancer. In this way, a biopsy provides information about

a patient's chances of survival or quality of life while disease is present. In the case of liver disease, a biopsy can detect how much iron has collected in the liver, the extent of cirrhosis or fibrosis, and the presence of cancer. Liver biopsy remains the only way to determine the magnitude of disease in the liver.

It is now well accepted, based upon the reports of several investigators, that persons who are C282Y homozygotes with serum ferritin less than 1,000 ng/mL, no hepatomegaly (i.e., enlargement of the liver), and normal liver enzymes (ALT, AST) have less than a 1 percent chance of cirrhosis. Most patients will opt out of having liver biopsy as a means of diagnosis in favor of other less invasive ways to diagnose HHC.

Liver biopsy is no longer necessary to diagnose hemochromatosis.
—*IRON2000 USA Scientific Conference*

Liver Biopsy Described

Liver biopsies may be performed during upper abdominal surgeries, either open or traditional, with large incisions, or minimally invasive and laparoscopic. Such procedures are performed by general surgeons or surgical subspecialists who limit their practice to liver, biliary, and pancreatic surgery. However, most liver biopsies are performed with needles that are quickly (within one second) inserted through the skin, between the lower ribs on the right side, and that remove a small bit of liver (typically weighing 0.02 to 0.05 grams or ~1/1000 of one ounce. Such biopsies are usually performed under local anesthesia and conscious sedation by gastroenterologists, hepatologists, general surgeons, or intervention radiologists.

Liver biopsies undergo processing sectioning a very thin (~5micron) tissue sample, which is stained and then examined by pathologists who are trained to recognize microscopic abnormalities.

If iron overload is suspected, a portion of the biopsy should also be sent to special laboratories for quantitation of liver iron concentrations and for calculation of the hepatic iron index (HII). The HII is the liver iron concentration, expressed in micromoles of iron per gram of dry liver, divided by the age of the subject in years. HII greater than 1.9 confirms hemochromatosis, or iron overload.

Pathologists can also detect iron by staining a section of the tissue obtained from liver biopsy with a special stain. The sample is examined under a microscope, where excess iron appears as dark blue spots. Without such a special stain, small or moderate amounts of iron could not be seen. Staining the tissue sample confirms the presence of iron, whereas drying and weighing the tissue sample, and then analyzing it for iron content, establishes the concentration of iron contained in the tissue.

Liver biopsies are generally performed on outpatients and are safe, although there is a chance that the patient will experience pain or leakage of blood or bile after biopsies. There is about one chance in 1,000 that the patient may need hospital admission and perhaps a surgical operation to stop the leakage of blood or bile.

The liver biopsy experience depends on the patient and the clinician performing the procedure. Some patients are prone to anxiety about certain procedures; others have little to no hesitancy. A skilled physician can perform the procedure with little to no discomfort for the patient, although transient pain after the biopsy may occur even after the most skillful biopsy procedure.

Alternatives to Liver Biopsy for Diagnosis of Hemochromatosis

Today's physicians have several noninvasive and cost-effective ways to confirm hemochromatosis diagnosis, such as quantitative phlebotomy, specialized MRI, and genetic testing. There are also situations in which hemochromatosis might be not be suspect but is diagnosed because of abnormal test results, preexisting disease, and most important, informed patients.

Quantitative Phlebotomy

In standard phlebotomy, about one pint or 450 to 500 mL of blood is removed, which contains approximately 200 to 250 milligrams of iron. In quantitative phlebotomy, the total amount of iron ultimately removed is calculated to determine whether the total body iron load was increased. In general, 4 grams of iron are found in about 16 to 20 pints of blood. Individuals who have 4 grams or more of mobilizable iron by quantitative phlebotomy are considered to have had iron overload. A conclusive diagnosis of hemochromatosis cannot be made in this way, but hemochromatosis can be highly suspect in such individuals. In such cases, genetic testing should be considered.

Magnetic Resonance Imaging

Specialized magnetic resonance imaging (MRI) can detect the presence of iron in organs such as the liver, heart, lungs, pancreas, and brain. An MRI can even detect iron in small glands such as the pituitary. Iron appears as dark areas on the MRI. A trained radiologist can distinguish the difference between darkness caused by a tumor and darkness caused by iron. Specialized MRI is emerging as the preferred, noninvasive way to confirm the presence of iron in all major organs of the body. An MRI, however, when performed before sufficient time has passed for significant iron overload to occur, may be normal in people with HHC.

"MRI cannot be stressed enough for people with hemochromatosis."
—*Dr. James Connor, professor of anatomy and neuroscience, Pennsylvania State University, and member of the Iron Disorders Institute Medical and Scientific Advisory Board*

The MRI requires a fairly large piece of equipment. A patient must lie on a table, which slides automatically into a tunnel-like cylinder that is actually a magnet. Radio frequencies interact with the magnet and provide information to sensors. As signals pass through the body, the sensors detect them. An increase in tissue iron decreases the intensity of a signal and results in a dark area on the final image. An MRI is different from an X-ray. MRIs do not use radiation to obtain an image, and unlike an X-ray, MRIs can see through a target organ such as the bone. A limitation of MRI scanning is that, as routinely done, it cannot differentiate between mild or moderate nonpathologic iron overload and severe dangerous iron overload. The reason is that even small amounts of iron cause organs to appear abnormally dark. This limitation can be overcome with the use of special algorithms for performing MRI scans, such as those offered by the FerriScan.

FerriScan

FerriScan technology is a novel, noninvasive diagnostic tool to determine liver-iron content to assist clinicians in the detection and treatment of iron-overload disorders such as HHC and thalassemia.

This technology, developed by Resonance Health of Australia, is cleared by the U.S. Food and Drug Administration for non-invasive diagnosis of individuals who would benefit from a definitive diagnosis of iron overload and as an effective means to monitor the liver-iron burden as part of phlebotomy or chelation treatment. The technology provides a safe alternative to liver biopsy and is fast becoming a valuable adjunct to gene testing for iron-overload diseases.

The FerriScan diagnostic test service uses existing MRI machines at radiology facilities worldwide that are configured to provide a suitable scan of the liver. The MRI data is transmitted electronically via a secure data process to the Resonance Health analysis center from anywhere in the world. Resonance Health uses its patented software to generate a liver-iron concentration result. The test requires no new equipment to be purchased by the MRI center and adds ~15 minutes to the standard MRI procedure.

Ferritometer

A Ferritometer employs technology called superconducting quantum interference device (SQUID). The SQUID is the world's most sensitive magnetic-flux detector. It is often referred to as a cryogenic or superconducting magnetometer, and indeed the measurement of extremely small magnetic fields is one of its most important applications. The devices, available from Tristan Technologies of San Diego, use magnetic fields to measure the amount of iron stored in the liver. The method is a very accurate way to measure iron through radiological studies.

The SQUID procedure is noninvasive and takes less than fifteen minutes to complete. Noninvasive liver-iron measurements using a Ferritometer (or SQUID) are currently available at two locations in the United States: Children's Hospital and Research Center in Oakland, California, and New York–Presbyterian Hospital in New York. There is also Ferritometer equipment in Torino, Italy, and Hamburg, Germany.

7
Benefits of Screening for Hemochromatosis

Screening for a disease is a technique used to detect the disease before it causes symptoms or organ damage. Examples of screening include the Pap smear, which can detect cervical cancer at a curable stage; the rectal exam, for occult blood and prostate enlargement, which can help detect colon or prostate cancer; cholesterol levels, to detect atherosclerosis and potential heart attack; and genetic testing, for disorders such as sickle-cell trait, Rh status, and spina bifida. The most common screening test in use is the measurement of blood pressure, an attempt to find and treat high blood pressure before it causes congestive heart failure, stroke, or other blood vessel damage.

Some screening measures are used often to check for disease potential, either at birth with genetic testing or at given intervals, such as pediatric checkups, scheduled visits with the physician (such as for school immunization), annual checkups, and work physicals. Other screening can be on a volunteer basis, such as colonoscopy to determine the presence of colorectal cancer, mammography for early detection of breast cancer, and the iron panel screening under way at an increasing number of medical facilities.

Before 1998 serum iron (SI) and total iron-binding capacity (TIBC), together with key liver enzymes, were included in executive panels (widely used blood tests). This provided a measure of screening for those with hemochromatosis. Back then, elevated serum iron and elevated liver enzymes in both asymptomatic and symptomatic individuals prompted physicians to investigate further until reaching the proper diagnosis of hemochromatosis or iron overload.

Changes in the Medicare reimbursement policy resulted in the removal of this type of screening mechanism from executive panels. Reinstatement of these crucial tests will not happen overnight. Changes in reimbursement policies take months to implement and months to rescind or change. At the IRONUSA 2000 Scientific Conference of May 2000, hosted by the Iron Disorders Institute, the chair of IDI's Medical and Scientific Advisory Board, Dr. Herbert Bonkovsky, and the vice chair, Dr. P. D. Phatak, submitted a letter to the U.S. Department of Health and Human Services. This action was in response to the Health Care Financing Administration 42 C.F.R. Part 410 Medicare Program, which negotiated rule making proposed changes. The changes regarded coverage and administrative policies for clinical diagnostic laboratory services and reimbursement for specific tests such as serum ferritin reflected in the proposed rule HCFA-3250-P.

Drs. Bonkovsky and Phatak's proposed wording would provide for reimbursement for the cost of serum ferritin for those with elevated fasting TS percentage.

Screening for Hereditary Hemochromatosis

What makes routine screening for hemochromatosis, an iron-overload disorder, a good idea? Saving lives and money are compelling enough reasons. Iron-overload disorder also meets many of the criteria for population-based screening:

- Iron-overload disorder is common.
- A sensitive screening test, TS percentage, exists and allows for detection during a long presymptomatic phase.
- A safe, effective treatment is available that can eliminate morbidity (having the disease), reduce deaths, and reduce health costs.

Iron accumulates in the liver, heart, pancreas, pituitary gland, and joints. Iron can interfere with the proper functioning of most of these organs; moreover, iron is a key nutrient for microbial and cancer cells. If an iron-loading disorder can be detected before accumulation has caused organ damage, the costs of treatment can be minor. The following illustrates the estimated costs for treating a person who has developed iron-overload disease.

Hemochromatosis screening and preventive maintenance might include a trip to the family physician, the cost of blood work, and a series of phlebotomies, depending on the level of accumulated iron, for an estimated onetime expense of $2,557 per person. That amount is far less than treating a lifetime (perhaps an abbreviated lifetime) of debilitating chronic disease.

About one million Americans have the genetic predisposition for HHC and hence the potential to develop significant iron overload. When potentially affected compound and simple heterozygotes are included in the population at risk, those numbers increase dramatically. However, when diagnosed and treated in time (i.e., before irreversible organ damage), the savings are obvious. The maintenance phase of HHC treatment costs approximately $600 per year, while treating conditions that result from iron overload can cost many thousands of dollars a year, not including the costs of lost time at work, pain and suffering, and the potential of premature death.

The age to begin screening is based on the age when TS percentages generally start to increase in individuals with the HFE genotype. Mayo Clinic experts recommend that all adults have a TS percentage test at least once during their lifetime, preferably as a young adult.

The Iron Disorders Institute recommends that family practice physicians consider screening for HHC using TS percentage by the age of eighteen or earlier in high-risk families in which an iron-loading condition has been established.

Genetic testing as a means of screening for hereditary hemochromatosis is not a practical or cost-effective way to identify individuals with the condition. Genetic testing can be expensive, and testing for mutations of HFE currently misses 15 percent of cases of significant iron overload.

According to the iron-overload and hemochromatosis expert Dr. Paul Adams, of London, Ontario, "The most established screening test for haemochromatosis is transferrin saturation which is raised in most, but not all, C282Y homozygotes.... The sensitivity of transferrin saturation for the detection of C282Y homozygotes has been reported to be 94 percent in the population screening study from Busselton, Australia[;] however[,] it was only 52 percent (TS% threshold > 50) in the large study from San Diego."

Total iron-binding capacity (TIBC) and unsaturated iron-binding capacity (UIBC) are elevated in anemias and low in iron overload. At one time, UIBC was less expensive than transferrin saturation because it is a one-step biochemical process where calculating the transferrin saturation is a two-step process. However, advances in laboratory technology have significantly lowered the cost of many blood tests for iron.

The U.S. National Institutes of Health Hemochromatosis Iron Overload Study HEIRS study on iron overload and hemochromatosis used UIBC to calculate transferrin saturation. Dr. Adams was one of the principal investigators of the study.

8

The HFE Gene

To understand what the terms *homozygote*, *heterozygote*, and *compound heterozygote* mean with respect to hereditary hemo-chromatosis, it is useful to keep in mind a few basic facts about human genetics. The genetic material (DNA) that constitutes human beings is arranged into forty-six chromosomes.

One-half, or twenty-three chromosomes, are inherited from each parent. Twenty-two of the twenty-three chromosomes are autosomes, and the remaining chromosome, the X or Y chromosome, is the sex chromosome, because the arrangement of the X and Y chromosomes determines whether an individual is a male (XY) or female (XX). Therefore, every human being, with rare exceptions, carries two copies, called homologues, of each of the twenty-two autosomal chromosomes and either an X and Y chromosome, or two X chromosomes.

The HFE gene, which when mutated causes hereditary hemochromatosis (HHC), is located on the short arm of chromosome 6. Hereditary hemochromatosis is considered an autosomal recessive disorder because both copies of the HFE gene, which reside on the two homologues of autosomal chromosome 6, need to have a particular mutation for the disorder to present itself. To date, several different mutations in the HFE gene have been described, but two in particular, when present in the appropriate arrangement, can lead to the development of hemochromatosis.

The major factor causing mutation is a replacement of the amino acid cysteine with a different amino acid called tyrosine. This mutation is referred to as C282Y. The second factor causing mutation is replacement of the amino acid histidine with another amino acid called aspartic acid. This mutation is referred to as H63D. There are additional mutations within the HFE gene, such as S65C and C282S. It is not yet known how significantly those mutations contribute to abnormal metabolism of iron. Studies have been undertaken to determine penetrance of these mutations. Depending on a person's inheritance pattern, he or she is a heterozyote, homozygote, or compound heterozygote.

Heterozygote: If an individual has only one mutated chromosome with any of the HFE mutations (e.g., C282Y, H63D, S65C, C282S), that person is referred to as a heterozygote. The remaining nonmutated (good copy) HFE gene is sufficient in most carriers to prevent the onset of symptoms.

Homozygote: If an individual has the C282Y mutation on both chromosomes, that person is referred to as homozygote for the C282Y mutation. Such individuals have a very good chance of developing hemochromatosis. An individual can also have the H63D mutation on both chromosomes; that person would also be called homozygous for this mutation. In the United States, approximately 83 percent of all HHC patients are homozygous for the C282Y mutation.

Compound heterozygote: If an individual has the C282Y mutation on one chromosome and the H63D mutation on the other chromosome, he or she can sometimes develop hemochromatosis. When two different mutations are found together in the same individual, the arrangement is referred to as a compound heterozygote. Approximately 77 percent of compound heterozygotes have the C282Y/H63D combination.

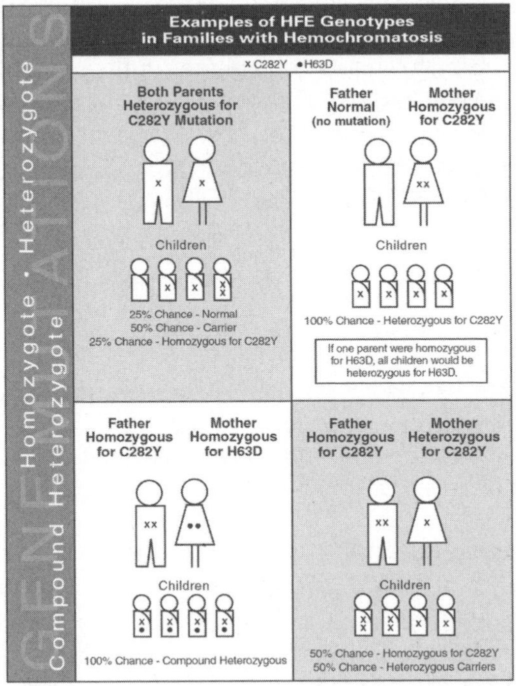
GENE MUTATIONS
Homozygote • Heterozygote
Compound Heterozygote
Examples of HFE Genotypes in Families with Hemochromatosis
x C282Y •H63D
Both Parents Heterozygous for C282Y Mutation
Children
25% Chance - Normal
50% Chance - Carrier
25% Chance - Homozygous for C282Y
Father Normal (no mutation)
Mother Homozygous for C282Y
Children
100% Chance - Heterozygous for C282Y
If one parent were homozygous for H63D, all children would be heterozygous for H63D.
Father Homozygous for C282Y
Mother Homozygous for H63D
Children
100% Chance - Compound Heterozygous
Father Homozygous for C282Y
Mother Heterozygous for C282Y
Children
50% Chance - Homozygous for C282Y
50% Chance - Heterozygous Carriers

It was formerly believed that heterozygotes were not at high risk of developing disease, especially if they had one of the lesser mutations of HFE, such as H63D or S65C. Since the discovery of yet another mutation, C282S, scientists have concluded that this particular mutation is associated with severe iron overload. Discovery of additional mutations will likely result in more people who were formerly classified as heterozygotes being classified as compound heterozygotes.

Homozygotes of the C282Y mutation are generally Caucasian. In one study at Self Hospital in Greenwood, South Carolina, the molecular laboratory investigator and IDI Medical and Scientific Advisory Board member Dr. John Longshore examined the cord blood of one thousand births. He found the HFE incidence of C282Y in the Piedmont region of South Carolina to be 1 in 121, which is higher than in many other regions of the United States. This prevalence is similar to that in Ireland, which is among the highest in the world at 1 in 80. Longshore also made the interesting finding of a C282Y-mutation African American homozygote.

More than 90 percent of people diagnosed with hemochromatosis who are of northern European descent are homozygotes for the C282Y mutation of HFE.

—A. Pietrangelo, "EASL International Consensus, Conference on Haemochromatosis," Journal of Hepatology, 2000

"There is ample evidence that C282Y/H63D heterozygote[s] are at high risk of developing hemochromatosis."

—John Feder, PhD, HFE Gene Discovery Team and former board member of the Iron Disorders Institute Medical and Scientific Advisory Board, at the IRONUSA 2000 Conference

Genetically testing a patient for the presence of C282Y and H63D mutations of HFE is a good noninvasive way to diagnose hereditary hemochromatosis. New mutations of HFE and other iron regulators continue to be discovered periodically. Some of these will become commercially available to the public, while other discoveries will remain available only to clinical researchers.

9

Role of a Genetic Counselor

Consulting with a genetic counselor before undergoing DNA testing is a wise investment in one's health. Genetic counselors are trained professionals with specialized degrees in medical genetics and counseling. They work as members of a health-care team to provide information, risk assessment, and support to families with a variety of genetic disorders. A genetic counselor can help individuals and families with hemochromatosis in numerous ways: by explaining the pattern of inheritance, by identifying at-risk family members, by reviewing testing options, and by explaining and coordinating genetic testing. These professionals can also point out the benefits and possible consequences of genetic testing as part of informed consent, which is the legal right of a patient to be informed of the possible consequences of a procedure. You can locate a genetic counselor at the websites of the National Society of Genetic Counselors (www.nsgc.org) or the American College of Medical Genetics (www.acmg.net).

Anyone considering genetic testing should be aware of the potential benefits and risks. Informed consent can illustrate some of the consequences, such as the fact that once mutations are identified, the information is part of your medical history for the rest of your life. Employers and insurance companies may scrutinize individuals with such mutations. To this effect, Congress has passed the Genetic Information Nondiscrimination Act (GINA), which was signed into law on May 21, 2008. The act provides individuals with federal protections against genetic discrimination in health insurance and employment based on family history and genetic test results. The health insurance provisions of the bill begin on May 21, 2009, and the employment protections begin on November 21, 2009. The act does not provide protection for life insurance coverage and long-term disability insurance. Additional information about GINA can be found at the Genetic Alliance website (www.geneticalliance. org/policy.discrimination).

Genetic testing offers invaluable information. Results can provide a long-sought-after diagnosis for those with hemochromatosis. Many people with HHC suffer from multiple health problems.

Genetic testing that reveals the presence of both mutations of HFE does two things. It provides a solid diagnosis of hereditary hemochromatosis, and it provides a great sense of relief and comfort to patients whose previous diagnoses included hypochondria. Knowing one's HFE status can alert an individual that he or she is in the highest risk category for iron-related disease. If detected early enough, iron-related diseases can be prevented. A simple blood donation two or three times a year and modest dietary changes might be the only preventive measures that such individuals need to observe to avoid potential disease.

"There is no doubt that genetics will revolutionize medicine, but citizens need to be well informed about any procedure that has long-lasting ethical, legal, and social implications. Numerous privacy and discrimination issues are still not fully addressed."

—*Elizabeth Thomson, PhD, Ethical, Legal, and Social Implications Research Program program director, Human Genome Project, National Human Genome Research Institute*

The National Human Genome Research Institute is one of the federal agencies in the United States charged with taking the leadership on the international effort to map and sequence all human genes, the Human Genome Project. The institute's Ethical, Legal, and Social Implications (ELSI) Research Program addresses the ethical, legal, and social implications of genetic testing. The purpose of ELSI is to examine the implications of new developing technologies and information while studying the basic science, the biology, and the actual mapping of the genome.

The intent of ELSI is to ensure that genetic technologies are integrated in an appropriate way into clinical and non-clinical settings, and to ensure that genetic information is used appropriately and not to stigmatize or to discriminate against people.

The National Institutes of Health's National Heart, Lung, and Blood Institute funded a major $30 million, five-year, multicenter clinical trial to look at phenotypic and genotypic screening for hereditary hemochromatosis and other iron-loading conditions. The study screened over one hundred thousand adults from very diverse populations who were being seen in primary care settings. One of the potential risks that could occur as a result of such screening is that people could be identified with HFE mutations and assumed to have hereditary hemochromatosis, when they are and may continue to be healthy. Dr. Elizabeth Thomson pointed out, "The day may come when there are enough genomic screening tests that each one of us will be identified to have or be at risk for one genetic disorder or another, putting us at some risk to become uninsurable in our current healthcare system."

10
Who Is a Candidate for Genetic Testing?

Hemochromatosis offers the possibly once-in-a-lifetime opportunity to explore and resolve the many issues that accompany genetic testing. Hereditary hemochromatosis is the poster child for this type of testing because it is so common, it is treatable, and early detection of HHC can result in prevention of disease. Moreover, HHC can provide the framework for the ethical, legal, and social implications of genetic testing while people benefit from its simplicity as a diagnostic tool.

Education is key. The Iron Disorders Institute believes that the HFE genetic test is an important and powerful tool. Its application is appropriate when the patient fully knows the benefits and clearly understands the risks. Physicians must be sensitive to the proper and improper use of this diagnostic breakthrough, and patients must have reliable information about genetic testing.

Genetic testing can settle issues of whether an individual has hemochromatosis. The test confirms the presence of the HFE mutation in 85 percent of people who have an iron-loading condition. These are remarkable statistics. Genetic testing helps a physician eliminate hours of guesswork and costly lab work, and it may reduce the need for invasive procedures such as liver biopsies. The patient most definitely benefits.

Family-Based Detection: How Genetics Can Save Future Generations

Jack Cluster and his two remaining sisters decided to undergo genetic testing. Two of their siblings had already died of suspected hemochromatosis: one from liver cancer and the other from bleeding esophageal varices, a liver disease–related condition. Their parents had been healthy and had lived well into their eighties. Jack and his two sisters were all found to be C282Y homozygotes. Jack believes that both of his parents were carriers and that all five children inherited both mutations of HFE. Three of those children were confirmed homozygotes; two died of causes commonly associated with undetected hemochromatosis.

Another example is that of Laura and Dick Main, both of whom are carriers. Laura's father was the first known member of the family to die of undetected hemochromatosis. Laura and Dick's twenty-four-year-old son Christopher was, hopefully, the last member of their family to die prematurely of HHC-related problems.

Genetic testing of couples who are planning a family to determine their carrier status is strongly recommended. An estimated 32 million Americans of European descent are carriers of HFE mutations. This means that the children of two carrier parents have a 25 percent chance of inheriting both mutations and developing health problems.

Genetic testing can identify patients before symptoms begin; this is especially helpful in the case of women who are still menstruating.
—*IRON2000 USA Scientific Conference*

Menstruation

When Jen's grandmother died in 1976, Jen was told that her death was due to myocardial infarction. Nothing else was ever mentioned; no autopsy was performed. All Jen remembers from that terrible time was thinking, "She's too young to die. She had just turned sixty-nine."

Over the years, Jen had experienced a number of symptoms, but not until 1991 did she suspect a connection between her symptoms and her grandmother's death. Jen's severe muscle pain, inability to conceive, heart arrhythmia, chronic fatigue, and elevated iron levels still did not result in the correct diagnosis.

Not until a genetics test revealed that she was a compound heterozygote did Jen receive a diagnosis and begin therapy.

Had the test been available a decade earlier, Jen's story might have a different ending. At forty-four, she is still young enough to have children, but she and her husband are not certain that they will choose parenthood at this late date.

A woman's risk of inheriting hemochromatosis is the same as a man's, but the onset of symptoms is usually later in life. Menstruating women have a slightly different iron loading rate from men: monthly blood loss through menstruation provides the benefit of monthly iron loss and therefore a slower rate of iron accumulation.

When Hemochromatosis Has Been Identified in the Family

When hemochromatosis has been identified in the family, all family members are at an increased risk of having HFE mutations or of being carriers. Brothers and sisters (siblings) of an individual with an HFE mutation have the greatest likelihood of previously undetected hemochromatosis. Parents and children are at an increased risk of carrying a single mutation in the HFE gene (i.e., of being carriers). Rarely, carriers may have increased iron stores. Individuals who are eighteen or older and have an elevated fasting TS percentage are good candidates for genetic testing in this situation. Checking iron levels periodically can help a person determine whether iron is accumulating, but genetic testing will confirm the diagnosis, eliminate doubt about the presence of the condition, and allow for early therapy once iron levels begin to rise—hopefully early enough to avoid disease.

Genetic testing is one of the most powerful new diagnostic tools of the century. Physicians and patients will benefit from the simplicity of the tests, but occasionally genetic testing can cause problems. Patients need to be aware of any negative consequences of genetic testing and whether or not their individual circumstances will be affected by new laws designed to protect them from genetic discrimination (see chapter 9). These matters can be discussed with their physicians or genetics counselors.

Informed Consent

Joint pain, chronic fatigue, persistent cough, and arrhythmia prompted Tim to see his company's physician. Tim's iron levels were elevated, and he was diagnosed with iron-overload disease. The company doctor started Tim on phlebotomies in the local hospital system. Tim's boss thought nothing of the periodic blood extractions; he found the notion of too much iron humorous, often making jokes about it. During a follow-up exam, the physician casually suggested that Tim get genetically tested, and Tim agreed. Results showed that Tim was a C282Y homozygote. Thinking that this was "interesting" news, Tim told his boss that he had a genetic condition called hemochromatosis. Within weeks, Tim was fired, lost his insurance, and had no way to pay for phlebotomy treatment. Had he known the consequences of telling his boss about the genetic outcome, Tim may have never mentioned it to him. The physician's attempts to illuminate Tim's boss about genetics and about how Tim would actually have improved health following phlebotomy all failed. The Genetic Information Nondiscrimination Act would now provide protection for Tim (see chapter 9).

The important thing to keep in mind about genetic testing is that having it done should be a personal and individual decision. Circumstances are different for every man, woman, and child. There is no reason a well-informed person should not be genetically tested if that person perceives a benefit from doing so.

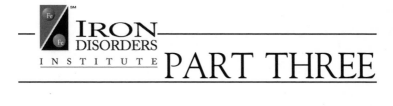

PART THREE

Hemochromatosis and Body Systems

11

Liver, Spleen, Gallbladder, and Pancreas

"The liver is a principal target for iron toxicity because it is chiefly responsible for taking up and storing excessive amounts of iron."
—H. L. Bonkovsky and R. W. Lambrecht, "Iron-Induced Liver Injury,"
Clinical Liver Diseases 4 (2000): 409–29

"Of all the organs, the liver serves as the most important 'landfill' for the disposal of excessive iron. In untreated HHC, for example, the liver iron concentration reaches 50 [to] 100 times that of normal figures. A similar proportional increase occurs in the pancreas."
—T. H. Bothwell, R. W. Charlton, and A. G. Motulsky, "Hemochromatosis," in
Metabolic Basis of Inherited Diseases, ed. C. R. Scriver et al., 6th ed. (New York:
McGraw Hill Information Service), 1433–62

"The liver serves as a principal depository for dangerous quantities of iron. Unaddressed excessive iron in the liver will eventually lead to cirrhosis as a result of fibrosis or scarring of liver tissue. Cirrhotic tissue provides a fertile ground for the initiation and promotion of cancer cell growth. Iron is a well-recognized mutagen and can cause development of liver cancer even in non-fibrotic tissue. Therefore, prompt treatment of any liver iron excess, even when mild, is prudent and integral to the patient's continued good health."
—Gene Weinberg, PhD, Exposing the Hidden Dangers
of Iron (Nashville, TN: Cumberland House, 2003)

Liver

Besides the brain, the liver contains the greatest amounts of ferritin, the primary containment vessel for excess iron. The liver also produces hepcidin, a protein that helps to regulate iron. The main effect of hepcidin is to lower the iron content of blood by trapping iron inside macrophages and by inhibiting the transfer of dietary iron into the blood from duodenal intestinal cells. An HFE genotype can interfere with the production of hepcidin and the proper regulation of iron in the body.

The liver has more separate functions in the body than any other organ except the brain. Situated on the right side of the body beneath the ribcage, the liver weighs about two and a half to three and a half pounds and is eight to nine inches wide and about six inches tall. It is concave underneath and covers the stomach, part of the small intestine, gallbladder, right kidney, and right adrenal gland. Among its functions, the liver produces bile, which emulsifies fats. It also metabolizes carbohydrates and filters harmful substances such as ammonia, alcohol, drugs, and toxic chemicals. The liver stores cholesterol, vitamins, and clotting factors. It contains macrophages called Kupffer cells, which are scavengers of harmful bacteria and old red blood cells from the bloodstream. The liver also provides for the elimination of waste products such as bile pigments, bilirubin, excess cholesterol, lipids, drugs, and poisons.

The liver processes everything we eat or drink, as well as supplements and many medications. In addition to its metabolic, filtering, defense, storage, and excretion capabilities, the liver has the remarkable ability to function when portions of it have been cut away. A liver can be surgically resected—the removal of a lobe for the purpose of transplantation—and the remaining portion will not only compensate in function but also generate new cell growth.

Pain in the upper-right quadrant of the abdomen is one sign of liver injury and possible disease. Pain in this area is a frequent complaint of hemochromatosis patients.

Other symptoms of liver disease include unexplained weight loss, nausea, vomiting, jaundice, ascites (fluid and swelling in abdominal area), and in some cases itching hands and feet

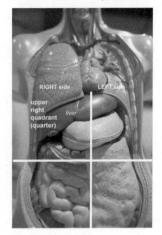

(which eventually spreads all over), mental confusion, difficulty concentrating, and out-of-character aggressive behavior.

Medical findings such as elevated liver enzymes, serum ferritin levels greater than 1,000 ng/mL with accompanying elevated TS percentage, the presence of the hepatitis B or C virus, elevated alpha-fetoprotein levels, or abnormal total and direct bilirubin may all be signs of liver disease. Abdominal pain, hepatomegaly (enlargement of liver), and unexplained weight loss with unexplained mild fever can also be signs of primary liver cancer. A liver biopsy can rule out primary liver cancer.

The liver can become diseased in several ways. Liver damage is commonly associated with viral hepatitis infection, alcoholism, drugs, exposure to toxic chemicals, excessive consumption of fats, nonalcoholic steatohepatitis (NASH), diabetes, and excessively high copper or iron levels (copper or iron overload.)

Hereditary hemochromatosis is the leading known cause of iron overload. Regardless of the cause of iron overload, the liver is the major site for storage of excess iron in the body. Excess iron accumulates in the functional cells of the liver called hepatocytes. The disproportionately high levels of hepatic (i.e., liver related) iron can result in cirrhosis or fibrosis. Any process or organ dependent on liver function is compromised in the presence of excess iron.

If a diagnosis of hemochromatosis is made after cirrhosis has developed, the chances that the patient will also proceed to hepatocellular carcinoma (liver cancer) are increased by 20- to 200-fold. At the current rate of detection, approximately 40 percent of patients with hemochromatosis and cirrhosis will eventually develop primary liver cancer. For most people with liver cancer, death is inevitable, unless transplantation with a donor liver can be performed.

The extent of damage to the liver is determined by liver biopsy. This procedure is currently the only way to absolutely assess liver damage, particularly the presence and degree of scar tissue (cirrhosis, fibrosis); however, there are reports of other noninvasive tests that are in the research and development stage. In analysis of the biopsy, liver iron is seen with a special stain (see the dark clusters in the liver-tissue sample image).

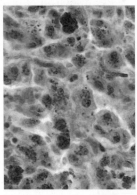

In addition to the toxicity of large amounts of iron, there is growing evidence that only mildly increased, relatively small amounts of iron can cause or worsen liver injury in the presence of fatty liver, elevated LDL (low-density lipoprotein, or "bad" cholesterol), low HDL (high-density lipoprotein, or "good" cholesterol), chronic viral hepatitis, chronic hepatic porphyria, and/or alcoholism.

Viral Hepatitis and Iron

More than fifteen years ago, scientists began to notice a correlation between elevated iron levels and chronic viral hepatitis. Some speculate that iron is released from liver cells injured by the presence of hepatitis virus.

Dr. Baruch S. Blumberg was among the first who noted that patients on dialysis with low serum ferritin levels cleared the infection sooner than did those with elevated ferritin levels. Dr. D. H. Van Thiel and colleagues were first to observe higher iron levels in association with poor responses to interferon treatment of chronic viral hepatitis. Until recently, interferon was the only treatment available for patients chronically infected with viral hepatitis B or C.

Most patients with hepatitis A and 95 percent of hepatitis B cases realize full recovery and build antibodies against future infection. However, 5 percent of those with hepatitis B remain chronically infected. There is no treatment for hepatitis A, and approximately one hundred Americans per year die of type A viral hepatitis. There are vaccinations against hepatitis A and B. However, for hepatitis C, which typically remains with a person for a lifetime, there is no vaccine. Moreover, long-term response to treatment for chronic hepatitis C is poor; only about 15 to 40 percent of people improve.

Dr. Van Thiel and colleagues studied seventy-nine patients, all of whom had chronic hepatitis. Serum iron, TS percentage, and ferritin for the patients were measured, and all patients underwent liver biopsy. All the patients were treated with alpha-interferon, but only 50 percent responded. Van Thiel noted that, in the patients who did not respond to treatment, liver-iron content was twice as high as levels of iron in responders to interferon.

Dr. Herbert Bonkovsky, and colleagues Dr. Barbara Banner and Dr. Alan Rothman, suggest that patients with viral hepatitis B and C respond to interferon better when ferritin levels are at about 15 to 20 ng/mL. Further, the iron metabolism experts Bonkovsky, Dr. A. M. DiBisceglie, and Dr. Bruce Bacon studied iron-reduction therapy in those with chronic viral hepatitis C. They noted that the liver enzyme alanine aminotransferase (ALT) was significantly reduced in response to interferon treatment when administered following a series of phlebotomies to reduce ferritin.

Alcohol Abuse

Patients with iron overload have increased susceptibility to liver-cell damage by alcohol. Hepatic-cell uptake of iron may increase in the presence of alcohol. Twenty to thirty percent of alcoholics, including many who have the HFE genotype, absorb twice the amount of dietary iron than do nonusers of alcohol. Alcohol overuse inhibits the body's ability to produce several very important and protective antioxidants and can contribute to the development of fatty liver disease. Furthermore, metabolism of alcohol can result in the release of iron from ferritin, resulting in enhanced production of reactive radicals that can cause oxidative damage to tissue and DNA.

A study conducted by Dr. Charles Lieber, of Mt. Sinai School of Medicine in New York, observed that drinking even moderate amounts of alcohol can lead to cirrhosis. In his study, participants were given diets supplemented with minerals (including iron) along with a daily dose of alcohol that was less than the amount needed to produce intoxication. After eighteen days, subjects developed an eightfold increase in liver fat, a precondition of cirrhosis.

Cirrhosis

Cirrhosis is the scarring of liver tissue. Alcohol misuse is but one cause of cirrhosis. Viral hepatitis B and C, cryptogenic cirrhosis (today, generally referred to as nonalcoholic steatohepatitis, or NASH), and hemochromatosis or iron overload also can cause cirrhosis.

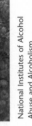

National Institutes of Alcohol Abuse and Alcoholism

Some patients with cirrhosis develop esophageal varices within the wall of the esophagus (varicose veins in the lower part of the esophagus). Blood pressure builds in the portal vein, which carries blood from the digestive tract to the liver. This pressure can result in a condition called portal hypertension, which causes blood to back up into the esophageal veins. Engorged or bulging veins can rupture from pressure or be torn by severe coughing, which results in bleeding. The varices can sometimes bleed profusely, leading to anemia; an untreated patient with this condition can bleed to death. Patients with bleeding esophageal varices must seek emergency help immediately. An endoscope can verify the presence of engorged veins.

The primary treatment for esophageal varices is to stop the bleeding. This may be achieved with high-blood-pressure drugs (beta blockers) to reduce pressure in the portal vein. Other approaches to stop bleeding include ligation, in which an elastic band is placed around the swollen vein, or endoscopic injection of a solution directly into the varices to dissolve them. A nonsurgical approach is a portal-systemic shunt. This device, called a transjugular intrahepatic portal-systemic shunt (TIPS), can be used with patients who are experiencing internal bleeding caused by variances due to cirrhosis of the liver. This device is also useful for those awaiting liver transplantation. With TIPS, a needle with a balloon catheter is threaded through a vein in the neck into the liver. Except for a moment when it cannot be seen, a contrast dye is used to track the location of the catheter. When the catheter is in the liver, a pathway between blood vessels is created to reestablish blood flow through the liver. Individuals with a portal-systemic shunt are highly susceptible to excessive accumulation of iron. Liver failure and brain disease (encephalopathy) are due to a buildup of toxins normally filtered out by the liver. The toxins pass through the shunt and into the bloodstream; functioning normally, the liver would have filtered out the toxins. In general, TIPS is used when other treatments have failed; it is also a temporary measure in patients waiting for liver transplantation, which may be a last resort for patients with advanced liver damage.

Assessing Liver Health

Liver function tests (LFTs) help to assess how well a person's liver is working. The tests include measurements of liver enzymes, bilirubin, prothrombin time, lipids (cholesterol and triglycerides), albumin, globulins, and total protein.

Bilirubin is a brownish yellow substance also called a bile pigment. Bilirubin is produced when the liver destroys (breaks down) old red blood cells. When the liver is damaged, bilirubin can leak out from the liver into the bloodstream. Eventually, excess bilirubin levels can be detected with visible signs. Jaundiced (i.e., yellowish) skin or sclerae (i.e., whites of the eyes), pale or very dark or black and tarry stools, and dark-colored urine are some signs of excess bilirubin. The liver and spleen should be examined to rule out disease.

Prothrombin time is a blood test that measures how long it takes blood to clot. Normal clotting time is ten to fifteen seconds; a long prothrombin time suggests bleeding or liver disease.

Lipids (cholesterol and triglycerides) are naturally occurring fats. At normal levels, these fats are necessary for metabolism. A cholesterol test measures low-density lipids (LDLs), the most harmful type of cholesterol, and high-density lipids (HDLs), the most beneficial type. Triglycerides are a type of fat in the bloodstream and fat tissue. Often, high triglycerides occur along with high levels of cholesterol, another type of fat. Triglycerides are measured along with cholesterol as part of a blood test. Levels greater than 200 are considered high. A total cholesterol test is a rough measure of all the cholesterol and triglycerides in the blood.

Albumin is the protein that transports many small molecules in the blood such as bilirubin, calcium, and medications. It also serves to control fluid from the blood leaking out into the tissues. Because albumin is made by the liver, decreased serum albumin may result from liver disease. It can also result from kidney disease, which allows albumin to escape into the urine.

Total protein test is a rough measure of all the proteins found in the fluid portion of the blood. Abnormal protein levels can indicate liver disease, some forms of cancer, chronic inflammation, and bleeding.

The phrase "liver enzymes" is commonly used to describe a group of enzymes abbreviated as AST, ALT, GGT, and ALP. These enzyme levels are routinely measured to isolate problems of the liver, gallbladder, large and small intestine, pancreas, heart, and bones.

Alanine transaminase (ALT) and aspartate aminotransferase (AST), referred to as transaminases, are made in the liver. If the liver is damaged or disease is present, these enzymes leak into the bloodstream.

The presence of alanine transaminase (ALT) in the bloodstream indicates inflammation of the liver (hepatitis), which may indicate liver damage (e.g., cirrhosis, tumor, cancer). If the liver is injured, high levels of ALT are released into the blood. This enzyme can be elevated by certain drugs, such as acetaminophen, antiseizure medications, cholesterol-lowering drugs, and antidepressants. Heart attack, infections such as mononucleosis, and pancreatitis can also produce elevated ALT. Elevated ALT levels are observed in hemochromatosis and iron overload, copper overload (Wilson's disease), nonalcoholic steatohepatitis (NASH), alpha-antitrypsin-1 deficiency, celiac sprue, or muscle-wasting disease. Sometimes ALT is referred to as serum glutamate pyruvate transaminase (SGPT).

Aspartate aminotransferase (AST) is an enzyme found in the

liver, heart, muscle, and bone. When cells of the heart, liver, or bone are damaged, AST is released into the blood. AST can help detect disease in any one of these organs and is most helpful in determining that a heart attack has occurred, as levels are elevated within eight hours of the heart attack. A few days after the event, AST then falls back into normal range. In chronic disease, AST remains constantly elevated. Sometimes AST is also referred to as serum glutamic oxaloacetic transaminase (SGOT).

Alkaline phosphatase (ALP) and gamma glutamyl transferase (GGT) are also known as cholestatic liver enzymes. The ALP enzyme is found in the liver, bone, kidney, and placenta. Injury to any of those organs will cause ALP to be released into the bloodstream. Elevated levels usually indicate an obstruction somewhere within the liver, such as gallstones. Elevated ALP can also be an indication of inflammation (hepatitis), bone disease, congestive heart failure, overactive thyroid, or liver cancer. Elevated ALP is normal in children, especially teenagers, who are undergoing rapid growth and physical changes, which includes bone growth. In these cases, a pediatrician can measure the GGT level, which will be normal if the elevated ALP is due to bone growth.

The GGT enzyme is found in the greatest quantities in the liver and biliary tract cells. It is also found to a lesser degree in the kidney, spleen, heart, brain, intestine, and prostate gland. Metabolic syndrome, obesity, fatty liver, medications, and excessive use of alcohol or supplements can affect GGT. The enzyme can also be elevated during heart attack, renal failure, chronic obstructive pulmonary disease, and diabetes. The GGT enzyme is most helpful in diagnosing an obstruction in the biliary tract.

When both ALP and GGT are elevated, it is generally due to liver disease. Also, GGT is very helpful in detecting chronic alcohol ingestion. The GGT enzyme is often elevated in people who have three or more alcoholic drinks per day. However, this is not completely reliable, as GGT can also be elevated in non-drinkers who are taking anticonvulsants or whose antioxidant production capability is compromised.

The levels of liver enzymes cannot provide a prognosis (i.e., expected outcome), and levels do not always correlate with the extent of liver damage. Patients with cirrhosis often have normal or only slightly elevated ALT or AST. The interpretation of liver enzyme levels depends on a complete clinical picture. Therefore, conclusions about the findings are best left to a physician who is experienced in evaluating liver disease.

The transaminases, ALT and AST, are the two most frequently evaluated liver enzymes in hemochromatosis patients. There are different types of hemochromatosis; the most common form is called the classic form or type 1. In type 1 hereditary hemochromatosis the transaminases are typically only mildly elevated (less than twice the normal range), often much less than those typically observed in patients with acute inflammation from viral hepatitis or alcoholic liver disease.

Alpha-fetoprotein (AFP) is a protein used with unborn children to detect defects such as Down syndrome and spina bifida. In addition, AFP is used to detect certain pathological conditions in adults, such as tumors. Increased serum AFP levels are found in up to 90 percent of those with hepatomas (i.e., liver tumors). Other conditions that can be suspect when AFP levels are elevated include cancers of the lung, stomach, colon, breast, and lymph. Often, AFP is used in hemochromatosis patients with a history of liver disease or who are at risk for liver cancer.

Gerry's experience as a liver transplant recipient illustrates the critical need to eliminate the knowledge gaps that persist even among top healthcare professionals. Even though Gerry drank in moderation, the fact that he drank at all was the cause attributed to his cirrhosis and the need for a new liver. After his transplant, Gerry's natural curiosity for numbers and evidence led him to examine his health records more closely. Something jumped out at him that would forever change his life. During more than three years of progressive illness, none of Gerry's three physicians (gastroenterologist, internist, and hematologist) ever checked his iron levels. Gerry's hematologist believed that he was suffering from a mild but chronic hemolytic anemia and was only curious as to why Gerry appeared able to maintain a year-round, all-over tan without going to a tanning salon. As Gerry had stopped drinking entirely at the onset of his illness, all three physicians believed that the persistent condition was not life threatening and would probably go away over time. They concurred that if there was indeed any liver damage, it would at worst remain stable because of his improved and healthier lifestyle.

None of his physicians had placed any significance on Gerry's rather sudden and unintended (though much welcomed) weight loss, his loss of body hair, and complaints of severe fatigue and depression, loss of libido, and diminished sexual function. Gerry just figured that this was all tied in to the aging process. Then suddenly one day Gerry almost bled to death as a result of hemorrhaging esophageal varices, a common sign of end-stage liver disease.

Gerry's iron levels were finally checked, but only after he was diagnosed with terminal liver disease. His iron levels were first measured when he underwent a pretransplant evaluation—too late to do anything about it. Gerry's serum ferritin measured 825 and his TS percentage was 65 percent. A genetic test later revealed that he was a C282Y heterozygote. Gerry said, "We must pay closer attention to the C282Y heterozygote. There are about 30 million C282Y heterozygotes in the United States; we cannot ignore this group because they do not fit the accepted profile of the highest risk group, C282Y/C282Y homozygote. It was terrible that someone had to die so that I could have a new liver, but worse, a person on the transplant waiting list had to also die; there just aren't enough organs to meet demands."

Gerry's liver could have been restored to good health if his iron overload had been detected early enough to be effectively treated. According to the American Liver Foundation, each year nearly seventeen thousand people in the United States are listed on the United Network for Organ Sharing (UNOS) waiting list. It often takes more than a year or two before they receive a liver, if they ever get one at all. Each year, about 6,500 people receive a liver transplant, and about 2,000 others die while hopefully waiting.

Gerry is now participating in a national clinical trial to test his tolerance for being weaned off of organ rejection drugs, and one of the top liver transplantation specialists in the world supervises Gerry's trial. Gerry is one of the first cases on record able to maintain normal liver function without the drugs. Gerry now works full-time encouraging healthcare professionals to understand and perform the proper blood tests for iron overload, since unfortunately there are few typical and visible signs of this metabolic disorder.

Many people die from iron overload, and too often the underlying cause of their demise is never detected—far more often than not, the death certificate memorializes only the final disease state. Cirrhosis with alcohol listed as a cause, cryptogenic cirrhosis (which is nonalcoholic steatohepatitis, or NASH), liver cancer, type 2 diabetes, or heart failure are generally, and belatedly, stated as the cause of death.

The Spleen

The spleen serves as the principal organ in the recycling of iron from spent red blood cells. In conditions of chronic hemolysis, such as beta thalassemia, sickle-cell disease, and congenital dyserythropoietic anemia, the spleen becomes overwhelmed, and surgical removal may be necessary to stop chronic hemolysis. Once the spleen has been removed, the patient is more susceptible to infections with germs such as pneumococci, meningococci, and *Haemophilus influenzae.* Daily doses of penicillin as a preventive measure are recommended for such patients. In contrast, patients with the classic form of hemochromatosis do not accumulate excessive iron in their spleens because the tissue mainly comprises macrophages. Stainable iron is usually present in the spleen but in lesser amounts than in the liver and pancreas. The splenic capsule frequently contains iron deposits that are calcified. In autopsies of newborns with neonatal hemochromatosis, there is little stainable iron in the spleen, lymph, or bone marrow but significant amounts in the pancreas, thyroid, and the liver.

When the spleen is enlarged (splenomegaly), which can be determined by touch or scan, a medical professional who specializes in spleen-related disease should examine the cause. Among the experts who may be consulted are gastroenterologists, hematologists, infectious disease experts, and internists.

The Gallbladder

There have been few studies of how hemochromatosis exactly

affects the gallbladder. Gallbladders of HHC patients are often removed because of cholelithiasis (gallstones). According to the Iron Disorders Institute's Patient Services Database, some HHC patients who have had their gallbladders removed report that the stones are "variable in size and black in color," possibly indicating the presence of iron in the bile. In a 1996 U.S. Centers for Disease Control and Prevention survey of 2,851 hemochromatosis patients, liver and/or gallbladder disease was reported by 9.5 percent of men and 5.2 percent of women aged seventeen to thirty-nine, 17.7 percent of men and 20 percent of women aged forty to fifty-nine, and 17.5 percent of men and 23.2 percent of women aged sixty to eighty-four.

High levels of iron can damage the sphincter of Oddi, which controls secretions from the liver, pancreas, and gallbladder into the small intestine (duodenum), the primary site of nutrient absorption.

According to Dr. Gene Weinberg's book *Exposing the Hidden Dangers of Iron*, "With specific attention to the sphincter of Oddi, French scientists examined 109 consecutive autopsies. These investigators concluded that chronic pancreatitis (which can be a consequence of excessive iron or chronic alcohol abuse), was more frequently associated with an abnormal sphincter of Oddi. At the University of Milan, 350 patients with alcoholic cirrhosis and hemochromatosis were studied. The incidence of cholelithiasis (gallstones) was three times higher in these patients than in non-alcoholic, iron normal controls."

12

Joints and Bones

Nearly 85 percent of patients with type 1 (classic) hereditary hemochromatosis experience arthropathy (joint disease). Hand, hip, knee, and ankle joints are most often affected. Joint pain is very common in the general population, and therefore not specific to hemochromatosis. Pain and enlargement in the knuckles of the second and third fingers (called iron fist) is an unusual feature of hemochromatosis. About 25 percent of people with hemochromatosis-caused arthritis have Heberden's nodes, which are bony growths in the joint nearest the tip of the finger.

Hemochromatosis arthropa-thy and accompanying joint pain may originate from a pro-gressive degenerative type of arthritis (osteoarthritis) with or without calcium deposits called chondrocalcinosis. Many X-rays of the hands of hemochro-matosis patients with arthritis 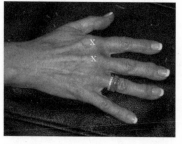 show calcium crystal deposits, osteophytes (bone spurs), and narrowing of the joint space. Some HHC patients are misdiag-nosed with rheumatoid arthritis.

Iron Disorders Institute image file

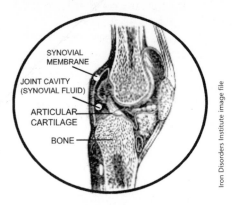

SYNOVIAL MEMBRANE

JOINT CAVITY (SYNOVIAL FLUID)

ARTICULAR CARTILAGE

BONE

Iron Disorders Institute image file

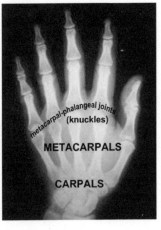

metacarpal-phalangeal joints (knuckles)

METACARPALS

CARPALS

Iron Disorders Institute image file

The same hand joints are also often affected by rheumatoid arthritis, but in hemochromatosis arthropathy, patients usually test negative for the rheumatoid factor in the blood. Rheumatoid arthritis generally attacks a multitude of joints symmetrically and produces a soft, warm, swelling joint. Typically a person will experience an hour or more of morning stiffness. Hemochromatosis arthritis can also be mistaken for gout because it sometimes affects lower extremities, especially ankles.

Primary or nontraumatic osteoarthritis is uncommon in the

ankle joint. Arthritis of the ankles and the knuckles is a clue that can prompt consideration of a diagnosis of hemochromatosis.

The X-ray finding of a white line of chondrocalcinosis in any joint is another clue indicating hemochromatosis. Chondrocalcinosis, or pseudogout, is a condition of chronic recurrent arthritis clinically similar to gout. In this type of arthritis, patients' arthritic buildup has calcium pyrophosphate dihydrate (CPPD) crystals but not urate crystals. The CPPD crystals can be observed with joint fluid aspiration.

Arthritis was recognized as a manifestation of idiopathic HHC in 1964 by H. Ralph Schumacher, who noticed the unusual combination of osteoarthritis-like changes at the metacarpal phalangeal joints (iron fist) and other joints less typically involved with ordinary osteoarthritis but typical of HHC-related arthropathy.

Joint effusions are usually noninflammatory, except when associated with CPPD deposition. Schumacher and his colleagues observed pathologic features of the joints, including the cartilage of five patients with hemochromatosis. In addition to the crystal or iron deposits, all had advanced degenerative changes in the cartilage. When iron was present, it was entirely intracellular (within the cell), and CPPD crystals commonly coated the surface of the eroded cartilage.

Percentage of persons in general population and in those with HHC who reported arthritic symptoms				
	Women		Men	
Age in years	General Population	HHC	General Population	HHC
17-38	5.9	10.3	5.2	8.9
40-59	23.4	34.9	14.7	22.2
60-84	51.1	42.8	33.8	31.5

McDonnell, S. M., P. D. Phatak, V. Felitti, A. Hover, and G. D. McLaren. "Screenings for Hemochromatosis in Primary Care Settings." *Annals of Internal Medicine* 129 (1998): 962–70.

Severe progressive arthropathy can occur or continue despite phlebotomy. Dr. Schumacher and his colleagues Drs. Pablo Straka, Margaret Krikker, and Andrew Dudley studied arthropathy in three hundred patients with HHC and joint pain. Their findings were based on responses from 159 cases as follows:

JOINT PAIN AFTER INITIAL PHLEBOTOMY	
WORSE	42
SAME	32
BETTER	27
PAIN DURING	15
PAIN AFTER	13

EFFECTS OF THERAPY ON JOINT PAIN	HELPED	DID NOT HELP
ASPIRIN	57	6
NSAIDS	32	10
HOT APPLICATION	154	5
COLD APPLICATION	33	109 WORSENED

Therapies to Relieve Pain

As there is no known cure for hemochromatosis arthropathy, patients can expect only to address the symptoms that are associated with joint disease. Pain is the No. 1 complaint heard from hemochromatosis patients with arthropathy.

Oral pain relievers such as nonsteroidal anti-inflammatory drugs (NSAIDs) can be used for pain, but problems associated with long-term use prompted a public health warning from the U.S. Food and Drug Administration in 2004. Some types of NSAIDs suppress the release of COX-1 or COX-2 enzymes, which contribute to inflammation. The FDA issued the warning because COX-2 selective agents, widely used by many arthritis patients, appeared to be associated with an increase in serious cardiovascular events (heart attack and stroke). The FDA warning included an increased risk for these events even from over-the-counter NSAIDs. All NSAIDs, including aspirin, have a tendency to promote bleeding in the stomach and intestinal tract.

Acetaminophen, another type of pain reliever, is not recommended for hemochromatosis patients because of the increased risk of liver damage that can result from this compound.

Intra-articular injection of glucocorticoid salts (steroids) or hyaluronic acid (HA) is another approach to treatment of osteoarthritis of the knee. In one meta-analysis of this therapy published in the *Journal of the American Medical Association*, authors stated that HA injection may not be as effective as had been stated in earlier reports.

Herbal remedies may be helpful because of their high antioxidant properties, but HHC patients should use these and other supplements sparingly, as excessive use, especially in concentrated form, can damage the liver. Before taking any over-the-counter product, discuss the matter with a pain-management healthcare professional.

Patients report that physical activity helps relieve pain, especially activities that include a range of motor exercises. Others report relief with hot compresses.

Other oral compounds with which patients experienced some degree of pain relief include the following:

- **Oral colchicine:** Colchicine is a medicine used to treat gout that dates back to the early 1800s; the FDA approved its use in the United States in 1939. The compound helps to suppress inflammation and may be most helpful in cases of CPPD crystal deposition.

- **Oral magnesium carbonate:** Magnesium carbonate has been used to prevent the formation of CPPD crystals. Some forms are used as antacid. The compound creates an alkaline environment, which is less conducive to the formation of CPPD crystals.

- **Glucosamine chondroitin:** Glucosamine chondroitin has sometimes been used to treat osteoarthritis. Some patients report relief with glucosamine chondroitin; however, the preliminary findings of a large study funded by the National Center for Complementary and Alternative Medicine at the National Institutes of Health demonstrated that the supplements are not effective. In a subsequent study, the Glucosamine/Chondroitin Arthritis Intervention Trial (GAIT), researchers continued to monitor 572 volunteers for an additional eighteen months and found that the supplements did not appear to slow the loss of cartilage, taken either alone or together with other compounds. The investigators found that arthritis worsened in 24 percent of participants who were taking the combination of glucosamine and chondroitin, which was an outcome similar to those taking the placebo.

Phlebotomy therapy will provide relief for some people, but patients in therapy to reduce excess iron levels often report no relief from pain. Some even report that the pain worsens with phlebotomy. This worsening effect might be a result of increased iron-generated oxidative stress on the joints. When transferrin-iron saturation percentages are elevated, the opportunity for iron to generate free radicals increases. These free radicals bombard cells, causing damage that leads to pain (for tips on how to counteract free-radical activity and oxidative stress, see chapter 37).

The mechanism by which excess iron causes some patients to develop arthritis has not been fully explained. Discoveries of the pathogenesis (origin of disease) of HHC arthropathy are beginning to emerge; with those discoveries, advances in pain management and early detection will follow.

Observations that tie the genetic influences of HHC to arthropathy are emerging. In one large population-based, longitudinal study (i.e., a study that studies lots of people for long periods of time), the H63D mutation of HFE was found to increase the early onset of arthropathy and increase early mortality in people who are homozygous for H63D. These findings emphasize the need for early detection and intervention with phlebotomy, excess iron reduction, and ongoing iron management.

Bone Health and Hemochromatosis

Patients with hemochromatosis often experience osteoporosis and osteomalacia. Both of these conditions are different from osteoarthritis, even though the names sound similar. Osteoporosis is a thinning of bone mass, osteomalacia is a softening of the bone, and osteoarthritis is a degenerative joint disease.

Joint pain is common with osteoarthritis, bone pain is common with osteomalacia, and people with osteoporosis often do not feel pain until a bone is fractured or broken.

Osteomalacia and Osteoporosis

Some patients with osteomalacia are misdiagnosed with fibromyalgia because of the similarities in pain sites. One key cause of osteomalacia is a vitamin D deficiency, due to lack of vitamin D or poor vitamin D metabolism. Hemochromatosis patients can experience osteomalacia with either normal or low vitamin D levels, which suggests another iron-related cause of the condition.

Osteoporosis is a bone-thinning disease. In its early stages, there may be no pain or noticeable symptoms. In advanced stages, people with osteoporosis can experience loss of height, spine deformity, severe back pain, and fractured or broken bones. Osteoporosis is more prominent in females, but it might simply be underdiagnosed in men. The condition can be detected with a bone mineral-density test, which uses imaging techniques such as X-ray, CT scanning, and ultrasound.

The role of excess iron in bone-formation abnormalities is not widely examined, but findings from the few studies of bone disease and iron are significant and provide sufficient evidence to prompt further large population-based investigation.

In one study, men with genetic hemochromatosis were assessed for bone mineral density (BMD) and bone remodeling (formation). All of the men had significant iron overload with very high liver iron concentrations (greater than 2.5). Of the thirty-eight participants, thirty-seven were homozygous for C282Y mutation of HFE; one was a compound heterozygote. Tests of BMD were performed on the lumbar spine (low back) and femoral neck (hip bone). Osteopenia (early mild bone loss) was observed in nearly 80 percent of participants and osteoporosis was present in 34 percent. The men's vitamin D levels were normal; and parathyroid function was normal except in the patients who had cirrhosis, in which case parathyroid hormone levels were decreased. Hypogonadism (which is responsible for hormonal deficiency) was found in 13 percent of the men. Femoral neck bone mineral density fell as hepatic iron concentrations increased. Investigators concluded that there is significant bone loss in HFE-related hemochromatosis that cannot solely be explained by hypogonadism or cirrhosis.

Although more evidence is needed, one theory offered by iron experts is that iron interferes with the development of osteo-blasts, the cells that form into bone tissue. In contrast, osteoclasts are cells that break down bone tissue. When osteoclasts are in excess, bone tissue destruction accelerates and osteoporosis is a consequence. Pharmaceuticals to slow or impair this destructive process are rapidly becoming commercially available.

Bisphosphonates (or diphosphonates) are a class of drugs that inhibit osteoclast action and the resorption (the breaking-down process) of bone. Bisphosphonates include alendronate (brand name Fosamax), risedronate (Brand name Actonel), and ibandronate (brand name Bonvia)—all are examples of oral bis-phosphonates approved for use in the United States.

Another bisphosphonate, Zoledronic acid (brand name Reclast in United States, brand name Aclasta in Canada and Europe) is approved for the treatment of Paget's disease, the second most common metabolic bone disorder. Additional studies are ongoing to examine the use of Reclast to prevent fractures following a hip fracture in men and women, treatment of corticosteroid-induced osteoporosis, and male osteoporo-sis. In a study reported in 2007 in the *New England Journal of Medicine* (May 3, 2007), in 7,700 women, Reclast reduced the risk of spine fractures by 70 percent and hip fractures by 41 percent. The drug is administered by injection once a year.

In July 2008 the National Institute for Health and Clinical Excellence (NICE) approved use of strontium ranelate for the management of primary and secondary prevention of post-menopausal osteoporosis. Strontium supplements may decrease bone resorption and stimulate bone-building osteoblast activity and new bone formation. Precaution is advised in patients with phenylketonuria, as strontium ranelate contains phenylalanine. Osteologix, an American company, has formulated a strontium-malonate combination that may also be promising.

13

Heart and Arteries

Heart muscle is one of the target tissues of iron overload, with resultant cardiomyopathy (heart disease) in some hemochromatosis patients.

"Regardless of whether iron overload in human beings results from transfusions in patients with thalassemia major, hereditary hemochromatosis or other causes, it (iron overload) impairs cardiac function and is a major cause of death."
—Yang et al. (Rammelkamp Center for Education and Research, Cleveland, Ohio), "Bimodal Cardiac Dysfunction in an Animal Model of Iron Overload," Journal of Laboratory Clinical Medicine 140 (2002): 263–71

The mean age of death for men who die of heart failure from undiagnosed or untreated hemochromatosis is fifty-eight, except for men who are routine blood donors. Family history of heart attack, history of early death by heart failure, or any of the symptoms of impending heart attack—especially arrhythmia—are good reasons to ask your physician to determine whether you have hemochromatosis.

Signs a person may be having a heart attack:

☐ pain that radiates up into the jaw and down the left arm
☐ irregular heart beat (arrhythmia)
☐ complaints of indigestion or feeling of heaviness in the chest
☐ fatigue
☐ swelling of feet and ankles
☐ shortness of breath
☐ ashen-gray color
☐ chronic cough
☐ sweatiness and anxiety

Iron Disorders Institute image file

Leading scientists continue to debate iron's involvement in heart disease. Here, though, it is perhaps helpful to distinguish heart disease or cardiomyopathy from coronary artery disease. What is commonly called heart disease can be either cardiomyopathy or coronary artery disease. The former is disease of the actual heart muscle; the latter is disease of the artery that nourishes the heart.

The Italian scientists Failla, Giannattasio, Piperno, Vergani, Grappiolo, Genetile, and Meles studied radial artery wall alteration in genetic HHC before and after iron depletion. They concluded that, in patients with HHC, arterial wall thickness increases before the onset of cardiovascular complications.

According to Claus Niederau, MD, Department of Medicine, St. Josef-Hospital, Academic Teaching Hospital of the University of Essen, in Oberhausen, Germany, "For hepatologists, and in particular for physicians and scientists who work in the field of hemochromatosis, and iron overload, the data reported by Monica Failla, MD, et al. are astonishing, and beg the question whether (and if so why) we have overlooked such an association for more than a century."

Niederau continues: "There is overwhelming evidence that cardiomyopathy occurs more frequently in patients with HHC than controls. However, there is also overwhelming evidence that this cardiomyopathy is not caused by coronary artery disease." Niederau also stated: "Recent literature does not support the hypothesis that iron contributes to atherosclerosis to a major degree although further studies are required to elucidate this association. There is overwhelming evidence that atherosclerosis, coronary artery disease and peripheral artery disease are neither prominent clinical features nor frequent cause of death in genetic hemochromatosis."

A study from 1979 to 1992 by the U.S. National Center for Health Statistics examined records in which hemochromatosis was listed as the cause of death provided data substantiating that "an association of cardiomyopathy (heart muscle disease) and hemochromatosis was increased about 4.8 fold over the expected ratio."

According to the First National Health and Nutrition Examination Survey Epidemiologic Follow-up survey, serum iron levels and TS percentages were not related to myocardial infarction. Other research has yielded various results. Importantly, researchers who have examined iron-reduction therapy in patients with hemochromatosis report that patients undergoing therapy express improved cardiovascular function once their iron levels are reduced (Gaenzer et al., 2002). Wolff et al., 2004, found that in patients with high LDL cholesterol, increased iron levels in the body were associated with carotid plaque buildup and atherosclerosis. Similarly, Mainous and Diaz (2009) found that men aged twenty to forty-nine with only moderately elevated iron stores (serum ferritin greater than 150 ng/mL) exhibited significantly decreased cardiovascular fitness during treadmill testing. They further observed that, when these findings are extrapolated to the American population, as many as 25 million men would likely be affected.

The Hemochromatosis Heart

According to the National Institutes of Health, restrictive cardiomyopathy is associated with hemochromatosis or iron overload. Restrictive cardiomyopathy is so named because the condition restricts the heart from stretching properly. While the rhythm and pumping action of the heart may continue to be normal, the stiff walls of the heart chambers keep the chambers from filling normally. So blood flow is reduced, and blood that would normally enter the heart is backed up into the circulatory system. Heart failure is the end result.

Another way that iron can contribute to heart failure is through free-radical activity, which results in oxidative stress or damage to cells that are involved. Oxidative stress causes cell death and can disrupt the conduction system or electrical impulses within the heart.

When iron disrupts these impulses, an arrhythmia can result. Arrhythmia is an irregular heart action caused by some disturbance in the discharge of electrical impulses between the sinus node and conductive tissues of the heart. The "lub" and "dub" sounds that help identify murmurs, arrhythmia, or pericardial friction are associated with the contraction of the ventricle, tension of the atrioventricular valves, and the impact of the heart against the chest wall. In a normal heart, "lub" is the first sound heard, followed by a brief pause and then the "dub" sound, which results from the closure of the aortic and pulmonary valves. In an arrhythmic heart, pauses are prolonged or erratic.

The heart's conduction system comprises a series of electrical impulses or discharges that flow through the heart at a steady and rhythmic pace, resulting in a heartbeat. An average heart beats about seventy-two times per minute. With each beat, approximately 80 milliliters (about a third of a cup) are pumped out of the heart and into circulation. When this system is unable to function normally, the result is a noticeably irregular heartbeat, or arrhythmia.

The conduction system can become impaired in several ways. The functional part of an organ comprises the parenchymal cells, and it is within these cells that iron can collect. Heavily burdened parenchymal cells can lead to cell death, which can interfere with the flow of cardiac electrical impulses. Another way the conduction system can be impaired is when there is rapid blood loss due to trauma, surgery, or possibly when iron is mobilized too quickly. Mobilization of iron occurs when blood is removed or infused.

People with chronic iron-loading disorders such as hemochromatosis and transfusion-dependent iron overload are especially at risk for heart failure. These individuals must be diligent with iron-removal therapy and keep iron levels within a safe range to protect their hearts.

Atherosclerosis

Coronary artery disease is the stiffening or narrowing of arteries as a result of specific contributing factors. One well-known factor is a cholesterol-containing component called low-density lipoprotein (LDL, or "bad" cholesterol). When a particular environment is made available to LDL, plaque may be produced within the artery's walls. Most scientists agree that deposition of plaques in the arteries requires oxidation of components such as LDL. And LDL has to be oxidized before unique foam cells can trap and process it. The walls of engorged foam cells gradually enlarge, slowly decreasing the size of the interior of the artery. Diminished blood supply is the outcome of this progression, and risk of heart attack is greatly increased. Some scientists speculate that iron, a known oxidant, catalyzes the oxidation of LDL and thus contributes to the atherosclerotic process.

Most scientists agree that arterial damage occurs relatively early in life. If iron reduction by phlebotomy is used to reduce serum ferritin levels, this damaging process can be reduced or averted in many people. In research conducted by the Department of Veterans Affairs, Zacharski et al. reported that patients younger than sixty-one years old with peripheral arterial disease (PAD) who were treated with phlebotomy were significantly less likely to die prematurely or undergo life-threatening strokes or heart attacks than were other PAD patients treated only with standard measures. It is noteworthy that the patients in this study were not hemochromatosis patients but had body-iron levels close to those considered normal in the general population.

When narrowed arteries deprive the heart of oxygen, damage to the heart can occur. Interestingly, the momentary lack of oxygen is not as detrimental as the restoration of the oxygen supply. When blood flow is cut off and thus oxygen deprived, biochemical conditions in the heart are altered. As oxygen reenters the cells, free radicals are produced. This causes iron to be released from its storage protein ferritin. Iron amplifies free-radical damage, causing potentially irreparable changes to cell membranes and DNA.

Cardiac diagnostic aids such as electrocardiogram (EKG) do not reveal iron in the heart. A highly skilled cardiologist using an echocardiogram can detect iron. Breakthroughs are allowing radiologists to observe iron in the heart with specialized MR imaging. The radiologist does not actually "see iron" using this technique. An increase in iron shortens the relaxation times of protons [H+] ions, which shows up on conventional MRI images as decreased signal or "blackness" of the iron-overloaded tissue.

> "There is nothing that creates this diffusely black area except high iron-period! In the new millennium it is clear that magnetic resonance imaging, amongst its many conquests, is going to conquer angiography."
> —David Stark, MD, IRONUSA 2000 Scientific Conference

Observing cardiac iron with MRI can provide invaluable information for the physician, but the method still cannot disclose how much iron is in the heart. Blood tests such as TS percentage and serum ferritin are needed to determine the amount of de-ironing necessary to prevent future damage.

Ferritin, an iron-storage protein, traps iron and protects vital organs against the destructiveness of the metal. The liver and brain produce the greatest quantities of ferritin, but the heart produces lesser quantities than these organs—possibly because the heart is a muscle, and muscles do not contain large amounts of ferritin.

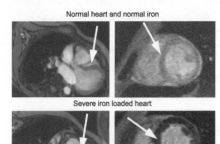

Normal heart and normal iron

Severe iron loaded heart

Images courtesy of Dr. D.J. Pennell, Cardiovascular Magnetic Resonance Unit, Royal Brompton Hospital, London

In early 2000, scientists at the Rammelkamp Research Center in Cleveland, Ohio, were studying how excessive iron affects the hearts of Mongolian gerbils. These animals have hearts very similar in structure to the human heart. Given large doses of iron dextran, the gerbils reacted remarkably like humans experiencing iron overload would. The animals suffered strokes and arrhythmia, and they died prematurely of heart failure, as do humans who die because of too much iron in tissues such as the heart.

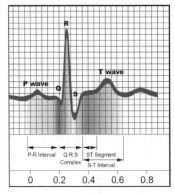

The gerbils were evaluated with EKGs. Long Q wave action was noted in the iron-loaded gerbils. The Q wave follows the P wave on an EKG and is usually not prominent. However, in EKG examples from iron-loaded gerbils, the extended Q wave can easily be seen. Upon autopsy, the scientists were able to determine that iron deposits were mostly in the left ventricle and epicardium (outer layer of the wall of the heart). Smaller amounts of iron were present in the right ventricle and atria and within the cells of the heart, but not in the interstitium (fluid space between heart cells).

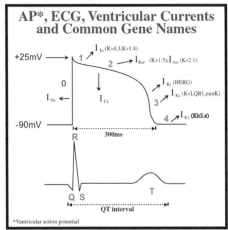

Chart courtesy of the Rammelkamp Center

14

Brain and Spinal Cord

"Excess or insufficient iron in the brain can contribute to neurological disorders. There is a possibility that the hemochromatotic brain may actually be iron deficient. Though portions of the brain are clearly capable of accumulating vast amounts of concentrated iron, the brain's ability to utilize this iron might be impaired in those with HHC."
—James Connor, professor of anatomy and neuroscience, Pennsylvania State University, and adviser to the IDI Medical and Scientific Board, at the IRONUSA 2000 Scientific Conference

The body's iron mismanagement is exceptionally clear with abnormal iron accumulation in the brain and nervous system, resulting in neurodegenerative diseases such as early-onset Alzheimer's, Parkinson's, Huntington's, amyotrophic lateral sclerosis (ALS, or Lou Gehrig's disease), epilepsy, Friedreich's ataxia, and multiple sclerosis. Symptoms of depression, seizures, and myalgias can be present when brain-iron distribution is abnormal.

Iron is stored in ferritin and transported to the brain and within the brain by transferrin. The management of brain iron is the same as in other organs. The brain, like the liver, makes its own ferritin and transferrin. Serum ferritin levels in the body are measured in a blood sample taken from the arm. However, brain ferritin levels are determined from fluid obtained from a spinal tap.

Depression is a debilitating psychological disorder that may result from an imbalance in the chemical substances (called neurotransmitters) that nerve cells use to communicate with one another. Brain and spinal cord studies have revealed that specific regions in the brain may also be involved in depression, supporting a biological explanation for this psychological disorder. There is strong evidence that depression associated with hemochromatosis may have common biological underpinnings.

Iron is required for the synthesis of some of the chemical communicators in the brain. Also, those regions in the brain that we know to be involved in motor skills and emotions are susceptible to iron toxicity. Although the long-established belief in the field of neurology regarding hemochromatosis is that most of the brain is protected against iron overload, the studies on which this belief is built were performed before recent technological advances (such as MRIs for living patients). In addition, the enhanced ability to detect iron in autopsy samples is now available. Also, scientists now know that there are two issues that are most important with respect to iron in the brain: there must be a balance of iron (not too much or too little), and the timing of iron delivery is critical. Even the right amount of iron delivered at the wrong time can be harmful.

The brain has an exquisite system for maintaining a timely balance of iron. All organs have access to iron in the blood, but blood iron is not immediately available to the brain because the blood vessels coursing through the brain are modified to form a barrier between the brain and the blood. This barrier is important for keeping harmful substances in the blood out of the brain. To get required nutrients such as iron and glucose across this barrier, the blood vessels in the brain have carriers. For iron, the blood vessels use transferrin receptors to carry iron in from the blood. Receptors recognize the blood iron-transport protein transferrin. Iron in the blood is bound to transferrin. In hemochromatosis (HHC), transferrin can be as much as 100 percent saturated with iron, unlike the normal saturation of roughly 30 percent. The high saturation of transferrin in HHC may fool the brain into thinking that plenty of iron is available, and the levels of transferrin receptors on the brain blood vessels may decrease to keep too much iron from getting into the brain.

The signals that are used between the brain and its blood vessels to determine how much (and when) iron should be transported into the brain must be discovered before this idea can be directly tested. A grant from the National Institutes of Health supported research for the scientists John Beard and James Connor 2003 to investigate this brain signal function. They proposed that the amount and timely delivery of iron to the brain in hemochromatosis is disrupted as the brain tries to read signals regarding the amount of iron in the blood. Poorly timed or inappropriate amounts of iron delivery to the brain directly affect the synthesis rates of the chemical communicators for nerve cells, and inappropriate levels of chemical communicators can be associated with depression.

The data supporting the idea that the levels of iron or iron-associated proteins (transferrin or ferritin) in blood can correlate with depression and other psychological illnesses are growing. Specifically with regard to depression, there is evidence that blood low in iron is associated with depression in some populations (e.g., iron-deficient women who take oral contraceptives), and depression was a reported side effect in a study using an iron chelator to treat individuals with thalassemia. In the brains of depressed patients, increased iron has been detected with MRI in specific regions. A popular therapeutic drug for depression, imipramine, can decrease the ability of a cell to obtain iron. These studies strengthen the argument presented previously for a greater understanding of the relationship between levels of iron in the blood and in the brain.

Finally, an interesting correlation between depression and activation of the immune systems has been noted. The relationship between depression and inflammation may be mediated by a decrease in the amino acid (i.e., a protein building block) tryptophan, which is required for the synthesis of serotonin. Serotonin is a major chemical communicator in the brain and is the chemical communicator targeted by the popular antidepressant Prozac. The synthesis of serotonin requires iron.

Under conditions of inflammation and immune response, the body tries to minimize iron availability to the invading pathogens by an action referred to as the iron-withholding defense. This is a system first described in the 1960s by Dr. Gene Weinberg, professor emeritus of microbiology, Indiana University, and Iron Disorders Institute Medical & Scientific Advisory Board publications chair. In addition, the cells of the immune system use iron to mount their own part of the defense response. Thus, an individual undergoing an immune reaction could get a double whammy of decreased tryptophan and iron withholding from the brain, which could have a significant deleterious affect on the ability to make serotonin, which could in turn lead to depression.

In conclusion, the role of iron in the synthesis of chemical communicators in the brain, and specifically of serotonin, is not disputed. The role of serotonin in mediating depression is becoming well established. Hemochromatosis involves a loss of iron balance in the body. Taken together, this information suggests a relationship between iron imbalance and depression. Aggressive, targeted studies aimed to understand the direct link between iron and depression are warranted.

15

Hormone-Producing Organs: The Endocrine System

Although the liver can tolerate large amounts of iron without disease or dysfunction, smaller amounts of iron can severely damage hormone-producing organs. The hormone-producing organs are part of a large group of ductless glands called the endocrine system, which includes the hypothalamus, anterior pituitary, thyroid, pancreas, gonads (testes or ovaries) and adrenals. The kidneys, though not part of the endocrine system, produce erythropoietin, a hormone that stimulates the bone marrow to produce erythrocytes. Problems with these delicate organs are displayed in signs and symptoms such as depression, moodiness, emotional outbursts, loss of interest, irregular menstruation, impotence, weight gain or loss, total body hair loss, excessive thirst or urination, poor sleep, and anxiety.

Too much iron in these organs leads to hormone imbalances, which can result in a number of health problems. For hemochromatosis patients, the most common known endocrine disorders are hypogonadism, diabetes mellitus, and hypothyroidism.

Diabetes Mellitus (Type 1 and Type 2)
Diabetes mellitus is a well-known consequence of excessive iron damage to the insulin-producing cells of the pancreas. People with HHC who have high iron levels are at increased risk of developing this type of diabetes. Reducing iron to a healthy level can have a positive effect on diabetes; in some cases, HHC patients who have completed therapeutic phlebotomy have reported the discontinuation of the need for insulin injections.

Diabetes mellitus is a group of disorders that have one common feature: abnormally high levels of glucose (sugar) in the blood. Normally, blood sugar levels are kept within a narrow range (70 to 125 mg/dL) by several hormonal and neuronal mechanisms, especially by the hormone insulin, which is produced by the beta cells of the pancreas. Beta cells are found in islet cells, specialized clumps of cells in the pancreas. When defects in insulin production, insulin action, or both, are present, high blood sugar can result.

Diabetes is usually divided into two broad categories: type 1 and type 2. Type 1 diabetes is caused by a deficiency of insulin production by the beta cells in the pancreatic islets possibly as a result of viral infections or autoimmune insulitis (i.e., inflammation of the beta cells). Type 1 diabetes is most common in children and young adults and is often called early-onset or juvenile diabetes. Type 2 diabetes is caused by a combination of reduced insulin effectiveness (insulin resistance); there is a concurrent increase in insulin production to compensate for its reduced activity. Individuals with type 2 diabetes initially have too much insulin in the bloodstream, or hyperinsulinism. Eventually, type 2 diabetes can result in pancreatic exhaustion and develop into insulin-dependent diabetes. The vast majority of adults with diabetes (about 90 percent) have type 2 diabetes.

Hypoglycemia—having too little blood sugar—can occur in either type 1 or type 2 diabetes. Insulin-dependent diabetics can experience low blood sugars when they administer too much insulin or fail to eat after injecting insulin. Type 2 diabetics can experience low blood sugars during the phase when insulin levels are abnormally high if other factors increase glucose utilization or decrease glucose production by the liver.

DIABETES	Type I	Type II
Age at onset	Early (before age 30)	Around age 40+
Symptoms	Frequent & abundant urination Thirst, weight loss Excessive hunger Ketoacidosis: abdominal pain headache, rapid feeble pulse, decreased blood pressure, flushed, dry skin, irritability, nausea, vomiting, air hunger/ shortness of breath, double or blurred vision	Frequent & abundant urination Thirst, weight change, itching Peripheral neuropathy
Therapy	Insulin & Diet	Diet, hypoglycemic drugs Possible insulin
Islet Cell Antibodies	Present at onset	Absent
Insulin in Blood	Little to none	Present
Body Weight	Normal/under	Obese (80%)
Blood Glucose	Elevated>200mg/dL	Elevated>200mg/dL
Symptoms of HYPOGLYCEMIA	Weakness, Tremor, Muscle twitching, Nausea, Vomiting, Pallor (paleness), Sweating, Confusion, Decreased blood pressure, Decreased heart rate, Palpitations, Air hunger (Shortness of breath, Sighing, Hiccups).	

Iron Disorders Institute image file

Although most mild or pre-diabetics have few or no symptoms whatsoever, symptoms of severe diabetes mellitus may include frequent and abundant urination, thirst, hunger, weight loss, and blurred vision. The cause of diabetes is not completely understood. Physical inactivity, obesity, and body fat distribution (especially in the abdomen) are all known risk factors for developing diabetes. The presence of diabetes in a family member also increases the risk of diabetes, which suggests that genetic factors play a role in causing the disease.

The connection between diabetes and iron is that iron can cause damage to tissues of vital organs by changing oxygen into free radicals, which leads to increased oxidative stress. Unopposed free-radical activity can wreak havoc on cells throughout the body. It may be that iron destroys beta cells, causing diabetes. Beta cells have very low levels of the enzymes that break down free radicals. Thus, agents that increase free-radical production such as iron could result in destruction of pancreatic cells.

The Pancreas

Absorption of nonheme iron depends on the pH value of the duodenum, the portion of the small intestine that connects to the stomach. When the environment is acidic, nonheme iron is more easily absorbed. When the environment is alkaline, less nonheme iron is absorbed. As part of the many naturally occurring iron-balance mechanisms, when excess nonheme iron is present, the pancreas (among its many functions) is triggered to secrete bicarbonate, which is alkaline and arrests overabsorption. People with impaired pancreatic secretions, such as in pancreatitis and cystic fibrosis, absorb increased quantities of iron.

The pancreas also secretes insulin to control blood sugar (glucose) levels. When blood sugar is high, insulin is secreted to lower the sugar. Sometimes the pancreas can overproduce insulin and the body becomes resistant to and cannot use the hormone to correct blood sugar levels (impaired glucose tolerance). Obese people and type 2 diabetics generally fall into the insulin-resistant group.

Patients with hemochromatosis who have excessive levels of body iron can experience reduced insulin production due to iron-damaged beta cells or insulin resistance due to pancreatic burnout, possibly from iron-mediated oxidative stress (free-radical damage). In either of these scenarios, diabetes mellitus can develop.

At this time, for those people with iron-loading disorders such as hemochromatosis, removal of excess iron from the body with therapeutic phlebotomy or periodic blood donation is the safest and most effective way to lower excessive body iron stores. If HHC is diagnosed before complications such as diabetes develop, maintaining a de-ironed status significantly diminishes the risk of diabetes and other disease. Research is under way to determine whether other (more expensive and complicated) methods for removing iron (called chelation) will benefit those with established diabetes-related neuropathy (caused by damage to the sheathing that protects nerve fibers).

"Chelation therapy—inactivation and removal of metals pharmacologically by special chemicals that bind iron tightly—has been shown to slow or even reverse peripheral nerve damage in experimental animals with diabetes," according to Drs.

Mingwei Qian of Baylor College of Medicine in Houston, Texas, and John Eaton, of the University of Louisville (2000). "It appears that, in diabetes, there is an accumulation of metals such as iron and perhaps copper bound to blood vessel walls. These metal deposits prevent the normal relaxation of blood vessels, which feed the nerves, and this slowly starves—and ultimately kills—the nerves. This explains why administration of chelators may be able to preserve nerve function even in advanced diabetes, at least in experimental animals."

Chelation therapy for humans with diabetes is still experimental and calls for additional research, such as the current U.S. study funded by the National Institutes of Health's Institute for Diabetes, Digestive, and Kidney Disease.

Upper Endocrine System: Hypothalamus, Anterior Pituitary, and Thyroid

The endocrine system is a highly complex and interdependent network of ductless glands. Glands are organs of the body that manufacture certain substances. The endocrine system discharges its product directly into the bloodstream in the form of hormones, whereas exocrine glands discharge substances to the outside of an organ to the epithelial tissue. Examples of exocrine system glands include salivary glands, mucous glands, the liver, sweat and tear glands, mammary glands, kidneys, the stomach, and the intestines. It is debatable whether the pancreas is part of the exocrine or endocrine system, as it contains both types of glands.

Principal glands that make up the endocrine system include the pituitary, adrenals, pancreas, parathyroid, thyroid, testes, and ovaries. The hypothalamus stimulates pituitary function, which in turn prompts other glands and organs in the endocrine system to produce hormones. Hormones are chemical messengers that regulate specific functions, and secretions from endocrine glands are destined for a singular target organ or gland. Properly stimulated target organs and glands support normal functions such as growth, metabolism, sugar balance, heart rate, breathing, and reproduction.

Sometimes referred to as the master gland, the pituitary produces key hormones. These include thyroid-stimulating hormone, prolactin, oxytocin, luteinizing hormone and follicle-stimulating hormone, growth hormone, and corticotropin. Two lobes make up the pituitary: an anterior (or front) lobe produces hormones that regulate growth and physical development. This lobe stimulates adrenal function, the thyroid gland, and the reproductive organs.

When the pituitary is damaged or its function impaired, hormones cannot deliver their chemical message. Then, organs that rely on adequate pituitary function are not adequately stimulated and cannot perform their intended functions. Abnormal adrenal function, hypogonadism, and hypothyroidism, three conditions caused by hormone imbalances, are prominently found in hemochromatosis patients.

Thyroid Function

The thyroid gland produces active substances that affect metabolism and reproductive function. When the thyroid gland is underactive, hypothyroidism results. Symptoms of hypothyroidism include chronic fatigue, loss of libido (sex drive), moodiness, depression, low blood pressure, slow pulse, reduced temperature, cool and dry skin, brittle nails, hair loss, weight gain, puffy face, dark circles under the eyes, ataxia (lack of coordination), aching muscles, joint stiffness and intolerance to cold, infertility, impotence, sterility, and irregular menstrual periods.

Endocrine System

The thyroid stimulates other glands to secrete gonadotrophic hormones so that reproduction can take place. In women, luteinizing hormone (LH) causes the release of follicle-stimulating hormone (FSH), estrogen, and progesterone, and it controls reproductive functions such as egg maturation and regulation of the menstrual cycle. In men, LH causes the release of testosterone and controls the quality of sperm and semen. Gonadotropins provide for the differences in sexual characteristics of men and women, such as voice, body hair distribution, and muscle formation.

Iron can be detected in the pituitary with MRIs, but it is not known whether iron can safely and completely be removed from the organ. Undiagnosed and untreated iron overload can cause permanent damage to the pituitary gland, resulting in irreversible hormone production. Hormones then must be replaced therapeutically.

Hormone replacement therapy is often suggested for patients with hemochromatosis. When hormone deficiencies are confirmed, replacement testosterone, thyroid hormone, androgen, or estrogen can stimulate normal reproductive organ function or treat symptoms. Testosterone is best taken as patch or slow-release application. Cases of polycythemia vera have been reported by men receiving testosterone by injection. Hormone replacement therapy should never be attempted without the supervision of a medical expert. Successful hormone replacement therapy can reverse infertility, impotence, and mood.

16

Skin, Nails, Hearing, and Vision

"Skin hyperpigmentation is characteristic of iron overload and presents in about 50 [to] 70 percent of the patients with hemochromatosis."
—Jacek Drobnik, MD, PhD, assistant professor of physiology and medicine, Department of Pathophysiology, Medical University of Lodz, Poland

In some of the earliest recorded cases of hemochromatosis, physicians noticed the bronze color of the patient's skin. Because these patients also had diabetes, doctors referred to the condition as bronze diabetes. The skin color changes observed in hemochromatosis patients (and others with iron overload) is called hyperpigmentation. The coloring can vary: coppery, reddish, tanned, ashen, or gray green (the color of some metals). In HHC patients, hyperpigmentation occurs all over the body, even in parts not exposed to the sun.

Melanin is a pigment found in skin, eyes, and hair. Hyperpigmentation in HHC patients is not fully understood, but it may be due to iron's ability to trigger free-radical activity. Melanocytes, the cells that produce melanin, would not function properly when oxidized or existing melanin might be oxidized. Whatever the process, the functioning of any system bombarded by free iron would be faulty.

Premature aging, loss of body hair and premature balding, scaly and dry skin, increased skin fungal infections, and koilonychia (a spoonlike indention in the fingernails) are attributable to high body iron levels. Koilonychia is a condition that may also be present in patients with chronic iron deficiency and is especially apparent on the first three digits: the thumb, index finger, and middle finger. One cause of koilonychia is increased erythropoiesis (red-blood-cell production), which depletes iron stores and leads to a thinning of the nail plate and atrophy of the distal nail bed. Nails produced under these conditions are misshapen. Patients with HHC might have koilonychia if they also experienced prolonged iron deficiency due to repeated phlebotomy.

National Institutes of Health MedinePlus

NOTE! buckling, shiny, raised or depressed areas on the nail surface

koilonychia

Another condition frequently experienced by HHC patients is porphyria cutanea tarda (PCT), which is characterized by blisters on the back side (dorsal) of the hand. About 40 percent of patients with PCT carry the C282Y mutation of HFE. The high iron levels serve to catalyze the formation of reactive oxygen species (ROS). According to the porphyrin metabolism expert Herbert L. Bonkovsky, MD, "ROS can enhance uroporphyrin formation by increasing the rate at which uroporphyrinogen is oxidized to uroporphyrin. Iron may also act indirectly to inhibit uroporphyrinogen decarboxylase activity by enhancing the formation of non-porphyrin products of porphyrinogen oxidation that are themselves direct inhibitors of the enzyme. Finally, iron can act to increase uroporphyrin production by inducing delta-aminolevulinic acid synthase, thus increasing the amount of delta-aminolevulinic acid, the precursor to uroporphyrinogen, present in the cell." (Lambrecht, R. W., and

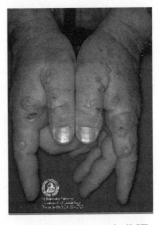

porphyria cutanea tarda (PCT)

Photo courtesy of Dr. M. Simon, Professor of Medicine, Dermatologische Universitatsklinik, Erlangen, Germany

H. L. Bonkovsky. "Hemochromatosis and Porphyria." *Seminars in Gastrointestinal Disease* 13 [2002]: 109–19.)

The PCT condition may accompany hemochromatosis; therefore, patients with skin discoloration, blisters, or complaints of pain from exposure to the sun should be further evaluated for hemochromatosis.

Hair Loss

Hair loss in HHC patients is a common observation. Some patients experience total body hair loss. Others may experience hair loss in selected areas of the body, such as the head, the pubic area, and outermost region of the eyebrow. Hair loss could be due to imbalances in hormones that stimulate the thyroid, adrenals, ovaries, or testes.

Gums and Teeth

Problems with gums, including swollen, spongy, or bleeding gums, are among the frequent complaints of HHC patients. Iron levels are higher in the gingival fluid and saliva, which can enhance growth of pathogens and increased free-radical activity. These effects contribute to the deterioration of the gums. In studies of harmful and benign strains of *Porphyromonas gingivalis*, a bacterium found in saliva, the harmful varieties needed less iron to thrive than the benign type. The harmful type therefore has greater potential to cause periodontal infections, which can result in tooth loss. The potential for tooth loss is worsened by bone resorption, a process that can also be caused by too much iron.

Lactoferrin (Lf), a protein that binds with free iron in serum, does so to withhold iron from harmful pathogens in body fluids, such as tears, saliva, breast milk, and semen. Lactoferrin also reduces oxidative stress from free-radical production, which can be triggered by free (unbound iron). Lactoferrin may play an important role in controlling gum disease. In a study of juveniles with localized gingivitis, investigators found that the level of bound iron in Lf is significantly reduced in those patients than in controls.

Hearing Loss

Elevated body iron increases the risk of hearing loss and possibly deafness in hemochromatosis. The cause may be due to the use of certain antibiotics. The antibiotic action of the aminoglycosides (amikacin, gentamicin, kanamycin, neomycin, netilmicin, streptomycin, and tobramycin) is not altered by iron. However, iron strongly increases the toxicity of these drugs for people who take them. In the series of hemochromatosis and iron-overload cases reported in 1980, about 30 percent of participants had hearing impairment. The drug-iron combination is thought to be dangerous because of its ability to generate the formation of free radicals (i.e., hydroxyl), which are very powerful cell-damaging oxidants. The tissues most likely to be harmed by iron-activated aminoglycosides are the hair cells of the inner ear and the proximal tubules of the kidney.

> "These results provide further evidence of the recently reported intrinsic role of iron in aminoglycoside ototoxicity, and highlight a potential risk of aminoglycoside administration in patients with elevated serum iron."
> —Conlon B. J., Smith, D. W. Supplemental iron exacerbates aminoglycoside ototoxicity in vivo. Hear Res. 1998 (Jan) 115 (1–2):1–5

Aminoglycoside drugs have been widely used since 1945, but the extent of hearing impairment in iron-loaded humans that might have been triggered by use of these antibiotics is not yet known. During the past half century, it has become apparent that the majority of useful antibiotics can combine with various metals, often specifically with iron. Hemochromatosis patients with high body-iron levels should discuss this potential with their healthcare provider and avoid taking such antibiotics.

Vision

Iron can damage vision in several ways. In a study in rats, exposure to cigarette smoke (which is high in iron contamination) was found to be toxic to lens tissue. The iron was deposited in the lenses of the animals.

"Iron retinotoxicity leads to a dysfunction of all layers but the changes may be reversible in the early period of the disease. The late period iron toxicity produces more severe damage to the inner retina than the outer retina."

—Imaizumi M., Matsumoto C. S., Yamada K., Nanba Y., Takaki Y., Nakatsuka K. Electroretinographic assessment of early changes in ocular siderosis. Ophthalmologica 214, no. 5 (Sept.–Oct. 2000): 354–59

As HHC patients age, they may be at increased risk for retinal iron overload, which predisposes them to age-related macular degeneration (AMD). According to reports by leading investigators of iron's role in AMD, in autopsies of individuals with AMD, AMD retinas had more iron in the photoreceptors. Also, iron levels were increased in AMD-affected maculae compared with normal maculae.

Hemochromatosis patients can lower their risk for any of these consequences with early detection and early and consistent therapy.

17

Lungs

Inhaling iron is an unnatural way to get iron. In contrast, the iron we get from food is the way nature intended us to get the nutrient. The iron that we get from food or supplements is absorbed, contained, or excreted. When we inhale iron, it enters directly into the lungs and accumulates there, increasing the risk for certain lung diseases, including cancer or damage to lung-cell DNA. Only small amounts of iron are exhaled. People with HHC are at risk of accumulating dangerous levels of iron from their diet because of faulty iron metabolism. However, people with HHC or people with normal iron metabolism share the potential to accumulate toxic levels of iron in the lungs. Interestingly, mutations of HFE provide some degree of protection from lung diseases such as tuberculosis or Legionnaires' disease because the pathogens that cause these two diseases can obtain iron from macrophages. People with C282Y mutations have very low macrophage iron; thus the pathogens that cause these two diseases cannot obtain iron to multiply. The degree to which we inhale iron depends on the environment. Environments in which a person is at increased risk for inhaling cancer-causing levels of iron include the workplace, home, and subway system. People who smoke or who are exposed to secondhand smoke are also at increased risk for inhaling dangerous levels of iron.

Workers who remove iron-silicate asbestos (the magnesium silicate is not known to be harmful), people who mine coal or iron ore, and people who work in iron smelters and do not wear protective masks are constantly inhaling iron.

Another source of airborne iron is underground subway or train systems. People who work in or travel daily by these systems are constantly exposed to iron filings generated from the grinding of train or subway wheels on the rails.

In a 2004 report of an ongoing pilot study of New York City airborne metal exposure, particulates were collected from a surface street location and from an underground subway station. Airborne concentrations of three metals—iron, manganese, and chromium—were observed to be more than a hundred times greater in the subway environment than in home indoor or outdoor settings in New York City.

Gene Weinberg, PhD, adds, "In a similar study conducted in Stockholm cultures of human lung cells exposed to airborne particles were monitored for oxidative stress and DNA damage. [The] lead investigator on the study, H. L. Karlsson, reports that '…all particles tested caused DNA damage and those from the subway caused more damage than the other particles likely due to redox-active iron.' The air particulates collected from the subway station were four times more likely to cause oxidative stress in the cells and were eight times more damaging to lung cell DNA. Moreover, the particle concentration per unit of air in the subway location was 5 [to] 10 times denser than that of the street location. Thus the actual increase in toxicity of the underground air was estimated to be 40 [to] 80 times that of the surface air."

The health hazards of tobacco smoking are clearly and abundantly documented. It is common knowledge that inhaled smoke from tobacco is a known cause of lung cancer. What some people may not know is that tobacco is loaded with iron, and iron is a booster for cancer cells and other lung diseases. Harmful pathogens like cancer cells or the bacteria that cause pneumonia or tuberculosis need iron to thrive just like any other living thing. When you smoke, you can overwhelm the body's defense system of macrophages, white blood cells contained in our body that scavenge harmful debris such as excess or unnatural sources of iron. To make matters worse, the tar and gas phases of cigarette smoke contain chemicals that promote the release of stored iron from the macrophages.

The body has several intricate mechanisms for balancing

iron in the body. The iron-withholding defense system (IWDS) described by Gene Weinberg, PhD, is an elegant system that withholds iron from harmful invaders. When this system is activated, a person experiences a mild drop in hemoglobin. If serum ferritin is not checked, this condition can be mistaken for iron-deficiency anemia. Once the harmful invader is gone, hemoglobin returns to normal (for more about this defense system, see chapter 18).

Inhaled iron collects in lung cells called alveolar macrophages. These are the cells that help fight against infections and cancers in the lungs. When heavily burdened with iron, these cells cannot protect a person against opportunistic infectious disease. Also, cancer cells thrive on iron. Mainstream tobacco smoke is estimated to contain as much as 60,000 picograms of iron per cigarette smoked. Thus a pack-a-day smoker could inhale more than 1 million picograms of iron per day. In a number of reports, alveolar macrophages of smokers have been found to be brimming with iron—in many cases, in amounts sufficient to prevent the alveolar macrophages from killing cancer cells and pathogenic microbes.

Ironically, the C282Y mutation of the HFE gene disrupts the loading of iron in macrophages. People with this mutation may be spared lung diseases such as tuberculosis. African Americans generally do not have HHC (although approximately 2 percent do carry a single HFE gene). However, they can inherit other genes that cause them to absorb and accumulate dangerous levels of iron, creating a condition called African siderosis. In this disease, iron does load in the macrophages, dramatically increasing the risk for tuberculosis in African Americans.

Scrubbing rust off metal objects such as automobiles, patio furniture, and so on, can increase the inhalation of iron oxide dust. The Swiss physician Julian Dreyfus reported one of the first and most dramatic accounts of inhaled iron in 1936. On December 6, 1934, a forty-four-year-old mother of two was admitted to Hôpital de la Chaux-de-Fonds, in Switzerland. She was experiencing shortness of breath and chest pain. Her family history of illness was not unusual, but the attending physician found a nodule, which he determined to be cancerous; so he removed it surgically. Shortly after the operation, the woman's condition worsened. She complained of pain in the left side of her chest; a lung tap produced more than a liter of red liquid. Three weeks later, another tap produced a liter of yellowish red-brown fluid. Now feeble, barely able to breathe, and with a faint heartbeat, the woman was admitted to the hospital. More lung taps were done, and tumor tissue was found in the fluid; she was diagnosed with metastasis of a lung carcinoma—and she died three weeks later.

Barely nine months after her death, her thirty-six-year-old brother was admitted to the same hospital for prolonged bronchitis. He was diagnosed with pleurisy. Four months later he returned to the hospital complaining of bronchial pain. An X-ray showed a poorly defined shadow in the lower third of the right lung, directly above the diaphragm. He was treated but developed a severe cough and eventually returned to the hospital. A pleuropuncture (tap) brought forth the same yellowish red-brown liquid as that of his now deceased sister.

Fluid extracted from his lungs also contained tumor tissue; he was diagnosed with metastasis of a lung carcinoma—the same as his sister. The patient was given radiotherapy, which seemed to have favorable effects.

Rarely had the doctor seen lung cancer in patients so young. The occurrence of lung cancer in relatively young individuals from the same family prompted the doctor to ask more detailed questions about the family's history. Conversations with the patient revealed that, when he was a child, his mother worked at home polishing screws for a watch factory. She used a rotating steel disk onto which she continuously dusted a red polishing powder.

From birth until the boy was twelve and his sister twenty, both siblings were often in the room where the mother worked with this powder. Initially they were present as spectators, then as helpers. It followed that another sister had spent eight years away from the family. She was still in good health. The brother however, only thirty-six, died within a year following the death of his older sister. Curious, the physician contacted the watch factory and was told the powder was iron oxide. The doctor obtained a sample of the powder and had it analyzed to be certain. Indeed, the polishing dust contained iron.

Both siblings had been exposed to prolonged inhalation of iron dust. That they died of lung cancer would be no surprise to someone who knows about HHC and iron overload. What may come as a surprise is that the children did not need to have HHC to have iron-loaded lungs.

DID YOU KNOW

The story of the Swiss brother and sister who died of lung cancer lay among papers in the office Eugene Weinberg, Professor of Microbiology, Indiana University, for decades. The original 1936 document was published in German. Dr. Weinberg knew the basic contents of the story, because a colleague who spoke German translated the article for him. In 1998, David Garrison's German teacher Georgia Williams, Wade Hampton High School, Greenville, SC, translated the entire paper, and wrote the translation out in longhand, which was nine pages long. The handwritten words were so beautiful and precise that this version remains the only known translation, just as she wrote it. The original paper and other scientific papers are used as reference material by Iron Disorders Institute.

Iron Disorders Institute image file

18

Immune System

People who have the common mutations of HFE are somewhat protected from certain types of infections but at increased risk for others. Pathogens (commonly used to refer to infectious organisms) invade our body in different ways. We can inhale them, ingest them, or they can gain access directly into the bloodstream. Pathogens get traction in iron-rich environments or iron-rich hosts. Common pathogens include cancer cells, fungi, protozoans, bacteria, and viruses.

Because too much iron can be lethal in the presence of harmful invaders, nature provides us with multiple systems to keep iron away from them. The HFE mutations alter some of these systems. Oddly, in doing so, HFE protects us against diseases such as tuberculosis but increases our risk for potentially fatal bacterial infections, such as by *Vibrio vulnificus*.

One naturally occurring iron-balance mechanism is the iron-withholding defense system (IWDS). First described by Gene Weinberg, PhD, in the early 1980s, this system is triggered when harmful invaders penetrate the human body. When the system is activated, hemoglobin and TS percentage drop to low or below normal, allowing just enough iron for proper functioning, while ferritin rises rapidly to capture and withhold the extra iron from the invaders. Once the invaders are identified and eradicated, the hemoglobin and TS percentage levels rise to normal and serum ferritin levels fall to normal. This temporary anemia should be allowed to persist until the threat is eliminated. (For more about anemia of chronic disease, or anemia of inflammatory response, read *The Iron Disorders Institute Guide to Anemia*).

In concert with the IWDS, an army of white blood cells is dispatched. White blood cells called macrophages are scavengers that find and engulf pathogens to render them harmless. White blood cells generate free radicals in the cell to serve as benevolent warriors to destroy the trapped dangerous invaders. Once the pathogen is contained and unable to do harm, the white blood cell is consumed by the spleen, which expels the now-harmless debris into the body's means of elimination: urine or feces.

"Iron is the metallic ion that presently appears to be most critical in determining whether an infectious agent is to be permitted to multiply in mammalian host tissues."

—*Gene Weinberg, PhD, "Roles of Metallic Ions in Host-Parasite Interactions,"* Bacteriological Reviews 30 (1966): 136–51

In Gene Weinberg's book *Exposing the Hidden Dangers of Iron*, Weinberg writes, "By 1966, medical microbiologists had learned that infections due to bacteria, fungi, and protozoa are greatly intensified by the presence of excessive iron. Nearly all pathogenic microorganisms need iron for survival, growth, and multiplication. None are able to bring in to the body of the host an adequate supply of the metal for their further multiplication. Accordingly, the microbial invaders either must acquire iron from the host or die. As is the case for cancer cell invaders, the preferred tissue sites for microbial cell multiplication are those that contain elevated or easily acquired iron."

Pathogens use one of four strategies to acquire iron from their hosts. *Escherichia coli* can break open red blood cells and extract iron from hemoglobin, while *H. pylori* can withdraw iron from human lactoferrin. At least one pathogen, the spirochete that causes Lyme disease, has evolved to bypass the need for iron and uses manganese instead. Apparently the spirochete is able to withdraw manganese from human transferrin. Some bacteria, such as those that cause ehrlichiosis (deer-tick fever) or Legionnaires' disease, are not able to extract iron from body fluids. Instead they grow only inside host macrophages that provide readily available iron. Although the mycobacterium that causes tuberculosis can develop slowly in body fluids, it grows best when inside iron-loaded host macrophages.

As early as 1870, A. Trousseau, a noted Parisian professor of clinical medicine, warned his medical students against feeding iron preparations to patients with quiescent (latent) tuberculosis. He was certain that this procedure could trigger clinical episodes of the disease. In recent years, numerous studies in animals have validated Trousseau's judgment. In 2001, in a study in humans, elevated dietary iron was associated with a 3.5-fold increase in cases of active tuberculosis.

Some pathogens have little or no ability to acquire host iron and are therefore dangerous only to people with severely iron-loaded body sites. A good example is that of the bacterium *V. vulnificus*, which lives in coastal, marshy areas and is often a contaminant of shellfish. This pathogen can obtain growth-essential iron from transferrin only if the protein is burdened with abnormally high amounts of iron.

The normal range of TS percentage is 25 to 35 percent. In untreated HHC, that can rise to 100 percent. In one study, none of eight strains of *V. vulnificus* could grow in the presence of transferrin with 30 percent saturation; nearly all could grow with transferrin at 100 percent saturation. In normal mice, an injection of 1 million bacterial cells of *V. vulnificus* was needed to cause a lethal infection. In mice injected with iron, only one injected bacterial cell resulted in death!

> # WARNING!!!
>
> DO NOT EAT RAW SHELLFISH *and*
>
> TAKE CARE WALKING ON THE BEACH
>
> Some shellfish contain a bacteria called Vibrio vulnificus, which can be fatal to a person with high iron levels

Accordingly, people who develop septicemia due to *V. vulnificus* generally have an iron-loading condition and are found to have either a wound associated with coastal seawater or to have recently eaten raw shellfish. Any type of iron loading can contribute to septicemia, including alcoholism, African siderosis, chronic hepatitis, hemochromatosis, and thalassemia. Even some of the millions of carriers of the HFE gene mutations have elevated iron values and are susceptible to lethal infections from *V. vulnificus*. As recommended in "Part Six: Taking Care of Yourself," all people in danger of iron loading are warned to avoid ingestion of raw shellfish or walking barefoot on beaches where contaminated shells may be present.

Another potentially lethal infection that occurs only in iron-loaded people is caused by *Capnocytophaga canimorsus*. This impaired pathogen is carried in the saliva of about 15 to 25 percent of healthy dogs and cats. Persons with normal iron values who are nipped or bitten by the contaminated healthy animals heal without medical treatment. In contrast, iron-loaded people must have prompt antibiotic therapy to avoid development of fatal septicemia.

With the human immunodeficiency virus (HIV), particularly in its more advanced stages, iron consistently has been observed to accumulate in bone marrow, muscle, the liver, the spleen, and brain white matter. Hereditary hemochromatosis is not known to be the main cause of this form of iron loading. Instead, it is the patient's chronic recurrent inflammatory response that attempts to withhold iron from invading opportunistic bacterial, fungi, and protozoan pathogens.

Warning: Hemochromatosis patients with TS percentage levels above normal are at increased risk for certain potentially deadly infections. Keep iron at a healthy level with a balanced and measured maintenance plan. Learn more about iron and infections in *The Iron Disorders Institute Guide to Anemia.*

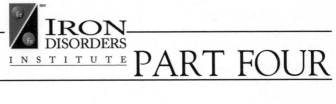

PART FOUR

Challenges

19

Frustrations of Getting the Diagnosis—Part 1

"Symptoms were experienced for an average of [nine and a half] years and more than three physicians were consulted before the complete diagnosis of HHC was made." —1996 Centers for Disease Control and Prevention (CDC) Hemochromatosis Patient Survey

The following stories represent some of the more challenging journeys that hemochromatosis patients have taken. Not all patient stories are as difficult as these examples. At the Iron Disorders Institute (IDI), we reach out to and talk with thousands of patients with positive stories to share. We also know many fine and caring healthcare professionals in the United States. They are genuinely eager to learn and make every effort to keep current with best practices. Our reason for emphasizing these challenging stories over the positive ones is because the stories exemplify the lack of awareness about hemochromatosis and how the IDI could reach out, educate, and make a difference in the lives of these patients.

There are more than nine hundred thousand physicians in the United States and millions of people with classic or nonclassic hemochromatosis. Our work has just begun, and we still meet challenges, especially when trying to sensitize a physician who has never diagnosed a case of hemochromatosis or a relative of a diagnosed patient.

According to Vincent Felitti, MD, former Director of Kaiser Permanente's Preventive Medicine Department in San Diego, where more than two hundred thousand individuals have been screened for HHC, "Statistically, a family practice physician will likely see one case of homozygous hemochromatosis every two weeks."

Dr. Tracy Coe, Welch Cancer Center, Sheridan, Wyoming, exemplifies the willing attitude needed to assure that patients receive a consistent approach to diagnosis and therapies that address the individual's case, including diet concerns. She writes about a particular case:

> "My patient had such impressive non-specific symptoms that it drove me to do a literature review. The Iron Disorders Institute (IDI) actually gave me more helpful information than my old internal medicine textbooks, and provided a great springboard to further my own education. Since we live in such a huge HHC area, I hadn't been previously exposed to such large numbers of patients before moving here and needed to start somewhere. *The Hemochromatosis Cookbook* has the most amazing introduction, and even as a specialist I learned loads, which helped me further help this patient and the other less-severe cases in our state."

> *Tracy L. Coe, MD, FACP; director, Medical Oncology;*
> *Welch Cancer Center; Sheridan, Wyoming*

20

Frustrations of Getting the Diagnosis—Part 2

Brad—Hemochromatosis, a Long Odyssey

With his wife's insistence, thirty-year-old Brad finally goes to his family physician. Brad has been suffering for several months with joint pain, mostly in his knees, which he attributes to years of running. He is also suffering from chronic fatigue. His doctor prescribes over-the-counter pain medication and attributes the fatigue to job-related stress.

His parents are at least C282Y heterozygotes or carriers for hemochromatosis, but Brad isn't aware of this; neither are his parents. His parents have been relatively healthy, and they are unaware they carry a potentially life-threatening genetic mutation. Brad has inherited one mutation from his dad and one from his mom, which makes him a C282Y homozygote—but he still knows nothing about HFE and its mutations. Neither does his physician.

Brad's chances of being a homozygote are one in four (25 percent). His siblings—two brothers and a sister—also have a 25 percent chance of being a homozygote, a 25 percent chance of being normal (i.e., no mutations), and a 50 percent chance of being a carrier themselves. Many carriers of the HFE mutation do not manifest symptoms, though there are some who do. It is possible that these individuals possess other contributing genetic abnormalities not yet identified.

Years pass and Brad gets progressively weaker, and he has pain in his ankles and knuckles. He makes an appointment to see his family doctor. He does not see his regular doctor but a new partner, who asks Brad about his family history. This offers few clues since Brad's two younger brothers, one sister, and mom and dad have no remarkable health issues. When his physician hears nothing out of the ordinary by way of disease in his parents or siblings, he asks Brad about his grandparents. Brad remarks, "Oh yes, my grandmother had diabetes," which leads the physician off track. The physician asks Brad about frequent urination or thrist and Brad remarks that he has experienced this to some degree. His doctor orders tests to measure Brad's blood glucose because of Brad's frequent thirst and family history of diabetes. The doctor orders a rheumatoid factor test because Brad has complained of joint pain. Blood work reveals slightly elevated glucose and is negative for rheumatoid arthritis.

Since diabetes is common and Brad's grandmother had diabetes, and he is symptomatic of the condition, Brad's physician makes the diagnosis of diabetes and misses the underlying cause in Brad's case, which is hemochromatosis. Brad is instructed to take an over-the-counter pain reliever for the joint pain, which this physician also believes is stress related. He gives Brad a prescription drug for glucose control and a copy of a diet, and he tells him to reduce the stress in his life. He tells Brad that he can control his sugar levels through diet and medication, but if problems persist, he will make arrangements for Brad to see an endocrinologist, a physician who specializes in diabetes.

At first Brad does well on his diabetes diet, but after several months he begins to struggle. Within two years he is completely off his diet and not exercising. Unbeknownst to Brad, other conditions advance unchecked. Iron proceeds to accumulate in Brad's vital organs. Liver cirrhosis has begun and his heart is being damaged irreversibly. His essential glands such as his anterior pituitary, gonads, and thyroid are filling with iron—leaving him impotent and depressed. To round things off, Brad is beginning to lose body hair, but it is the loss of hair on his head that bothers him most.

Desperate for relief, he calls his family doctor and asks for a referral to the endocrinologist. Two months later, with the specialist, Brad complains that his diabetes must be out of control. He has lost his libido and admits to being impotent. He complains about his hair loss and remarks that his fatigue and joint pain is worse.

His endocrinologist tells Brad that his symptoms are probably not related to diabetes and that he suspects hypothyroidism; he tests Brad's thyroid function. The endocrinologist runs several other tests as well, including for blood glucose. When test results confirm that he has an underactive thyroid, Brad is relieved. Hair loss, chronic fatigue, and loss of libido are symptoms that can be associated with hypothyroidism. His doctor solves yet another mystery and prescribes thyroid-hormone replacement therapy for Brad, but the hemochromatosis continues to evade detection.

Within a few months of taking the thyroid replacement hormone, modest improvement by way of increased energy and libido fools Brad into thinking his problems are over—unfortunately, they are getting worse. Brad's fatigue returns. His libido begins to fade, and he develops abdominal pain, shortness of breath, chest pain, and irregular heartbeat.

Brad feels that the endocrinologist can no longer help, so he calls his family doctor and is referred to a cardiologist for the heart trouble and a gastroenterologist for the abdominal pain. Because Brad is having chest pain and is concerned about a heart attack, he makes an appointment with the cardiologist first; he gets an appointment right away.

The cardiologist gives Brad a very thorough physical exam, complete with stress test, blood work, and EKG. Brad experiences no heart arrhythmia during this exam. "These things never seem to take place when a doctor is in the room," comments Brad. His EKG is normal, but because he is slightly overweight, the cardiologist puts him on a low-fat diet and an exercise program of daily walking.

Brad tries faithfully to follow his new diet and exercise program. But ten days into his new routine, profound fatigue overpowers him. His motivation evaporates. He musters the strength to contact the gastroenterologist. He is so discouraged at this point that when the scheduling nurse asks if he prefers a morning or afternoon appointment, Brad hisses in response, "I don't give a damn! Just give me anything!" By now he is a physical and emotional wreck. His skin has darkened. Brad appears to have a tan, though he has not been in the sun. There are dark lines in the creases of his hands and dark circles under his eyes. He is still in pain; his head is pounding. He is depressed, overweight, short of breath, and still having irregular heartbeats. He is impotent and has no interest in sex, and he watches in horror as far too many clumps of his hair swirl down the bathtub drain.

Brad's wife turns to the Internet and finds several resources. She contacts Iron Disorders Institute. In response to her request for information and support, materials are mailed to Brad; these include physician educational materials that have been developed by the Iron Disorders Institute Medical & Scientific Advisory Board. Brad is relieved and feels more confident now that he has trustworthy literature to share with the doctor. After apologizing profusely to the scheduling nurse for his outburst, Brad's TS percentage, serum ferritin, and liver enzymes are measured. The gastroenterologist suspects that Brad's symptoms are related to HHC. He notes that Brad's liver is enlarged (hepatomegaly). When the test results come back, Brad finally gets the pieces of the puzzle that were missing. His fasting serum ferritin is more than 3,000 ng/mL, his TS percentage is 97 percent, his liver enzymes are mildly elevated, and he is told he needs a liver biopsy to confirm diagnosis.

Although Brad undergoes a liver biopsy, the procedure is not necessary to diagnose hemochromatosis, but it is necessary to assess the extent of liver damage, as Brad's serum ferritin was in excess of 1,000 ng/mL. The biopsy clearly shows Brad's cirrhosis. The good news is that he does not have liver cancer. When diagnosis of hemochromatosis is made after cirrhosis has developed, the chance that the patient will develop liver cancer later increases 20- to 200-fold.

Another way Brad could have been diagnosed is through genetic testing; later, he opts to do this. It is no surprise that he is C282Y homozygote. Brad immediately begins calling his siblings. One brother refuses genetic testing fearing that he will lose his job.

Another brother is tested right away and is also a C282Y homozygote. His sister is considering the genetic test.

Brad starts therapeutic phlebotomy and his iron levels are restored to normal. Some of his symptoms improve and some worsen, but he knows the cause of his years of pain and suffering. It has a name: hemochromatosis.

Brad goes back to his family physicians to share what he has learned. He carries with him some print materials, which explain how two simple tests, TS percentage and serum ferritin, would have likely resulted in an early diagnosis. From the time of Brad's first symptoms and initial doctor's visit to his final discovery, eleven years had passed and he had seen five different physicians.

For some patients with HHC, Brad's story sounds quite familiar. False assumption can set a patient up for a series of misdiagnoses, possible mistreatment, and a seemingly unending cycle of symptoms, treatment, temporary relief, new symptoms, another diagnosis, and so on. When eventually Brad sought help and found a physician who was informed about hemochromatosis, the complete diagnosis was made and proper therapy begun.

Jack—Hemochromatosis and Delayed Detection Despite Clues

Jack had been in agony for more than ten years because of severe pain in his hip and finger joints. He was often very tired but thought it was because of stress from the constant pain. Repeated trips to his physician ensured him a prescription for the newest arthritis drug, which offered temporary relief. However, within a few weeks of beginning a new drug, Jack's liver enzymes would become elevated and he would have to discontinue the medication.

Having exhausted the list of prescription pain relievers, Jack's physician decided to consult with a colleague, a gastroenterologist, who suggested measuring Jack's iron levels. For Jack, this triggered a memory of a physical three years earlier, where his serum iron had been elevated. Seemingly unimportant at the time, there was no follow-up to retest for serum iron. The significance of this earlier abnormal level was a sobering detail for Jack. An older brother and one sister had just died, within a year of each other. His older brother Don had died of bleeding esophageal varices and his sister Grace had died of liver cancer. "I wonder whether they would still be alive today?" Jack thinks. "I also wonder if my arthritic pain would have become so intense. One thing for certain, I would have needed fewer phlebotomies," Jack concludes.

Jack's physician, who was not the attending physician three years earlier when abnormal serum iron occurred, ordered a complete iron panel, and Jack was properly diagnosed with hemochromatosis. He was able to help two sisters who went immediately to their physicians with IDI's information for doctors and patients. Both sisters were diagnosed with hemochromatosis. All three were genetically tested and found to be C282Y homozygotes. All received therapeutic phlebotomy and are doing well. Jack's diagnosis was too late to save his other siblings. He is convinced they had hemochromatosis.

Eastman Family—Hemochromatosis in One Family
Everyone in the Eastman family sat around the Thanksgiving dinner table. Logs crackled in the fireplace; the beautiful fall colors filled the window. Familiar holiday smells of nutmeg and cinnamon floated from the kitchen, where pumpkin pie, fresh from the oven, cooled. Norman Rockwell could not have painted a more normal and familiar scene. But things were anything but normal for the Eastman family; they had endured years of seemingly unrelated health problems without knowing the cause. Everyone in the family had some degree of poor health, but it would be nearly thirty years before Nancy Eastman could put it all together. Now on this Thanksgiving Day, her family gives thanks to be alive. Even though symptoms varied from person to person within the family, eventually the connection was made.

Nancy was the first person in the Eastman family to be diagnosed with hemochromatosis, followed by the diagnosis of her two sons, two brothers, one nephew, and one sister. Across the table is Nancy's mother, who was diagnosed thirtysome years earlier with diabetes. Bypass surgery a few years ago was just the beginning for Nancy's mother. She had terrible sores on her feet that would not heal; and she fell, breaking a leg in the process. Nancy thought about her dad; he had died nearly twenty years earlier of a heart attack at the age of fifty-seven.

He had cancer and gallbladder problems, and his autopsy showed an enlarged heart and brown residue in his liver.

She glanced over at her sister, who had erratic periods and had tried for twelve years before she got pregnant. Eventually she had a hysterectomy. A liver biopsy as a result of Nancy's diagnosis revealed mild cirrhosis and provided the diagnosis of HHC. She was tested genetically and carried only one mutation of HFE gene, C282Y.

Her older brother experienced his first heart attack at the age of forty-five and within one year had five bypasses. Now at the age of fifty-six, he is on full disability. His two sons, Nancy's nephews, have high blood pressure. Her younger brother had been severely depressed for years. When his iron was finally checked, his TS percentage was 62 percent; his serum ferritin was more than 300 ng/mL. After phlebotomy treatment, he seemed better. His twenty-one-year-old son has a TS percentage of 52 percent; his daughter is anemic. Nancy's youngest brother is thirty-six; he has no symptoms yet, but she is concerned about him.

Nancy thinks back on her own situation. Two difficult births, toxemia, and high blood pressure seemed all a part of being pregnant. At the age of forty-four during a routine physical, the physician noted that Nancy's skin looked like that of a person who had hemochromatosis. That was the first time she had ever heard the word. No tests were done to determine whether she indeed had the disorder. Four years later, Nancy returned to her doctor with complaints of abdominal pain, chronic fatigue, joint pain, and depression. This time the doctor mentioned hemochromatosis as a real possibility. He tested liver function and ran an iron panel. Nancy's liver enzymes were elevated, her TS percentage at 62 percent, and her serum ferritin at 1,223 ng/mL. Nancy was referred to a gastroenterologist for a liver biopsy. Hemochromatosis was ruled out. Nancy was given a letter saying so, and she was told to check back with her family doctor in one year, but Nancy did not accept this diagnosis, or lack of one.

Nancy began to attend a local hemochromatosis support group meeting. She was encouraged to persist in her efforts for answers. After some effort, she obtained the original biopsy slides and took them with her biopsy result letter to another physician, who examined the slides and diagnosed her immediately. Nancy was glad she had challenged the liver biopsy findings in the letter, especially when the doctor remarked, "I hope we got this before liver cancer." She began therapeutic phlebotomy. After thirteen extractions in twelve weeks, Nancy developed tightness in her jaw and chest. She remembers her doctor saying, "You're too young to be having a heart attack!" A cardiac catheterization revealed an ischemic region (dead tissue) on the inferior (lower) wall of her heart, 50 percent blockage in one artery, and 65 percent in the other. A stent was installed and she was given medication. The pain in her feet (especially her toes), kidney infections, red spots on her face, and scalp problems did not seem related to hemochromatosis—but after phlebotomy, these symptoms improved or disappeared entirely.

Nancy misses her dad, but she looks around the Thanksgiving dinner table and gives thanks that the family knows the underlying common denominator of their health problems, hemochromatosis. She also expresses her gratitude for the literature published by IDI and given to her at one of the meetings because she feels it helped her entire family.

21
Women Don't Get Hemochromatosis, Do They?

Clara

"You don't need to be tested for hemochromatosis," her physician remarked. "It's rare and it doesn't occur in women," he concluded and closed her file, which was now several inches thick. Clara looked at her doctor, trying to remain civil. "Just humor me, and do the tests."

Clara had been searching for answers about her health for more than four years. Her extensive reading had led her to believe that she might have hemochromatosis. Her father had died at the age of fifty-nine of a sudden heart attack. He had other problems, which were not mentioned openly while he was alive. Clara's mother eventually admitted that her husband, Clara's father, had often been depressed and drank heavily, especially at bedtime. He had lost all interest in sex and was so exhausted that he missed work frequently. She was ashamed to tell anyone that her husband was an alcoholic. Besides, he would often have emotional outbursts that worked well as a deterrent for telling anyone about his condition. She was shocked when he died of a heart attack; she had thought his liver would fail long before his heart.

Clara wasn't certain that her father died of hemochromatosis, but her own personal battle with unresolved health issues made her think it could be possible. Besides, she rationalized, a TS percentage test wasn't very expensive, and if her suspicions were true, whatever the cost, it would be worth it.

Clara's TS percentage was indeed elevated. Her repeat fasting TS percentage was 48 percent, and her ferritin was 137 ng/mL, not sufficiently high enough, according to her physician, to order a phlebotomy. She asked for genetic testing and was found to be a C282Y/H63D compound heterozygote.

Gayle

Gayle graduated from nursing school in 1965. She barely remembers the word *hemochromatosis* or the term *bronze diabetes*. She became a regular blood donor and learned that she was O positive, but it wasn't her blood type that made her curious. While other donors gave blood and left within ten or fifteen minutes, her donation was taking up to forty-five minutes to complete.

In the late 1980s, Gayle's younger brother, Thomas, had just returned from a three-month job in the Middle East. On his return, he had a battery of tests, which included ferritin. Tom's level was 4,000, and the physician told him he suspected hemochromatosis. Tom's eyes widened. "That's what my father-in-law died of!" he exclaimed. The physician asked whether Tom's wife had ever been checked for hemochromatosis, explaining that it was inherited. They may want to know for the sake of their children.

Tom's wife, Jill, had blood work, and they both had a liver biopsy, which confirmed hemochromatosis in Tom and Jill and early cirrhosis in Tom.

Meanwhile, Gayle was still having difficulty with her blood donations, though she continued to go regularly. She was certain that since her brother had been diagnosed with hemochromatosis, she would be too. She knew her slow-moving, "thick" blood was somehow related. But when she was tested, the doctor told her he saw no signs of the disorder. All he found was somewhat-elevated hemoglobin. Her physician told her to stop smoking and the hemoglobin level would drop.

Three years later symptoms of fatigue, dry and itchy skin, hair loss, and weight gain landed Gayle a diagnosis of hypothyroidism and a prescription for Synthroid. "I pestered the doctor to test my ferritin," comments Gayle. "Finally he gave in; my ferritin was 400." The doctor told Gayle not to be concerned about hemochromatosis; her liver enzymes were normal and she had no symptoms. Gayle insisted that her ferritin be checked periodically. She watched it steadily rise until, within a year, her ferritin was up to 800. She asked to be referred to a gastroenterologist. When Gayle heard the gastroenterologist say, "You have no symptoms." She repeated, "I have a ferritin of 800, my brother has hemochromatosis, and my hemoglobin is high. What about a liver biopsy?" The gastroenterologist agreed and performed the biopsy. As Gayle puts it, "Much to everyone's surprise but my own, my liver contained 3+ iron!"

After two years of therapeutic phlebotomy under the gastroenterologist's supervision, Gayle changed doctors. She felt the gastroenterologist had lost interest in her. She pointed out that during her two years of therapy under his supervision, he hadn't even palpated her liver. Gayle switched to a hematologist but as joint disease developed she had to consult with an orthopedist.

Her first twinge of arthritis began in the base of one thumb. Arthritis advanced to the point of needing joint replacement surgery on the entire right hand. Gayle's therapy now includes injections of cortisone into joints in her hands three times a year. She wears a splint on her hand, writes with "Dr. Grip," and uses "Big Grip" kitchen utensils. She is taking high-blood-pressure medicine and often wonders about a paternal aunt who died at the age of forty-nine of cirrhosis. Most of the family suspected that the aunt might have been a drinker, until they had a personal experience with hemochromatosis. None of Gayle's children has high iron levels; she believes they are carriers.

Editor's note: as a rule, hemochromatosis patients do not have elevated hemoglobin.

Jennifer

"Iron overload disease first showed up in my life in 1971; I was eleven years old," begins forty-year-old Jennifer. "Our family physician diagnosed me with viral hepatitis, as my liver counts were off. The hepatitis went away, but my liver counts never reverted to the 'normal' range. My physician at the time even wrote 'hemochromatosis?' in big red letters on my chart. The chart went into his folder, and my physician never thought to follow up on his hunch. My mother never thought to question it either, as the doctor assured us things would be 'just fine.'

And somehow, the ball was dropped, and we went back to our normal lives. Meanwhile, I was storing iron every day."

Jennifer's sister Joyce was hospitalized at the age of forty. After passing out in the street as a result of high blood sugar, she was diagnosed with type 1 diabetes. Although Joyce exhibited many of the same symptoms as Jennifer (arthritis, stomachaches, headaches), no one made a connection between the sisters' conditions. Also, not one physician thought to check Joyce's iron levels.

It wasn't until after Joyce was released from the hospital that a family friend suggested that maybe Joyce and Jennifer had a basic systemic problem. The friend gave Joyce the name of a new physician, which resulted in Joyce's diagnosis of hemochromatosis, iron-overload disease. Joyce was put on a schedule of phlebotomies almost immediately. Jennifer continued her very busy schedule and promising career.

The word *hemochromatosis* was foreign to every member of the family. They all thought, "Poor Joyce!" Little did they know that this is a hereditary disease. Although Joyce's diagnosis was confirmed, no physician suggested that her siblings be tested. It was at least four months into Joyce's treatment when one of her phlebotomists told her that hemochromatosis was very much an inherited condition. The entire family started reading.

By this time, Jennifer had moved from New York City to Los Angeles. The move, compounded with losing both a job and a fiancé within weeks of each other, was highly stressful. She was still not menstruating and still had arthritis, which had now been present for three and a half years. Her arthritis had even required surgery on her feet the year before. The surgeons attributed her arthritic feet to an athletic childhood. A connection between her own symptoms and her sister's diagnosis of hemochromatosis had still not been made.

Finally, research compiled by the family on hemochromatosis paid off. They realized the necessity of testing each member of the family. "We all got tested immediately, along with our mother, Louise."

Of Louise's five children, two had full-blown hemochromatosis, Joyce and Jennifer. Joyce's ferritin was 2,900. Jennifer's was more than 4,900; her TS percentage was 98 percent.

"Being diagnosed with a disease when you are not feeling 'sick' is a weird thing. It's very easy to just deny it. Yes, I had arthritis and no periods, but I was feeling okay most of the time. I was definitely not prepared for having a 'disease,' especially one that required any kind of treatment! But I took the time to speak to someone more knowledgeable than myself. I eventually found a hematologist at UCLA who suggested a liver biopsy to confirm the diagnosis. I agreed, as a part of me was still sure that I didn't have this 'disease'!"

"Biopsies don't lie," continues Jennifer. "I had hemochromatosis. And to my surprise, apparently so did my father, Tom. He had died at age fifty-eight due to heart and liver failure. He had hemochromatosis all along, and the iron had slowly killed him. Joyce and I had inherited hemochromatosis from our father. But we have learned since the gene discovery that Mom had to be at least a carrier. My sister and I made a promise that we wouldn't let it hurt us the way it had hurt him [referring to their father]. He had spent years in and out of hospitals with multiple health problems. All the problems we now know to be associated with HHC."

Jennifer, at the age of twenty-six, began therapy; she endured a long and difficult two years of weakness and problems with anemia and eventually had to give up her job in Los Angeles and move back home. The last portion of her treatment was the toughest. She endured forced-sustained anemia to ensure that the deep, residual tissue iron was removed. Jennifer felt this was an important part of her therapy.

"I was still not having periods; the doctors had put me on heavy doses of estrogen, in the hopes of 'jump-starting' my reproductive system. The downside to this was that I put on about twenty-five pounds in no time flat! On my worst days, I'd complain that I was not only sick, but I was sick and fat. Mind you, I was 110 pounds at five foot seven before the added weight; not exactly a blimp."

Then a miracle happened. "I woke up one morning, and I was having a period! I never thought I'd be happy to be menstruating, but let me tell you, I was jumping for joy. I was returning to being a normal, healthy functioning human being! It took about a year for my periods to return fully. By this time,

I was living back in New York City. I continued to have regular tests on my iron levels as well as my hormonal levels. I had been told by more than one physician that I would not be able to have children, as I was not making any 'follicles,' even following a round of trying out the fertility drug Perganol. This devastated me, but I resigned myself to this being a part of God's greater plan. I was thankful to be healthy for the most part, and decided that I would build the best life I could."

Jennifer's job in New York eventually enabled her to return to her hometown in Florida when her company relocated to the area. Her new office was within five miles of her mom. Two weeks after arriving back in Florida, Jennifer met a handsome, charming man. They married and several months later, Jennifer experienced what she calls another miracle.

"I woke up feeling very queasy one morning, thinking I had the flu. It lasted for three days until my husband, Wayne, finally came home with a pregnancy test. The test was positive. I told him that was impossible, and he went out and bought four more—each a different brand. Four confirming positive tests meant one thing: I was pregnant! I immediately ran off to the doctor, and she confirmed it. It was the happiest day of my life—until the day nine months later, when my son Adam was born."

"Somehow, my life was given back to me in full, and there's not a day that goes by that I am not eternally grateful," recalls Jennifer. "Adam has given me more joy than I could have ever imagined. He is now grown, and he is as healthy as a horse! He surfs, plays golf, tennis, hockey, skateboards, snowboards, fences, and a bunch of other things. My son has also given me the role of a lifetime—being a mother. And lucky me, I had the best model to learn from—our mom. Thank you, Mother. Adam and I think of you every day, and we spend our lives living in ways that would make you proud."

Ellie

Ellie is a wife, mother, medical technologist, and clinical laboratory science instructor. She would spend twenty-one years trying to get the proper diagnosis of hemochromatosis. Her ordeal began with the first hint of iron overload at age twenty-five when she experienced her first miscarriage. Her second miscarriage took place two years later. Ellie had struggled with infertility, a possible sign of hemochromatosis, but in time became pregnant after taking Clomid, a fertility drug. Her obstetrician prescribed prenatal vitamins and iron supplements. Soon after starting the iron supplements, she began having intestinal cramps and stopped taking the iron. While pregnant, her hemoglobin remained around 15 g/dL. "My obstetrician remarked that my body seemed to do well being pregnant," remarks Ellie.

"My first actual symptoms appeared when my two children were toddlers. I had recurring bouts of extreme sadness, muscle pain, and fatigue. The fatigue challenged me the most. Considering my lifestyle, it was not surprising that I was tired, even exhausted, on a regular basis. I worked full-time while my husband completed his PhD. I pursued my master's degree in Health Sciences in the evenings and continued to care for our two young children."

Then Ellie began having heart palpitations and symptoms of irritable bowel syndrome (IBS), while the aching in her muscles and joints continued. Her family practice physician was the first in a long line of doctors to try to pick at the pieces of her disease. Ellie would see eight different doctors before she got the complete diagnosis.

In the early 1990s, one physician noticed slightly elevated liver function tests (LFTs) and apparent borderline hypothyroidism. Since elevated LFTs are a sign of possible liver damage, the physician monitored these levels closely. Ellie was told the elevated LFTs were due to a fatty liver.

"The most frightening experience in my search for a diagnosis occurred when a gastroenterologist shocked me with his comment: 'You either have hepatitis, cirrhosis, or liver cancer. I don't think you have hepatitis because you are not sick enough. If you have liver cancer there isn't much we can do for you anyway, and to confirm the cirrhosis, we will have to do a liver biopsy. If we do the liver biopsy, there is the danger of hemorrhage.' When I asked him what a liver biopsy would feel like, he replied, 'Like a horse kicked you.' Needless to say, I was not comfortable with Dr. Seven. I agreed, nonetheless, to repeat the blood tests. I did not want to have a liver biopsy—particularly by this physician. Due to my aversion to the biopsy, the doctor ordered a CT scan. I waited, fearful the results would reveal some type of liver cancer. The CT results were normal and an MRI was ordered immediately. I waited again, frightened by the possible results. Nothing was found. Hemochromatosis was never seriously considered in this process. I am not sure it was even mentioned."

The eighth physician was the first to mention hemochromatosis. He explained that this disease was probably more prevalent than we realized and could be treated with phlebotomies. He announced that the only definitive test for this disease was a liver biopsy. Ellie shared her fear of the procedure, and he told her that as long as her iron levels were monitored and she continued to have menstrual periods that the biopsy could be postponed, but that she should be prepared to have the biopsy in the future.

In the summer of 1997, Ellie visited family, including her cousin, an internal medicine physician. Prior to the visit, Ellie's mother shared with her that this cousin was compiling family information about depression.

"When I questioned him, he clarified that it was not the depression he was researching, but instead the family's liver problems. Our grandfather had died of liver cancer, and my cousin himself had just recently learned that he was a hemochromatosis patient. My husband's response was immediate, 'Isn't that what Dr. Eight thinks you might have?' The referral to the eighth physician had occurred about two to three years prior to this revelation. Suddenly, it clicked! The answers to the puzzle were clear. The elevated LFTs, fatigue, joint pain, heart palpitations, thyroid problems, miscarriages, infertility problems, fibromyalgia, irritable bowel syndrome, and depression were all a part of the same picture. I was certain I had hemochromatosis!"

By this time genetic testing was available, and it revealed that Ellie was C282Y homozygous for hemochromatosis.

"Looking back on this journey, one key piece of the puzzle that was missing during all those years of assessments was my extended family medical history. If my memory is correct, the medical form that inquired about family medical history asked about parents and grandparents—it did not include aunts, uncles, and cousins. On the paternal side of my family, my father died of pancreatic cancer at sixty-six. He lived longer than either of his siblings. One of his brothers died of primary liver carcinoma, and the other brother died of a massive heart attack in his late forties or early fifties. My grandparents did not die of illnesses attributed to hemochromatosis, so an abbreviated family history did not pick up the problem that is evident in our extended family."

"People with HHC get frustrated when it is obvious that something must be wrong, but no one can give a justifiable diagnosis. Even when HHC is diagnosed, the correct treatment plan is vague. Guidelines for screening must be determined and extended family histories reviewed. Carriers, as well as those of us homozygous for the disease, need regular monitoring. We want to be confident that the plan for monitoring this lifelong disease is valid. We want all of the medical staff to understand our disease. I am confident our frustrations will lessen, or even disappear, as educational opportunities on hemochromatosis occur. With hemochromatosis, as with other diseases, early detection prevents serious consequences, and means that our quality of life improves dramatically—sooner rather than later," concludes Ellie.

Allison and Meredith

Identical twin sisters Allison and Meredith are C282Y homozygotes, but they are not yet aware of this genetic status. Before each receives a definitive clinical diagnosis, they both will continue to suffer debilitating yet different symptoms and multiple miscarriages. The disparity of their symptoms, even as identical twins, is true of many HHC patients and is still not understood. Their subsequent and varied responses to similar treatment plans following diagnosis is also emblematic of HHC patients and again is not largely understood.

The impetus for each sister to aggressively pursue a clinical diagnosis of hemochromatosis was that one of their middle-aged brothers, at the advice of his family physician, was exploring the possibility of HHC, given symptoms of extreme fatigue, joint pain, and sleeplessness. Not surprising, but dismaying, is that both sisters, while exhibiting a variation of these symptoms and more, would continue to struggle for the support of a similar diagnosis from their own family physicians and medical specialists. This is even despite the fact that one identical twin, twenty years prior at the age of twenty-two, before the availability of genetic testing for hemochromatosis, was advised by a hematologist to donate regularly, as her elevated iron levels suggested that she was a candidate for hemochromatosis.

Allison's final diagnosis of hemochromatosis began with random symptoms and fertility issues. In her quest for answers, she sought help from a family physician, naturopath, and hematologist, without a complete diagnosis.

Allison had experienced two miscarriages, two successful pregnancies, and three subsequent miscarriages in attempts for a third child, when symptoms of dizziness, weakness, thirst, breathlessness, and arrhythmia became too great. Her family doctor diagnosed her with a viral infection but, at her request, agreed to refer her to a cardiologist. The cardiologist performed an EKG and echocardiogram, which he reported was normal. Dissatisfied with the lack of conclusive information and continued ill health, Allison continues to seek answers. The speculation of hemochromatosis in her brother's case and her past candidacy for the condition, leads her to aggressively pursue a similar diagnosis. At her next visit to the gynecologist, she asks for an iron panel and genetic testing for hemochromatosis. The test results reveal she has elevated iron levels and hemochromatosis. Phlebotomies are started but overdone. After eighteen phlebotomies in one year, Allison becomes iron avid, a condition where the serum ferritin is normal or low but the TS percentage is elevated.

Running parallel to Allison's story is her sister Meredith's experience. Meredith, however, is suffering from more physically debilitating symptoms, which include joint pain in her hips and knees, tightness in her chest, constipation, and overall fatigue. She is repeatedly given the same diagnosis: prearthritic symptoms aggravated by iliotibial band syndrome (IT-band) or runner's knee issues and exercise-induced asthma. Eventually other symptoms emerge. Meredith becomes severely lactose intolerant, which results in abdominal pain, vomiting, diarrhea, and increased tightness in her chest; she also experiences an early-term miscarriage. A colonoscopy is performed, which is normal; she is given an inhaler and placed on a dairy-free diet.

With her brother and sister both speculating that she has hemochromatosis, Meredith seeks out the advice of a genetic counselor and eventually is diagnosed by her physician with type 1 hemochromatosis. Most interesting in Meredith's case, compared to that of her identical twin sister, is that Meredith experienced much more physically debilitating symptoms, despite the fact that her iron levels were within the "prescribed" range at the time of diagnosis.

Meredith's story does not end with the genetic diagnosis. Although her iron levels were within in the range, she was advised and opted to undergo therapy. Immediately, she felt relief from her symptoms. She is now sleeping more soundly, the chest pain and joint pain are almost gone, and her memory and clarity of thought improves. Her phlebotomy schedule, however, is so rigorous that she too is overbled and becomes iron avid. She is now plagued by extreme fatigue, light-headedness, and irritability. Her family physician prescribes iron pills—50 milligrams of ferrous sulfate—three times a day. Within three weeks, Meredith's symptoms begin to abate. Her ferritin climbs from 7 ng/mL to 87 ng/mL. Both sisters learn from the Iron Disorders Institute about iron avidity; they postpone phlebotomies and eventually begin to feel back to normal—but it takes Meredith thirty-two weeks to recover from overbleeding.

In their pursuit of a diagnosis, the difficulties each sister encountered could largely and "understandably" have been attributed to the general lack of knowledge of either the existence of hemochromatosis or the difficulty of clinically diagnosing HHC because of the elusive nature of its symptoms. This was, however, not the case for either sister, as each woman repeatedly, on the basis of her familial history, asked whether HHC was a contributing factor in the medical status. Each woman struggled at length for a definitive diagnosis principally because HHC continues to be proclaimed and viewed as a condition that primarily affects middle-aged men. This is simply not true. The fact is this: hemochromatosis is not gender specific or gender biased; at this point, it is only more clinically apparent in middle-aged men. That does not mean that it does not affect persons of various ages and of both sexes.

Meredith and Allison share their story for a multiple of reasons. First, they wish to dispel the myth that HHC affects only middle-aged men. Second, they hope that their being identical twins with different symptoms accentuates the fact that HHC does not present specific symptoms. Third, they hope that people give strong consideration to the effects and course of treatment—both of these things will vary among patients. Finally, they want more attention to be paid to the link between HHC and infertility in women.

22
Heterozygotes and the Other Homozygote

Jen

When Jen's grandmother died in 1976, Jen was told that her death was due to myocardial infarction. Nothing else was ever mentioned; no autopsy was performed. All Jen remembers from that terrible time was thinking, "She's too young to die. She had just turned sixty-nine."

Over the years, Jen had experienced a number of symptoms, but not until 1991 did she suspect a connection between her symptoms and her grandmother's death. Jen's severe muscle pain, inability to conceive, heart arrhythmia, chronic fatigue, and elevated iron levels still did not result in the correct diagnosis.

Not until a genetics test revealed that she was a compound heterozygote (C282Y/H63D) did Jen receive a diagnosis and begin therapy.

The Other Homozygote: H63D/H63D

Cindy began having symptoms when she was in her late forties. She was a mother and had a demanding job working for a U.S. senator. It seemed reasonable to attribute some symptoms—especially of fatigue—to the long hours and demands of a working mother. After fatigue, she struggled with aches, pains, poor sleep, and weight gain. Her primary care physician referred her to an ob-gyn, who told her she was likely going through early menopause. Not satisfied, she asked to be referred to another specialist. Cindy would see six more doctors without any conclusive results. In a chance encounter, she met a patient who had hemochromatosis and suggested that she contact Iron

Disorders Institute (IDI), which she did. She was given literature, which she took to her physician, but he tossed it to one
side and told her that it was not likely hemochromatosis but
that he would do a genetic test anyway. Cindy called patient
services at IDI to report the outcome of the genetic test. She
began by saying, "Well, it's not hemochromatosis; the doctor
says I don't have it." Cindy reported that physician had not
ordered the entire iron panel to determine both ferritin and
iron saturation. She emphasized that, because she did not have
the genes for hemochromatosis, she would just have to live
with her symptoms until someone could figure out the cause.
The IDI patient-information contact asked if she would mind
sharing the results of the genetic test, which she was happy to
do. Her results revealed that she was an H63D/H63D homozygote. A subsequent complete iron panel revealed TS percentage of 67 percent and 450 ng/mL serum ferritin.

23

Emotions Crowd Out Reason

Karen—Hemochromatosis, a Misguided Treatment

Karen was in a panic. She wanted to know why her thirty-year-old husband was severely anemic after a series of phlebotomies, when in fact his ferritin had been higher than 650. It seems her husband had been suffering from chronic fatigue, among other symptoms. Doctors had been baffled, unable to reach a diagnosis. Karen had searched "frantically for answers," as she put it. "The Internet offered the only real hope, and her husband's doctor was ignorant!" she added.

Ironically, the only thing ignorant about her husband's physician was that he allowed himself to be persuaded to perform phlebotomy on this persistent woman's husband, and he did not order sufficient tests. The husband did indeed have an elevated ferritin, but his TS percentage had not been checked.

Believing that she had the correct and necessary information to get her husband diagnosed and treated, her persistence was intimidating. The physician—probably fearing consequences, such as a lawsuit—did exactly what Karen insisted, which was to begin therapeutic phlebotomy on her husband.

Unfortunately, the man became severely anemic as a result of repeated phlebotomies. His hemoglobin reached a dangerously low level of 5.0 g/dL before the phlebotomies were stopped (that level of hemoglobin is what Elaine reported—it is the lowest known hemoglobin value at which a patient has survived). It's a small wonder that the woman's husband didn't die of heart failure from unnecessary bleeding.

What Karen did not learn in her early search for information was that elevated ferritin alone is not enough to warrant phlebotomy. It is, however, a signal to investigate further. In this case, a simple TS percentage test most likely would have ruled out iron overload as the cause of her husband's symptoms. Elevated ferritin does not always indicate iron loading. Clearly, Karen was a victim of the recently recognized phenomenon of cyberchondria—an unfounded anxiety about health problems due to reading about medical issues on the Internet. Karen was given information about hereditary hyperferritinemia, an inherited condition of early-onset cataracts. Serum ferritin can be very high in patients with this condition. Diagnosis can be made by an ophthalmologist. Karen admitted that her husband had cataracts.

Charlene—Neonatal Hemochromatosis, an Emotional Assumption

Charlene shouted at her pediatrician that her newborn was going to die without a phlebotomy. Hemochromatosis had been diagnosed in her family, and her newborn who had been genetically tested was a C282Y homozygote. On one trip to the family doctor, she convinced the doctor to test for TS percentage and serum ferritin on her newborn. When the infant's iron levels came back elevated, the woman panicked. The family doctor admitted he did not know much about hemochromatosis in children and referred Charlene to a pediatrician.

When Charlene demanded a phlebotomy for her newborn, the pediatrician was both horrified and dumbfounded at how this woman could have ever reached such a conclusion. With Charlene and her baby still in his office, the doctor contacted the Iron Disorders Institute. We faxed information about pediatric iron levels provided by IDI's Medical and Scientific Advisory Board. The information explained that newborns have naturally high iron levels during the first few months of life. Some infants can have a TS percentage as high as 90 percent. Infants can also have high serum ferritin levels during this time. It is critical that adequate iron be available for the rapid growth and development that takes place in the first months of life. Without sufficient iron, a child can experience developmental delays and cognitive impairment, perhaps even mild retardation. Eventually, the pediatrician was able to calm Charlene and help her realize that pathological iron overload in newborns is rare. Among materials sent to the pediatrician was the consideration to test the child at age three for the possibility of an iron-loading condition and every five years thereafter until an iron-loading pattern might be revealed. Materials were also sent to Charlene about the naturally high iron levels in newborns and about hemochromatosis and breast-feeding.

Mothers can become quite agitated, especially when they believe that their children are at risk of developing a life-threatening disease. When they hear the term *neonatal hemochromatosis*, they don't realize that it is a totally different condition from HFE-related hemochromatosis. When they learn that neonatal hemochromatosis is fatal in most cases, mothers can leap to the possibly incorrect conclusion that their newborn's life is in jeopardy. Visit our website for additional information about neonatal hemochromatosis and pathological iron overload in children: www.irondisorders.org.

Charlene learned that her highly charged emotional assumptions would have had dire consequences had not her level-headed pediatrician consulted IDI for more information to clarify the differences between HFE-related hemochromatosis and neonatal hemochromatosis. Charlene's pediatrician recognized cyberchondria and dealt with it accordingly by seeking more information to soothe Charlene's anxiety.

24

The Wrong Diagnosis

Inflammatory Disease Masquerades as Iron Deficiency

Paula was ten years old when her doctor told her she was anemic and needed to take iron pills. Her doctor wanted to remove Paula's tonsils, but her anemia first had to be corrected. Since Paula's fifth birthday, tonsillitis was a frequent condition for her that necessitated several rounds of penicillin. Paula wasn't looking forward to a tonsillectomy, but if it would help her fatigue and weakness enough so that she could be with her friends, then she would not mind having her tonsils removed. Attempting to get her hemoglobin level high enough for surgery, Paula ate iron-rich foods and took a prescribed 325 milligrams of iron two times a day. Improving her hemoglobin consumed her summer. While her friends romped and splashed in community pools, Paula watched remotely, not wanting to expend too much energy. Her tonsils were removed during Christmas break, but her symptoms didn't improve.

On a surgical follow-up examination, Paula wondered how long she would have to take supplemental iron. She asked her doctor, who responded, "How long do you intend to live?"

At thirty-five, Paula began having joint pain, she never seemed to have energy, and her colon was a constant source of trouble. Still, she dutifully responded to the local Red Cross blood center's call for blood donation. She had been a regular blood donor for thirteen years, but elevated liver enzymes prompted a letter from the Red Cross telling her that she could no longer donate blood.

Two years later her joint pain worsened. Paula heard about a physician who knew a great deal about iron; she made her appointment. Her doctor measured her iron levels and because they were high, he explained iron overload to her. Diagnosed with suspect hemochromatosis, Paula knew that the forty-two years of taking iron pills had been slowly poisoning her. Without thirteen years of regularly donating blood, which had kept her tissue iron levels in check, Paula's story would have had a possible lethal outcome. She speculates about the diagnosis of anemia when she was ten. Since hemoglobin can drop slightly when infection is present, Paula wonders whether her constant tonsillitis was the real reason for her lower than normal hemoglobin.

If diagnosed with anemia, request an entire iron panel that includes serum ferritin, TIBC (total iron-binding capacity), and fasting serum iron. Follow up with your physician to identify the underlying cause of inflammation. Never take iron pills until iron-deficiency anemia is confirmed.

The Wrong Treatment

Bob and his son Mark were both tested for genetic hemochromatosis. Bob was a C282Y homozygote; his son Mark had no mutations. Mark's mom Sally asked the IDI patient-information services coordinator how that could happen. The coordinator explained that Mark was an obligate (no other choice) carrier since Bob had two mutations and that Mark should be retested, since errors do occur with genetic tests—unless of course Bob was not the biological father. Sally insisted that he was the father, declined to retest her son, and chose not to be genetically tested herself. She proceeded to get an iron panel for her husband Bob and her son Mark. Bob's serum ferritin was nearly 4,000; his TS percentage was more than 100 percent saturated. The son's ferritin was 60; his saturation percentage was 31 percent. The same gastroenterologist was seeing both Bob and Mark. He started the father on monthly phlebotomies and ordered a liver biopsy for the son. Bob got progressively worse with fatigue, abdominal pain, heart arrhythmia, mood swings, and depression, and he developed diabetes. Mark's liver biopsy came back with mildly elevated iron, and the doctor started weekly phlebotomies. After a few weeks, Sally called in a panic to report that Mark had become so weak that she feared hemo-chromatosis was going to take his life. She reported that her son's hemoglobin had plummeted to 9 g/dL and that he had fainted during his last phlebotomy. With her permission, the IDI faxed a letter to the physician suggesting that he consider Mark sufficiently de-ironed. In the letter, we mentioned that Bob might benefit from a liver biopsy and increased frequency of phlebotomies, possibly to twice a week if he could tolerate it. Bob's liver biopsy confirmed advanced cirrhosis and 4+ iron. Mark's phlebotomies were discontinued.

25

Multiple Symptoms That Can Prompt Diagnosis

Clues: Depression and Mood Swings

Larry had considered suicide; his depression had gotten so bad that he could not function. He slept, missed work, and refused to be social. He screamed at his wife, berating her for minor issues. She was intimidated by her husband's fits of rage; she was extremely stressed because she never knew when an outburst would occur. She loved her husband but felt helpless to make his life better; she admits that she considered divorce. She blamed herself a lot and reasoned, If Larry has been to so many doctors, how could they all be wrong? Every one of them told him that he needed a psychiatrist. She did her best to be tolerant and held on to their history together. Earlier in their marriage, Larry had been a very successful salesman. His father had died of a heart attack when he was fifty-eight; prior to his death, he drank and exhibited many of the characteristics now emerging in Larry.

It was another year before Larry obtained his complete diagnosis. At wit's end, on the brink of taking his life, Larry was persuaded to try one more physician. Larry did not know where to begin, but determined, he looked for a physician who would listen. He was fortunate; he found a persistent, patient, and kind doctor who believed that Larry's problems were not just related to mental health. The physician kept searching until a liver biopsy finally provided enough information to confirm hemochromatosis. Larry's liver biopsy revealed 2+ iron, and fortunately for Larry, there was no cirrhosis. His serum ferritin was slightly less than 1,000 ng/mL, his TS percentage was at 88 percent, and a genetic test revealed that he was homozygous for the C282Y mutation.

During therapeutic phlebotomy, Larry's depression began to fade. "I cannot pinpoint when exactly the depression left; I just remember waking up one day and realized I was happy for the first time in years." Later it was confirmed that he had an under-active thyroid and low testosterone; with hormone replacement Larry's moods became more stable. Larry eventually reached normal iron levels, but he remains faithful to his maintenance schedule of one blood donation every two months.

Clues: Impotence, Joint Pain, and Hair Loss

Lucia, a medical technologist, was particularly tenacious in her struggle to discover the cause of the extreme fatigue and pain that sapped her husband Terry's energy. Persistent pain began to insinuate itself into Terry's life during his late teens, particularly in his joints, sides, and legs. He suffered from fatigue and other vague symptoms. But his family doctor could find nothing wrong.

"Doctors just passed the symptoms off as 'I don't know, but you're young and look healthy enough, so it can't be anything major. We'll run a few blood tests,'" Lucia says.

Everyone thought Terry was a hypochondriac, and without a definitive diagnosis as to the cause of his distress, he began to believe he might be. He stopped seeing a doctor and seldom talked about his chronic pain. Eventually his joints hurt nonstop. A rheumatologist performed routine blood work and found that Terry's liver enzymes were slightly elevated. However, the doctor dismissed the results and gave him a clean bill of health. Terry was a member of a fraternity at a university, and the doctor assumed that the elevated levels were due to heavy beer drinking.

As the pain grew worse, another problem arrived. Terry was having trouble getting and holding an erection. He and Lucia did not think the cause was medical. His father had died suddenly at the age of fifty-five of a pulmonary embolism, and Terry and Lucia were living with his mother to help her deal with his death. Their bedroom was directly above his mother's, so they thought his impotence was due to stress and the awkward location of the bedrooms. But as the year passed, the pain grew worse, the impotency remained, and exhaustion consumed him.

"One night, Terry said to me, 'I'm dying; I feel like I'm dying,'" Lucia says. At the hospital, she arranged to have his blood drawn and asked for every test on the lab-order sheet. She had no idea what to look for or what she would find. She did find that his liver enzymes were slightly elevated again. A hospital pathologist suggested that he might have hepatitis. After all, Terry was a housekeeper at the hospital, and could have been exposed. Although the test for hepatitis came back negative, it provided the first clue to the cause of Terry's constant physical misery. The test showed Terry's iron levels were elevated.

The technician who ran the ferritin test showed it to the laboratory pathologist. The level was so high that the instrument couldn't read it. The blood had to be diluted ten times to get a reading. The value was 3,600 ng/mL—normal is up to 200.

"Our laboratory pathologist came to me and said, 'Your husband is very sick,'" Lucia recalls. "The first thing that occurred to both of us was, 'At last, some answers.' Terry wasn't crazy."

The pathologist made an appointment with a liver specialist. Within a week of the appointment, Terry was undergoing a liver biopsy. "The doctor told us Terry would have died had I not run those tests," Lucia says.

Doctors and technicians conducted X-rays and myriad other tests to discover how much damage had been done to his body. The toll was grim. At twenty-four years old, Terry had liver damage, arthritis, and nonfunctioning adrenal glands. He was bloated and had blue dots on the insides of his legs from ankle to midcalf and dark circles under his eyes. He lacked facial and body hair, and his skin color was gray. But he was alive.

Terry began phlebotomy treatments, but it was two years before his iron levels returned to normal. In the first year after his diagnosis, he was hospitalized four times. He'd often catch colds, which then led to bouts with bronchitis and pneumonia.

Today Terry is tall and handsome. His libido is back, and the gray skin color and circles under his eyes are gone. His adrenal functions are normal, and he has a beard and some body hair. Yet he is in constant pain. He still catches frequent colds, which lead to bronchitis. His arthritis is bad, and he continues to have pain in the liver area. Terry now undergoes phlebotomies about once every two months. He absorbs iron so fast that it is difficult to establish a regular maintenance program.

He's prone to episodes of pulmonary embolisms; he's already experienced two. The first destroyed the lower third of his left lung. "I was told I was extremely lucky that I wasn't dead or at the very least a vegetable," Terry says. The second came five years later in the form of multiple blood clots in the right lung. Doctors don't know whether the embolisms are related to his iron disorder, and Terry must take blood-thinning drugs for the rest of his life.

Lucia works in the blood-bank laboratory at the hospital and tries to educate patients about iron disorders, particularly HHC. She is angered when she hears of cases of high iron test results that doctors don't take seriously. She firmly believes that people need to assume responsibility for researching the cause of their sicknesses if a diagnosis eludes doctors. And they should not be bashful about demanding tests if their symptoms point to a possible cause.

Clues: Diabetes, Heart Trouble, and Liver Damage

John straddled the snowmobile. The engine hummed, drowning out noises around him. Bending over, he scooped up a handful of snow, which he promptly ate. His thirst seemed insatiable; no matter how much water he drank, he could not overcome the persistent need for more water. Trips to the bathroom were now an around-the-clock occurrence. As snow melted in his mouth, John was unaware of a fellow snowmobiler barreling toward him from behind. "I vaguely remember the collision," says John. "Mostly I recall being airborne and a terrific pain in one leg, and my gut."

After a painful five-mile-per-hour jostling ride on a handmade pine-branch gurney, John was delivered to the emergency room, carried by friends who had seen the accident. Broken bones were of less concern to the emergency room doctor, who suspected internal bleeding. John was rushed to the operating room where the surgeon confirmed a ruptured spleen and noted cirrhosis, as well as a pendulant tumor. "I was conscious when a nurse shouted that my blood glucose was in the 600s, but I passed out at that point," recalls John.

John learned later that he had flatlined. "I'm only forty-one!" John remembers thinking when told the account of his near-death experience. Later in his hospital room, John woke to see his wife, Kay, and his two daughters crying. "I'm fine," John told them, but they cried even harder. John learned later from Kay, a registered nurse and director of hospice, that she had overheard a conversation in the cafeteria that "the McGruder biopsy was likely liver cancer; he's probably a heavy drinker." Kay was shocked at their casualness; she knew John was not a drinker. Kay continued her story: earlier, while John was on the operating table, one of the surgeons stepped out to ask her how much John drank. "Nothing," she had replied. "He is not a drinker." Kay felt that the physician didn't believe her. John eventually received his diagnosis of hemochromatosis because of the liver biopsy.

26

You Must Be a Drinker

"Are you a drinker?" is frequently a question that physicians ask hemochromatosis patients, especially during the process of diagnosis. Reactions from patients can range from strong denial to embarrassment, shame, or regret—if drinking was part of their lifestyle. Feelings of being judged or punished often filter into the mix of emotions that follow such a question.

Undiagnosed hemochromatosis patients often present with elevated liver enzymes, and some may have cirrhosis or fatty livers. These signs can prompt a physician to suspect alcohol abuse, especially when a doctor is unfamiliar with hemochromatosis.

"One of the saddest examples of this type of misunderstanding that I can recall is the story of Vester," begins Chris Kieffer, a founding director of IDI. "Vester regularly attended a hemochromatosis support group that I held in my home. At each meeting he talked about his many symptoms. His family history was filled with early deaths; all sounded suspiciously like hemochromatosis. The father and one brother died prematurely of cirrhosis; another brother died of heart failure. None of them drank, but all of them were so accused and told to stop drinking if they wanted to get well."

Chris continued: "I encouraged Vester to get his iron levels tested, which he tried to do. He went to five different doctors all of whom accused him of being an alcoholic—mostly because he had elevated liver enzymes and the family history of cirrhosis. I knew this man; he was not a drinker, not even socially. Concerned, I accompanied him to a local doctor who agreed to run the iron tests. Vester's iron was elevated, although not terribly high, but enough to start phlebotomies. Once the iron levels came down, Vester began to improve. Because he felt better, we all thought that he was going to be OK. But this doctor retired and the one who took his place did not see any benefit to Vester's phlebotomies. In time, Vester began to get sick again and go downhill rapidly."

Chris was able to find a doctor in Atlanta who knew about excess iron and cirrhosis. This doctor performed a liver biopsy on Vester and immediately diagnosed nonalcoholic steato-hepatitis (NASH), or nonalcoholic fatty liver disease. His iron level had climbed and his cirrhosis was so advanced that Vester needed a liver transplant, which he got—and he survived. Years later, three other members of this family were diagnosed with hemochromatosis; two of them also had NASH.

The leading NASH expert, Herbert Bonkovsky, MD, says: "Today, we know that excess iron in combination with a fatty liver increases the risk for cirrhosis. These patients can be wrongly accused of alcohol abuse, but there are questions and tests that clinicians can use to confirm suspicions."

"Vester eventually got help and is today doing very well, but what makes his story sad are the deaths," remarked Chris. "Two precious brothers died with family members and friends thinking that they were 'secret drinkers.' Someone else died because the liver that could have gone to them went to Vester. If his iron levels had been addressed early and managed better, he may not have needed a new liver."

27

Lost Opportunity: Elevated Serum Iron

After five physicians and ten years of trying to get a diagnosis, the suspense was unnerving. The sixth doctor would finally connect the dots. He glanced down at the lab results and looked up at his forty-year-old patient, Cliff, who was hopeful that this time he would hear something promising. This physician had been recommended by one of Cliff's friends, a nurse.

"You have a disease that is potentially fatal, if not caught in time," the doctor informed Cliff. The words had not had time to sink in before the doctor continued: "And we caught it in time. You have hemochromatosis, an inherited disorder of iron metabolism."

Cliff asked for more information. "Your body absorbs more iron than people with normal iron metabolism. It's very treatable," his doctor explained. According to Cliff, The doctor 'caught it in time' because, at the time, iron was part of many blood chemistry panels. Cliff's elevated iron prompted the doctor to suspect and further test for hemochromatosis. The doctor was familiar with hemochromatosis and suspicious of Cliff's vague, seemingly unrelated symptoms of joint pain, stomach problems, and elevated liver enzymes. When he ordered an executive blood panel for Cliff, his serum iron jumped out as abnormally high. He knew which tests to do next, fasting serum iron, total iron-binding capacity (TIBC), and serum ferritin.

Cliff told his physician that over the years, his mildly elevated liver enzymes had been referred to as perhaps some type of low-grade or chronic hepatitis. "Based upon these findings, one doctor suggested I cut back on alcoholic beverages," Cliff continued. "I like a glass of wine with dinner now and then, but I certainly would not consider myself a drinker."

Cliff's joint pain was diagnosed as arthritis. He was given a prescription pain reliever. The doctor told him that his bursitis was due to "too many bumps and bruises from an active lifestyle." Cliff loved being near the water, snow skiing, cross-country motorcycling, surfing, tennis, touch football—and he had been in two automobile wrecks. Again, the doctor said that his pain reliever should help.

Cliff was told that his stomach problems were most likely stress related; his job as a criminal prosecutor involved high-profile work that was often nerve-racking. The doctor prescribed Tagamet antacid, which did not work.

This physician was different: he listened attentively as Cliff continued the saga that led him to the present. "One doctor thought I had some illusive cancer. Another doctor noticed what appeared to be my year-round tan, except that I had no tan lines."

Cliff's TS percentage and ferritin were elevated, though Cliff only recalls that his ferritin was near 2,000 ng/mL. A scan of his liver helped confirm the HHC diagnosis. "No one considered my many ailments as symptoms of a single disease," Cliff adds. Therapeutic phlebotomies were ordered. Cliff went twice weekly at first, then once weekly. He reports that "the therapy has virtually eliminated" his symptoms.

This physician's proper diagnosis of Cliff led to the diagnosis of Cliff's younger thirty-five-year-old brother Chris, who, as it turns out, had a much more advanced case of hemochromatosis. Chris lived in the country, where he drank iron-rich water and cooked in iron skillets. He, too, had complained of symptoms similar to those of his older brother Cliff, but he never gave it thought there might be an inherited link. Chris's ferritin was 9,000 ng/mL when first tested. He was seen and treated by a different doctor than Cliff was.

At first, Cliff's insurance would not pay for the phlebotomies, even though the cost was minimal. Cliff concludes, "Thanks to the right factors being in place and coming to the attention of the right doctor, my family has been spared the tragedy of two brothers losing the battle to a potentially fatal disease. This is a battle that is needlessly being lost by others."

28

Ignoring the Doctor

Tug spotted his medical chart; it was within reach. He grabbed the folder, returned to his seat, propped his right foot on his left knee, dropped the folder on his crossed leg, and flipped open the file. His rationale was, "I pay the doctor to make these files. I'm entitled to see what's in them." The receptionist for the Parkway Family Practice glanced at Tug and smiled. She noticed he had picked up his chart.

He scanned down through several unfamiliar words. Some words were too large to venture attempted pronunciation, but one popped out at him. It was ferritin.

"Woooowheeee!" was Tug's response to the numbers beside the word *ferritin*.

His doctor came into the reception area in time to hear Tug's remark. He motioned for Tug to follow him to his office. "Your ferritin is 6,895; that's about 200 times more than normal. You have an iron saturation of 96 percent. Tug, you really should have had that liver biopsy," he concluded.

"I suppose you're right, Doc. I should have kept that appointment last year when you sent me to the gastroenterologist," Tug confessed. "I'm ready now."

This had not been Tug's first visit to the Parkway Family Practice physician. One year earlier he had asked his primary care physician if there was anything that could be done about his aching joints. Prior to seeing this doctor, Tug had suffered for more than fifteen years with painful joints. He had been to the Asheville Hand Center, since most of his pain was in the first two fingers of his hands. They had given him a prescription for pain medication, which Tug never filled. He took over-the-counter medications for pain, finally settling on Aleve. It worked to dull the pain, but nothing really made the searing ache go away entirely. Tug decided that the ache would become his constant, though annoying, companion.

An early morning phone call from his primary care physician was a delightful surprise for Tug. "What in the world are you doing calling people at six-thirty in the morning?" he asked his doctor. "You need to come in right away; today if possible," was the doctor's response. Tug complied.

The doctor told Tug that his iron levels were elevated and that he suspected hemochromatosis. He explained that hémochromatosis has as consequences joint pain, diabetes, liver disease, and heart trouble. He went on to tell Tug that this was out of his field and that a liver biopsy was needed to confirm diagnosis. Tug winced, but he trusted his doctor.

"Besides being a caring doctor, he is a gentleman, and an all-round good and kind man. If he says I need a liver biopsy, then I need one," said Tug.

The first available appointment with the gastroenterologist was not for four months; Tug confirmed the time slot. He turned to his wife, Barbara, who was five months pregnant, and remarked, "My appointment is right at the time of your due date." An interesting observation, since their son John Tyler decided to be born the same day as Tug's appointment with the gastroenterologist.

"I forgot everything!" Tug laughs. "Things were nuts; I didn't remember the appointment till weeks later. Then I just decided that high iron, so what? At least it isn't cancer. I actually thought it would just go away, like some disappearing act or something."

Tug's disregard for his iron levels allowed the metal to accumulate and add to his troubles. Excessive thirst and frequent trips to the bathroom at all hours of the day and night were also ignored. Tug was, however, scheduled to see a chiropractor, who checked his blood sugar levels. "My levels were sky-rocket high!" remembers Tug. The chiropractor advised Tug to get to his primary care doctor immediately. Hence the follow-up trip to Parkway Family Practice and the decision to keep the next appointment with the gastroenterologist.

Liver biopsy confirmed Tug's doctor's year-old suspicion. Therapeutic phlebotomy was started immediately on an initial schedule of once a week. This wasn't aggressive enough; Tug's levels were not moving, and he asked for more frequent extraction. The gastroenterologist was hesitant to step up the frequency and told Tug so.

Tug decided to get serious about this thing called hemochromatosis. He began to search for information. Among some of literature he found was Iron Disorders Institute's magazine and booklet describing therapy. "I read how the iron is pulled from ferritin to make new red blood cells. The IDI materials really inspired me to have another talk with my gastro man," Tug commented.

After convincing the gastroenterologist that he could tolerate more frequent phlebotomy, his extraction schedule was increased to twice a week. Tug tells his experience with treatment. "My hemoglobin was checked before each blood draw. It was always 14.5 or 15. No other tests were done until I nearly collapsed in the doc's office one day. My hemoglobin was still normal but my ferritin was only 9. When I reread the IDI materials I figured out I had been overbled. Believe me, it was no picnic. I learned the true meaning of being tired. I was weak as a newborn kitten."

Between the physician and his straight-talking, take-charge patient Tug, they agreed—no phlebotomy for a couple of months. Two months later, Tug was feeling somewhat better. His hemoglobin was back up to 14.7. He continues his phlebotomy treatments monthly at Mission St. Joseph Hospital Outpatient Treatment Center in Asheville, North Carolina, where he describes the service as outstanding. Tug believes that he feels better when his ferritin is in a range of 25 to 30, and he will work for iron balance now that he is on the home stretch.

Tug says he has learned several things with this experience. When asked what he might say to help someone who might have hemochromatosis, he advises, "Don't wait like I did; if your doctor suspects this, get on it, and stay with it!"

29

Ignoring Diagnosed Family Members

Grant was fifty-three when he got his diagnosis; he had been genetically tested and was homozygous for C282Y. His serum ferritin was 630 ng/mL and his TS percentage was 78 percent. He was relieved to get his diagnosis because he had suffered with terrible fatigue and joint pain for a while. After learning that his condition was inherited, he first went to the Internet to read what he could about the condition. He got worried when he read that hemochromatosis could be fatal. The more he read, the more concerned he got for his two brothers and sister. He called his sister first; she listened but did not sound convinced. He wanted to call his brothers, but unfortunately he did not get along well with either one, and he wasn't sure just how to go about letting them know that they might also have this condition. Their father had died at fifty-eight of heart failure, and Grant wondered whether this cause of death could have been hemochromatosis. The more he read, the more concerned he became. His concern made him very outspoken, something that was not appreciated by his siblings. He begged his mother for help, but she declined. (Later it was learned that his mother felt shame for having given her children a potentially deadly disease.) Grant kept trying. He called his sister, who told him that she had talked with her doctor and had been told that women don't get hemochromatosis. This frustrated Grant even more because he knew that his sister had gone through menopause and so her risk of loading iron was increased. Grant wrote letters and sent cards and e-mail but his brothers refused to pursue help. At a holiday gathering, Grant gave it one more try. His two brothers grew angry and walked away. For six more years, Grant tried to get his siblings to get tested. By now, one brother was experiencing heart arrhythmia, his sister was diagnosed with hypothyroidism, and the other brother was impotent. Even still, none of Grants siblings would pursue testing to see whether they had hemochromatosis.

30

One Woman's Legacy

Jim is one of the oldest known surviving hemochromatosis patients in the United States with no hemochromatosis-related health problems. Jim was diagnosed early, received appropriate treatment, and equipped himself to live in good health by staying informed. His sister Anna Marie died at twenty-eight; the final autopsy report listed hemochromatosis as the cause of death. The details of her autopsy were extensive; excessive iron deposits were found in her heart, liver, bile duct, skin, pancreas, spleen, intestinal tract, kidneys, lymph nodes, adrenals, and thyroid. It was also noted that Anna Marie had a history of amenorrhea (no menstruation). Her death resulted in the diagnosis for Jim and one other sister. Jim was in the navy at the time. Late in December 1978, he reported to "sick call" at the U.S. Naval Hospital in Orlando to request blood tests to determine his iron levels.

"Initially, the doctor felt my request was unwarranted, as I did not have any 'overt manifestations.' 'Your skin doesn't have a yellow cast to it,' he said after examining the front and back of my hands. Furthermore, the navy was experiencing an austere budget, and he felt he wasn't able to justify ordering expensive blood tests. Obviously, he needed more evidence, so I suggested he review my sister's autopsy report. Skeptical, he did order the appropriate blood tests."

The doctor immediately ordered a liver biopsy, along with several other tests. In 1979, a liver biopsy was considered the gold-standard measurement for a positive diagnosis of hemochromatosis. Jim's liver biopsy was performed in January 1979.

The pathology report confirmed the clinical diagnosis. "Excessive deposits of hepatocellular iron, consistent with hemochromatosis. No evidence of tumor, cirrhosis or granuloma."

"In early February, I began an aggressive de-ironing program lasting for twenty-one months. At first, my phlebotomies were conducted weekly; later they were reduced to biweekly visits. My doctor's—Lieutenant David Schneider, Medical Corps, U.S. Navy—stated goal was to remove the excess iron as rapidly as possible without causing anemia. He primarily used hemoglobin (Hgb) and hematocrit (Hct) as his guide in avoiding anemia since a blood test for serum ferritin was not available at the time.

"My phlebotomist, a navy corpsman, was excellent at inserting that monstrous 16-gauge needle into my arms! He introduced me to using a blood-pressure cuff rather than the standard narrow tourniquet, which allowed me to control the pressure during the phlebotomy and keep my fingers from becoming excessively numb and tingling. He also suggested that I take an aspirin the night before to help alleviate clotting in the needle. I continue to use both of his suggestions to this day, which have made my lifelong therapy more bearable.

"After retiring from the U.S. Navy on May 1, 1979, my family moved from Florida to Massachusetts in October. By this time, I had accepted without reservation that therapeutic phlebotomies would become an integral part of my life. I first realized the importance of maintaining good records of my medical treatment when I contacted the nearest VA hospital for treatment. I was immediately asked for a copy of my liver biopsy result. I'm glad I had my records, or I might have had to endure the unnecessary risks of another biopsy. Thereafter, I have kept a database of blood tests and phlebotomies, including penetration sites and extraction volume related to my treatment of hemochromatosis.

"Several years later, I recognized that although Anna Marie's death was akin to one door closing, I had not appreciated enough the fact that my children, and their children, were also impacted by hemochromatosis. I knew it, but at the same time I didn't know it. If it hadn't been for the discovery of the hemochromatosis gene in the mid-nineties, I may have failed to see that a new door of opportunity had opened. Now I could, at the very least, identify which of my children and also their children will potentially be affected. Here was a real opportunity to educate my family. I, along with my sister, Irene, could be the prime example that iron education and treatment would be the key to a healthy future free from iron-related disease for generations to come.

"Thus, I embarked on a personal quest to have all my children and their children identified as to the possibility of experiencing iron overload. Genetic testing and establishing baseline values would be the first step, and the cheek-swab method appeared to be the simplest. My results merely confirmed my diagnosis: a double mutation of C282Y gene. I did not have my children tested once my wife's results were normal for the C282Y and H63D genes. Their heterozygosity was a genetic certainty.

"Anna Marie's death also reminds us that it is our responsibility to continuously pass this knowledge on to future generations and to inspire to them to continue to do the same. This is her legacy."

Besides his community volunteer work teaching people how to use the computer, Jim continues to be a devoted volunteer helping to raise awareness about hemochromatosis. He makes regular financial contributions to any organization showing promise of getting the word out. During the years following his diagnosis, he has influenced thousands of patients and doctors to stay informed and to follow the Iron Disorders Institute guidelines for diagnosis and management of hemochromatosis. Anna Marie's complete story is told in the April 2001 issue of IDI's newsletter, which Jim undertook and wrote for more than four years as the Rusty Curmudgeon.

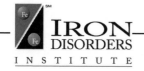

PART FIVE

Hemochromatosis: How It Was, How It Is, How It Must Be

31

How It Was

Before the discovery of the HFE gene, most health agencies and healthcare providers believed hemochromatosis to be rare, an older man's disease. Women were not believed to be at risk. Patients were often dismissed as hysterical, fanatical, or with mental health problems. During this time hemochromatosis was often diagnosed at autopsy; sparing surviving siblings in some cases. This chapter is about that past; it is important to share these stories to remind us and ensure that no one has to suffer or die prematurely because of hemochromatosis. For each of these families, a positive influence emerges that changes future events permanently.

Unnecessary Death

Rhonda Forman

Dolores and Rob Forman shared this story. "Hemochromatosis has claimed the health and lives of too many loved ones. Our beautiful daughter, Rhonda, would be celebrating life right now and possibly be married and have children. Instead, she died March 5, 1984, and was diagnosed at autopsy with hemochromatosis.

"Her death certificate reads 'congestive heart failure due to hemochromatosis.' Rhonda's autopsy report includes hemochromatosis involving heart, liver, cirrhoses, pancreas, spleen, kidneys, adrenal glands, salivary glands, thyroid glands, stomach and duodenum, lymph nodes, and brain.

"Seven years of elevated iron tests provided only one diagnosis: amenorrhea. How was Rhonda's proper diagnosis of hemochromatosis missed? All the experts in the world who saw her were not aware that amenorrhea is an important clue. If any one of these physicians had known this, our daughter may have been diagnosed. Instead, she was told to lose weight for her symptoms to improve.

"Rhonda gave so much in her twenty-three years; but she lives on in a way. As a result of her unnecessary death and this most sobering autopsy report, which cannot be denied, Rhonda will continue to help save many lives. We share this with you in the hope one of those lives might be yours, or that of someone you love as much as we love our Rhonda. She is missed by many."

Charlie Herr and Christopher Main

Medical books lay open on the table of Charlie Herr's hospital room; the pages on hemochromatosis were earmarked. Most of the medical staff had never seen this diagnosis on a chart. Many had never heard of it. Charlie's condition remained critical and then deteriorated. After fourteen days, the decision was made to take him off life support. He passed away peacefully with his family all around him. Hemochromatosis manifested itself in Charlie as arthritis, bronzed skin, and heart disease. He was twenty-three when he died.

"Dad donated blood regularly. Sometimes he was called in the middle of the night to give when O negative was in short supply because of an emergency where someone had been in an accident. We realize now that blood donations all those years acted as phlebotomy," notes Laura, one of Mr. Herr's six children. She continues, "Just before Dad's death, we learned from the doctor who diagnosed him, Dr. Michael Novena, that hemochromatosis (HHC) is hereditary. One person in eight can carry a single mutation of the HFE gene, and one in two hundred can carry a double mutation of the HFE gene. We believe Dad had a double mutation. Of the six children, five girls and one boy, some of us were tested immediately, including our mom. She and I tested positive for a single mutation; making us carriers. My brother Chip and sisters Missie, Debbie, Gretchen, and Marcie all were tested. Chip has both mutations; all the rest of us are carriers."

Since Laura was a carrier and knowing that hers sons might be at risk, her husband, Dick, was tested and found to be a carrier as well. Both sons were then tested and found to be homozygotes. Dick and Laura realized at that moment the vastness of HHC. Although they may never manifest symptoms or load iron to excess, their two sons, Chris (age twenty-three) and Matt (age twenty-one), inherited one mutation from each parent, placing them in the highest risk category for iron-overload disease. Chris and Matt both developed symptoms; both loaded iron.

"We learned about hemochromatosis any way we could; our local physicians wanted to help, but they didn't have much information about HHC. The most help came from Dr. Margit Krikker of the Hemochromatosis Foundation and the Iron Disorders Institute. Dr. Krikker helped us to locate doctors, and IDI supplied us with excellent educational materials about hemochromatosis. Prior to what we received from IDI there were no credible written materials, only photocopied and poorly done folded papers asking for donations.

"Matters were complicated for our sons because they lived out of state, one at college and the other working out west. Chris and Matt had difficulty finding physicians who understood hemochromatosis. One hematologist told Matt, 'Hemochromatosis is an older man's disease and should be of no concern to you now. Watch your diet and alcohol consumption and come back in six months to a year.' At that time, Matt's ferritin was 175 and his TS percentage was 63. The hematologist made no mention of the need for phlebotomies or further testing.

"Chris's was a different story. He was living in Denver, working at Columbine JDS, a computer software company servicing radio and TV stations throughout the world. Like most of his peers with careers foremost on their minds, health concerns were secondary, especially since Chris felt good. I thought back to when Chris was five. He had been experiencing heart symptoms that baffled his doctors. The odd symptoms followed him into adulthood and were rechecked periodically, but nothing conclusive was determined. Like Dad, who assumed that his arthritis was age related, the symptoms Chris credited to his being on the go were probably attributable to the insidious HHC damage under way.

"Chris realized the importance of getting treatment and did so. Initially, he required weekly phlebotomy. As his high iron count decreased, the intervals between blood draws stretched to a month with a level check at that time. The goal was to reach and maintain good levels and eventually stretch the treatments to every three months. A new evaluation would determine the frequency of phlebotomies required for the rest of his life."

Chris discovered that arranging for phlebotomies proved difficult for a traveler. Often clinics require detailed prescriptions for the draw, and the documentation is not standard everywhere. In some places there is a hefty fee for blood disposal, and in others, the service is free. "Thank you! Red Cross of Columbus, Ohio," interjects Laura. Chris always tried to arrange for his phlebotomy when he was at home.

Every Sunday night Laura and Dick knew that they could count on a call from Chris. This became an established habit and an opportunity for father, mother, and son to keep current with one another's lives. On learning that Chris was going to begin international travel, Laura reminded her son about updating his immunizations and flu shot and told him that in addition to his hepatitis A, he needed to get the hepatitis B series as well. Laura had learned through both Dr. Sharon McDonnell at the CDC and the Ohio State University travel medicine department that those series were critical.

Shortly before the city of Hong Kong was to be returned to the jurisdiction of the People's Republic of China, Chris accepted his first overseas assignment to Hong Kong. He was thrilled to have such an opportunity and to travel to a place where he could witness firsthand this historic occasion. Sunday evening after a tour on the mainland, he called home, excited about what he had seen.

But on Monday, Chris began to feel ill. He had been served a questionable meal on the tour. He wondered about contaminated food. His symptoms continued, so he called a doctor but could not get an appointment until Friday. In the meantime he drank lots of fluids (including orange juice from room service) and took ibuprofen for pain relief. He went to work each day. By midweek, the symptoms began to subside and he felt a little better, but he kept the appointment on Friday. When he saw the doctor, Chris didn't think to tell him that he had hemochromatosis. He only told the doctor that he had eaten something he thought might be contaminated and had gastrointestinal symptoms as a result, but by Wednesday he felt better. The doctor prescribed antibiotics and acetaminophen and said if he had any more problems to call back.

That night Chris called home and left a message on the recorder, "Mom, call me. I'm sick. I'll be in my room. Call back any time." Laura was the only one home when she heard the message. She immediately called Chris's room at the hotel. Someone picked up the phone, but there was only silence followed by a dial tone.

"I called back two more times. There was no answer. I called the hotel desk and after considerable pleading, persuaded the night manager to go into Chris's room to check on him. I asked him to call me right back. I waited, all the while knowing something was terribly wrong. The phone call came. The manager, Andy, told me as gently as he could, to sit down and breathe. He then told me that Chris was dead, that the police were in his room, and that I would have to call back on Monday."

Stunned and in disbelief, Laura called her husband. The entire event was surreal, as though they were participants in someone else's tragedy. The next two weeks were somewhat a blur for Dick and Laura Main as they went numbly through the motions of trying to get through each day. Complicated arrangements began with long-distance phone calls until the Mains could get to Hong Kong to claim the body of their son.

When Laura's father, Charlie, died, Dick was grief stricken. He loved Charlie and spoke of his death as "a great loss to [him], as he was the glue that held the whole group together. He was the one who quietly made things work on a day-to-day basis. He fixed stuff! He loved his grandchildren and all his accumulated sons and daughters-in-law. Even though he was color blind, he could still sell clothes in a men's clothing department. His loss just left a big hole in my life. I was able to move on, however, knowing that in time we all lose our parents in the natural order of things. Which is why I was dumbfounded, unable to comprehend the death of my son. It is not the natural order of things. It is an event any loving parent fears most but may not vocalize."

Dick continued: "As a dentist, I feel like I have a fairly professional look at diseases and disorders compared to a nonmedical person. So, in spite of the fact that complications of hemochromatosis have taken two people from my life, I am still able to look at the disorder in a fairly clinical way.

"Initially, we really didn't have the proper information to have our sons treated adequately; doctors just were not aware. It really makes Laura mad, but I understand that the medical community can't keep up with all the developments in every field. I tried to act strong; after all, I'm the father, husband, man of the family. But soon feelings of disbelief changed to a profound emptiness. I feel as if a part of me has been ripped out and a permanent void remains. I miss Chris every single day. I feel like a vital piece of my future has been stolen. I still find myself waiting for his regular Sunday-evening phone call. I don't blame anyone or hemochromatosis for the loss of my son. I just don't think that way. What I do know is that my relationship with my family has suffered. I'm no longer the positive force in their lives. Physically, I'm a mess. Weight gain, lack of exercise, loss of sex drive, and inability to sleep are problems I just can't seem to face and defeat.

"The only thing that I think will heal my open wounds is to stay away from reliving the dreaded events over and over. It just hurts too much to tell and relive the story. I guess I'm looking for distance and time to heal the hurt. I know that my life must go on, and I know that these events can never go away. I want to become me again, but that is impossible. The 'me' I want to be includes being a father to both my sons."

Matt is doing fine at this time. He misses his brother terribly; Chris was his best friend. Matt has many questions about hemochromatosis, and his brother's death is still, for him, unexplained.

Chip Herr, Laura's brother and Chris's uncle, remarks, "When I think of Chris today, how he died, so far from home, I'm filled with overwhelming remorse and anger. If I could just say to people, 'Above all else talk to your family physician about getting tested for HHC. If your doctor looks at you with a blank face, educate him or her! And if the physician is reluctant, force the issue! If that doesn't get results, it's time to look for a new doctor! The test to detect hemochromatosis is just too simple and inexpensive when you consider it might save a life." Chip also has hemochromatosis.

Laura Main is on the board of directors of the Iron Disorders Institute. Her sister Missie Kendall is a frequent volunteer for IDI events and programs. Laura speaks to groups every chance she can to convey the importance of awareness of hemochromatosis. In Ohio, her efforts have resulted in hemochromatosis being taught as part of the curriculum at Ohio State University, to a large population-based screening program where hundreds of people have been diagnosed with abnormal iron levels, and bringing two new board members to IDI: Mark Wurster, MD, to the Medical and Scientific Advisory Board, and Chad Bortle to the board of directors. It was Laura's level of knowledge and life experiences that resulted in Chad Bortle's hemochromatosis diagnosis.

Irene de Sterke: Mother, Wife, and Friend

Irene de Sterke shook her head vigorously, indicating she did not want to have a liver biopsy. Nearly twenty years of being examined, poked, prodded, and cut into without resolve had tarnished her faith in doctors. Liver biopsy seemed just one more unnecessary and invasive procedure. Irene had learned to live with constant chronic fatigue and pain in her fingers, feet, and knees. After seven major operations to correct ulcerative colitis plus hip replacement surgery, her prolonged illness had left her weary.

Beginning in the mid-1970s, Irene visited her family doctor because of joint pain and incapacitating fatigue. Her husband and children had been concerned about her constant state of tiredness and terrible arthritic pain. When visits to the doctor became a routine event and countless numbers of physicians were unable to get her well, her family began to consider her case hopeless. They wondered whether she might be exaggerating her symptoms—maybe the terrible pain she tried to describe was the consequence of something psychological. How could the family possibly know the life of Irene, wife and mother, was in danger? Irene, in fact, was not imagining her pain or fatigue. These symptoms were signals from her body that she was slowly and insidiously being poisoned to death.

Irene de Sterke's health continued to decline. "She became overwhelmed with the pain and fatigue," remembers her son Philip. "Family gatherings were tense. We hated seeing her suffering; it made us feel helpless and cruel for not knowing what was causing her health to be so poor. My sister, Dad, and I tried to comfort her, but we were not the ones experiencing the pain except superficially as bystanders and observers of her agony. We all wanted answers."

Exasperated, Irene finally was referred to a rheumatologist in a major hospital. "This doctor suspected my mother had hemochromatosis," Philip recalls. "But he was not going to treat her without confirmation by liver biopsy." At the time his mother refused to have the biopsy, her ferritin was 6,020 and her TS percentage was 97 percent. Irene was persistent in her denial of the procedure. Remarkably, her doctor declined to treat her unless she agreed to the biopsy.

Frustrated, scared, and angry, Philip wanted a better understanding of this rare condition called hemochromatosis and why his mother's doctor felt a liver biopsy was imperative for diagnosis. Enrolled as a student at the University of Amsterdam, Philip had access to and knowledge about how to search the library and publications. "I found little information about this 'rare' disease," he remembers. "But from the information I was able to find, I could tell that the biopsy would not be necessary to make the diagnosis and I told this to her doctor. He still refused to treat her without the procedure."

Knowing that his mother needed treatment, Philip persuaded her to have the liver biopsy. "I felt like I was taking sides with the doctor against my own mother. She was fearful of the procedure, knowing what it involved. I knew that without the liver biopsy she was not going to get treated. Here in the Dutch Netherlands nearly 99 percent of the population is covered by national insurance. Guidelines are very strict and physicians have to follow them closely to assure the same standard of care for everyone."

Results of Irene's liver biopsy were not surprising to Philip, who by now had read extensively about iron. Her liver was loaded; she had a 4+ iron content. This was exactly what her physician wanted, so that he could confirm his suspicion of hemochromatosis. Therapeutic phlebotomies were started, but because Irene had small veins, the large needles used in standard phlebotomy did not work. In the hospital where she was receiving treatment, some doctors were experimenting with an iron chelator called deferiprone, also known as DMHP or L1.

Chelators such as deferoxamine (brand name: Desferal) can be given intravenously for the purpose of removing iron from patients who have complications such as anemia and iron overload at the same time. Desferal is a chelator that can bind with iron in the bloodstream. Bound iron is then excreted from the body in urine. Deferiprone is a different chelator. It is less efficient than deferoxamine, but it has an advantage in that it can be taken orally.

"As the only alternative to phlebotomy, these doctors decided to give my mother this experimental drug. One and a half years later she died due to hemochromatosis. I could have sued the doctors, but I chose not to. I decided to help educate them instead," Philip continues.

The chelator deferiprone/DMHP/L1 has been approved for use by humans in the European market under the product name of Ferroprox. Several scientists, including Dr. Nancy Olivieri of Toronto's Hospital for Sick Children, have called into question the effectiveness of this drug. During human clinical trials using L1, Dr. Olivieri noted that her patients were demonstrating an increased incidence of cirrhosis and that death due to liver failure in patients being given deferiprone was higher than in controls.

"Knowing what I know today, I realize there were a number of choices other than chelation therapy that could have been offered to my mother. She could have had a chest port. A chest port involves the surgical implantation of a device through which blood can be removed or medicines administered. Used primarily by doctors for AIDS and cancer patients, it would have allowed doctors to de-iron her without concern for access to her veins. Mother certainly was a candidate for this procedure because of her extremely high levels of iron and inaccessible veins.

"She also could have had frequent extractions using a small-gauge needle like the butterfly needles used for children and the elderly. Removal of blood twice or even three times a week using this method would have de-ironed her and she might well be alive this minute."

"Also," Philip adds, "she never needed that liver biopsy; I have read about quantitative phlebotomy. Mom could have been diagnosed in this way."

One year after the death of his mother, Philip began to have his own experience with chronic fatigue. "Because of my mother's ordeal, I knew the right tests to ask for," Philip remarks. "My saturation percentage was 60 percent, but my ferritin was only 250, just slightly increased. I was suspicious that these slightly elevated iron levels could be causing my symptoms, but I too met with skepticism from my doctors. I got tested genetically, thinking this would give me the proof that my iron levels were significant. But as it turns out I am a just a carrier, a C282Y heterozygote.

"Still, my iron levels seemed significant to me. Maybe there were other mutations that contribute to iron-loading conditions. I wanted to know if my theory was correct. One thing for certain, regardless of what I might theorize, I knew I was going to have to convince my doctor much the same way I tried to do so for my mom."

Philip began his search for expert proof on the Internet. He remarks, "Not much was available on the subject, and further, what I was able to find was not always correct. I started to contact hemochromatosis patient advocacy groups around the world for advice. I read everything I could find. Some of the best print materials came from the Iron Disorders Institute. However, I wanted to talk face-to-face with an expert, and since I lived half a continent away from the United States, I continued to look for an expert close to home. Eventually my efforts paid off and led me to a professor, Dr. J. Marx, who specializes in hemochromatosis. Since he lived only twenty miles from me and had an interest in iron loading among HFE heterozygotes,

I consulted him. He did some extra tests, and then he agreed with me that some phlebotomies were the best strategy. The results were not major, but I was very happy that the excess iron was removed.

"I didn't know enough about hemochromatosis in time to save my mother, but I was determined to help others before they died like she did," Philip concludes.

Following the death of his mom, Philip de Sterke began an exhaustive and comprehensive search of the Internet and established a website with links to any possible information that might be helpful to people trying to learn about HHC. He went on to found Hemochromatose Vereniging Nederland, with a mission to raise awareness among physicians and government agents about hemochromatosis. You can access the Netherlands Hemochromatosis Society website by visiting www.irondisorders.org.

Philip closes by saying, "It is a mistake not to take the carrier status seriously. Dr. B. de Valk wrote a very good thesis on C282Y carriers and the risk of heart disease. I recommend everyone read it."

Sam Martin: Poet, Brother, Husband, and Son

Sam Martin was thirty-two when he died unexpectedly on December 31, 1998, from congestive heart failure caused by undiagnosed hemochromatosis.

After a six-day illness characterized by shortness of breath, lack of appetite, fatigue, and low blood pressure, Sam went to his family doctor on December 28. The doctor diagnosed a severe lung and ear infection and sent him home with antibiotics. Early on the morning of Wednesday, December 30, Sam agreed to let his family take him to the hospital.

Emergency room staff at St. Joseph Health Center discovered that Sam had congestive heart failure and an acute diabetic condition. He was transferred to the intensive care unit. Doctors were not sure of the cause of his illness but told family that they thought a massive infection was the most probable. Doctors told Sam's parents and wife late Wednesday morning that he might not survive, and the crisis escalated as more of his vital organs failed. A balloon pump was installed to keep his heart going. He was put on a ventilator and was heavily sedated.

On Thursday, one crisis followed another. Measures that helped one problem worsened others. After Sam's team of doctors discovered that his liver was failing, they began to suspect the hereditary metabolic disorder hemochromatosis. But a definitive diagnosis was not possible at that time; DNA tests would take twenty-four hours and Sam was too unstable for a liver biopsy. After a code blue on Thursday evening he was in a coma. Kidney dialysis worsened his heart failure. Sam died at 11:30 p.m., surrounded by his family. Days later, after a focused autopsy, doctors confirmed that Sam had hereditary hemochromatosis.

Following Sam's death it was found that his father and sister are carriers of the C282Y gene. His mother is a carrier of both the C282Y and the H63D genes, and his other sister carries the H63D gene. Sam was found to be homozygous for the C282Y mutation.

Hereditary hemochromatosis was not known to be present on either side of Sam's family. On both sides lived relatives who reached advanced age, and there was no history of early death to warn of this genetic time bomb. Sam's death struck his family like a bolt of lightning. When they learned how easily hemochromatosis can be diagnosed and treated, family members were left with much anger at the needlessness of Sam's death.

Sam was the Martins' oldest child and only son. As a boy, he seemed perfectly normal, strong, and healthy. He even won physical fitness events in Cub Scouts, and he set a new school record for pull-ups at his elementary school.

Although there were a couple of unusual aspects to his health history, nothing seemed especially serious. At ages three and four, he was evaluated at Children's Mercy Hospital for a heart murmur. After two thorough annual evaluations involving many tests, doctors pronounced his heart normal, just noisy.

Sam had an excellent pediatrician who noted high blood pressure during a football checkup when Sam was fifteen. Again he was referred for evaluation to Children's Mercy Hospital. Several days of testing revealed no obvious problems. Next, an arteriogram was recommended. But since Sam's parents knew him to be a somewhat tense person, they declined that risky procedure and opted for treatment by a doctor who helped Sam reduce his blood pressure through biofeedback training. In later years he took blood pressure medication.

Since Sam's death the Martins have learned that an EKG at that time showed some slight strain or abnormality, though they don't remember hearing about it then. They wonder, "Could that arteriogram have revealed his hemochromatosis?"

Sam's physical health as a young man seemed OK. Although he took blood-pressure medication and an antidepressant, he seemed to have normal physical health and energy.

Sam had several symptoms of hemochromatosis in his last year or two, but they were easy to attribute to other causes. The pain in his neck and back seemed to result from a rear-end auto accident, and his fatigue seemed related to his repeated attempts to give up smokeless tobacco. Sam was more likely to visit the health-food store seeking ways to help himself than to visit his doctor. He used herbs such as ginkgo biloba and ginseng. He underwent Rolfing treatments.

Sam's doctor for his last five years, an osteopathic physician, never ordered iron tests. Routine screening and diagnosis when he was much younger would have saved Sam's life and health.

Sam is survived by his parents, James and Sidney Martin; his wife, Lucinda Martin; and his sisters, Rachel and Hannah Martin.

Sam was a poet, photographer, gardener, stained-glass artist, bird lover, connoisseur of Mexican food, and an aspiring guitarist. He was a lifelong Kansas City resident and worked at a print shop. His family remembers him most as a loving brother and son, and the most kind and spiritual person they have known. Without him, the Martin family will never be the same.

The Martins are grateful to the St. Joseph Health Center doctors and staff, who worked heroically for forty-two hours on Sam's behalf and who treated them with compassion. But questions still plague them: Why did Sam die so young from hemochromatosis? Did he have a heart defect that contributed to his death? Did he accumulate iron faster through his diet or use of tobacco? Did other genetic factors hasten the development of the disorder? If hemochromatosis usually kills at age fifty or sixty, why did Sam die at thirty-two?

Sam's final diagnosis included the following:

1. End-stage dilated cardiomyopathy with congestive heart failure
2. Liver failure
3. Renal failure
4. Upper gastrointestinal bleeding
5. Disseminated intravascular coagulation
6. Hemochromatosis

Sam's autopsy states that he died from multisystem failure due to hemochromatosis. The autopsy report mentions a history of hypertension. Noted on the anatomic portion of the report are cardiac failure, hepatic cirrhosis, pancreatic insufficiency, renal insufficiency, coagulopathy, gastric hemorrhage, bilateral pleural effusions, and ascites. Also noted are an enlarged heart, gallstones, and an enlarged spleen. The report continues with a notation that all organs had a dark reddish-brown discoloration. There was marked iron deposition in the liver and heart consistent with advanced hemochromatosis.

Iron tests done the day Sam died showed Sam's percentage of saturation was 93 percent and his ferritin 99,465 ng/mL, the highest known recorded ferritin in the United States and probably in the world.

Jack Ritter: One of the First Documented Cases of Hemochromatosis

"Please! Hold the plane for us!" Bonne Ritter shouted into the phone. "We have a medical emergency! I have to get my husband to Mayo Clinic; it's urgent!" she emphasized. "What is Mr. Ritter's problem?" asked the Philadelphia Airport employee.

Nearly screaming, Bonne yelled back in response, "It's life or death! He has been given twenty-four hours to live. Please, I beg you, hold that plane!"

"I'm not trying to pry, Mrs. Ritter; we want to put a special attendant on duty if it would help."

Amid all the chaos, fear, and anxiety, here was a calm voice of a caring person offering a helping hand. Bonne explained the medical crisis the best she could under the circumstances. "I'll never forget her response," Bonne says, remembering that bitterly cold day in February 1968. "Drive carefully, we'll hold the plane."

These words quieted Bonne momentarily, allowing her to gather her thoughts. The Philadelphia Airport was fifty miles from the Ritters' home. Without the cooperation of the airport, Jack surely would have died.

Twenty-year-old Jack Ritter was an accomplished Franklin and Marshall College basketball player. During a heated and competitive game against the rival team, Dickinson College, Jack fell to the floor in what later would be determined to be a grand mal seizure. The team doctor, who had not seen the seizure but was familiar with such disorders, had carried Jack off the court. He suggested Jack go home for a complete examination by the family doctor.

Jack was a welcome sight to his mother. She had been ill and appreciated his company. His seizure experience became somewhat overshadowed by his mother's prolonged illness. She was being treated for an enlarged heart; her skin was very dark—just like Jack's. Her eyelids were the same color as the dark circles beneath her eyes. When Jack was finally able to see the family doctor, he was diagnosed with a mild heart attack, caused by a condition possibly inherited from his mother.

The diagnosis didn't keep him out of World War II, however. Expecting a classification of 4-F, everyone was surprised that the army accepted Jack. His new bride, Bonne, was certain Jack would never pass the physical exam. In boot-camp formation Jack collapsed three different times, yet he went on to serve his country on both the European and Pacific fronts without complaint.

Returning from war physically unscathed, Jack was greeted by his wife, Bonne. It was time to start building a new life. Within a year of his return, Jack and Bonne were expecting their first child, Tom.

One night, only three days before their third anniversary, Bonne was awakened by what she initially thought was an earthquake. The bed was shaking, and she heard noises she was too groggy to interpret. She rolled over toward Jack; his body was rigid. Bonne had witnessed seizures before, so she knew what was happening to her husband. Tom was only nine months old at the time. He slept in a crib in the same room as his parents and was awakened by the unfamiliar noises. Bonne remembers seeing Tom's tiny figure peering at her from the crib, and not knowing which one to comfort first. Her experiences as a schoolteacher had taught her to keep calm in a crisis. She gently held on to Jack so that he would not hurt himself, while she tried to diminish the look of fear in her child's eyes with soothing words of reassurance.

A new family doctor told the Ritters that Jack had probably just had a very bad nightmare. This was not uncommon among war veterans who often relived terrible war experiences in their dreams. It was 1947; the word *epilepsy* was never mentioned. Society thought it was disgraceful to have epilepsy. The Ritters referred to the experience using a word their family doctor had offered. Saying that Jack had convulsions seemed a bit less offensive than saying he had had an epileptic fit.

Later that year, Jack began to have joint pain and he continued to have seizures. The family doctor made several referrals to specialists, but the Ritters didn't know which doctor to see first—the psychiatrist, osteopath, or endocrinologist. The psychiatrist gained more out of an interview with Jack than the other way around. Jack's positive attitude and pleasant demeanor were not what this doctor expected to see. The osteopath offered that Bonne could use a good massage. She appeared tense while Jack seemed relaxed; he was accepting the events without complaint. It was the endocrinologist, however, who offered the greatest amount of torture. He suggested Jack needed his bile drained weekly.

Without a word of complaint, Jack submitted to the doctor's orders. His sweet nature and strong faith were obvious in the way he endured several difficult, some painful, procedures. Each week for months he lay with his head near the floor and his feet elevated on an exam table. A tube was run down Jack's throat to somewhere in his gut. He said nothing of the discomfort, though he gagged each time the tube filled with green-yellow liquid. Next came the spinal taps, too numerous to count, followed by an EKG and an EEG. Back then, there were no sophisticated MRIs or CT scans. Jack's EEG was performed with fine needles implanted into the skull. Each of the needles sank painfully into his skull. The electrodes embedded in Jack's head would send messages to a device that resembled a lie-detector machine.

As it turns out the EEG and EKG provided the first evidence of something tangible. Jack had an abnormality in the front-temporal lobe. He was prescribed Dilantin and phenobarbital. The physician concluded from the EKG that Jack had a pro-lapsed mitral value.

By now Jack was thirty. He had been seen by seven doctors and been in six different hospitals. It was only the beginning. For fifteen more years he continued to see the very best of physicians, including a specialist from London. The Ritters' lives revolved around medication schedules, paperwork from insurance companies, and trips to doctors.

Jack's attitude miraculously remained positive and he never complained, even though he had cause to do so. He was beginning to feel weak and too fatigued to keep up his usual twelve-to fourteen-hour workday. His skin was still dark; his seizures continued. He was hospitalized for blood poisoning. Joint pain, abdominal pain, and heart arrhythmia continued. Now his personality was changing. He was often confused or cross, immediately apologizing for his behavior afterward. Jack wanted to be a good husband and father; he would never intentionally hurt Bonne or Tom.

In 1965 Jack had five grand mal seizures in the same night, which led to a referral to a neurologist at Mayo Clinic. Three days in Mayo resulted in a diagnosis of epilepsy, possibly due to an injury to the front left lobe of the brain. By now the Ritter family didn't fear the consequences of using the word *epilepsy*. Years of trying to keep this deep secret only added to the imagination of the neighborhood gossip ring. Jack's medications were adjusted and he changed the time of day that he took them; the daily dose was left the same.

This worked for nearly two years. The Ritter family and his many physicians assumed that Jack's problems were all related to the epilepsy. They were wrong. That year, 1968, would prove just how wrong they all were.

Within a two-week period of time Jack lost forty-one pounds. He mentioned that his mouth was very dry. The family doctor said he thought Jack had become allergic to the Dilantin and instructed Bonne to discontinue the medication for a few days and see what happened. Bonne protested strongly, reminding the doctor that Jack had been on this drug for twenty years and stopping it abruptly might cause him to seize and never recover.

The doctor snapped back at her, "So, now, you're the physician!" Bonne took a deep breath, trying not to show her anger at such a demeaning remark. She quietly offered, "I have read about this medication and its precautions. I am simply concerned for my husband's well-being."

Numerous phone calls and an eventful trip to a dermatologist, who noted that Jack's liver was enlarged, began the cascade of events that would finally lead to proper diagnosis.

At 11:00 a.m., Bonne heard her name over the classroom intercom. She had an emergency call in the office. Adrenaline shot through her body as she raced from her room into the office where her caller waited on hold. "Hello, this is Bonne Ritter," she choked out. The family doctor, the same one who had talked with her days earlier, was on the other end of the line. "Bonne, it's serious. Four different specialists have no idea what is wrong with Jack, but they agree on one thing, that you need to get him to Mayo Clinic today." Emphasis was placed on the word *today*. A roar in Bonne's head nearly drowned out the rest of the message that three of Jack's vital functions had shut down.

It took her exactly eleven minutes to convince the airport employee to hold the plane. She raced to get Jack and rushed to the airport, a fifty-mile ride, where the Ritters made the flight that would save Jack's life.

It was nearly 9:00 p.m. when the plane touched down in Rochester, Minnesota, home of the Mayo Clinic. To Bonne and Jack's surprise and delight, there stood Dr. Frank Howard, Jack's neurologist, ready and waiting with his station wagon. His expression betrayed his attempt not to look shocked. It had been three years since he had last seen Jack. Once in the car, Dr. Howard instructed Bonne to turn on the dome light. Next he asked to see the palms of Jack's hands. Jack weakly turned toward the physician and offered his right hand with the palm upturned.

Bonne saw the doctor's shoulders rise as a result of a deep breath taken when Jack's palm obviously confirmed something he suspected. "I think they'll find hemochromatosis," said Dr. Howard. Neither of the Ritters had ever heard the word.

Jack was admitted to Methodist Hospital, where nine doctors soon surrounded his bed. They spoke in low tones consulting one another. Jack was semiconscious, drifting in and out of sleep. He was exhausted. One physician remarked that nearly all of Jack's body hair was gone. Another noted the dark skin, especially the lines in Jack's hands and closed eyelids. On the ninth day and with the sixteenth doctor, the Ritters were told Jack needed a liver biopsy. Dr. Howard held Bonne's hand; his gentle clasp offered consolation in this moment when she was trying to understand what was happening. "You mean to tell me that after all he has been through, you need a biopsy to confirm what sixteen different doctors agree is hemochromatosis?"

"We could all be wrong, Mrs. Ritter," the doctor replied softly. Bonne was moved by the humbleness of the physician.

Undeniable proof was provided with the biopsy. There was no cirrhosis, even though they said Jack's liver was so large it would fill a dishpan. It was a small miracle that there was no cirrhosis or cancer, considering the years of unchecked iron accumulation. Another shock as a result of the biopsy was that Jack had diabetes—a consequence of the hemochromatosis, the physician explained.

Bonne remembers being handed a sheet of paper with a single paragraph describing hemochromatosis. When she and Jack arrived home, the family physician had the same paragraph except that his included a line about prognosis. He informed Bonne that Jack probably had about nine months to live. Bonne called the doctor at Mayo, who told her the prognosis depended on how well Jack complied with therapy and followed his diet. At the time Jack was forty-six.

The next twenty-nine years would include meeting one of the finest physicians in the area of Reading, Pennsylvania, Dr. William Reifsnyder. With his help, Bonne saw her husband through excruciating arthritic pain, brittle diabetes, hip replacement surgery, numerous transient ischemic attacks (TIAs), and three heart attacks. In 1996 Jack was hospitalized with kidney failure.

Jack died September 19, 1996. He was seventy-three. Surviving twenty-nine years after his diagnosis, he remains one of the earliest documented cases of hemochromatosis in the United States. Always joyful and in good spirits, he was a model father, husband, and patient. He and Bonne had been married fifty-two years in August of that year. They celebrated in Jack's hospital room with a small cake and a cup of coffee toast to their years together. She and Jack had talked about starting a support group for people with hemochromatosis. "Honey," he had said, "if we save one person from going through what we have gone through, it would be worth it."

Bonne carried on Jack's hope to help people. She established and ran one of the best-attended HHC discussion groups in the United States for decades. Bonne continues to raise awareness distributing the Iron Disorders Institute's educational materials throughout her community.

Bridging Yesterday to Today

Unnecessary suffering and deaths of loved ones angered and motivated all of the individuals in these stories. Common to all of them was the desire to protect future generations by raising awareness about hemochromatosis. They faced long hours, little money, and a vast sea of need, but their motivation was too strong for them to give up. One volunteer expressing frustration about trying to inform physicians blurted out a phrase that would be repeated many times: "I feel like a gnat in a hurricane!"

Despite the tremendous odds, plans were carried out that would forever change the face of hemochromatosis. High priority was given to partnering with the CDC to educate physicians and to producing literature with medically reviewed content. Confidence was high that if these two priorities were met and successfully carried out, that unnecessary pain, suffering, and premature death because of hemochromatosis would be an exception rather than the rule.

A congressional budget line item funding hemochromatosis research and a partnership with the CDC and NIH was achieved. A panel of hemochromatosis experts was formed to serve as medical and scientific oversight for content in educational literature.

The *Annals of Internal Medicine* published a multipage supplement on hemochromatosis in 1999 that addressed diagnosis, treatment, and management. The IDI was given permission to photocopy the supplement to mail it out to healthcare providers. Volunteers and staff spent countless hours photocopying, collating, stapling, stuffing envelopes, and sticking mailing labels on envelopes to more than seven thousand healthcare providers in the Southeast (the Carolinas, Georgia, Alabama, Florida, Tennessee, and Virginia). Follow-up calls (and in some cases, personal visits) were made to ensure that the providers received, read, and found the material helpful. Achieving this objective was tedious but rewarding.

Through this pilot outreach program, the IDI learned the following: physicians are too busy to read long articles on topics that may not seem germane to their patient population. The attitude that hemochromatosis was a rare disease affecting older men prevailed because most of the physicians still had never diagnosed a case.

In a visit to the office of a key clinical investigator, Laura Main and Cheryl Garrison spotted the unopened envelope buried deep in a pile of "must read" materials. The physician admitted that he wanted to read the material but lacked the time. From these findings, IDI sought the help of its Medical and Scientific Advisory Board to develop a snapshot of the symptoms, reference ranges, diagnosis, management, genetics, diet, and resources for clinicians. In late 2000, IDI produced the first of its kind Physician Hemochromatosis Reference Chart, containing at-a-glance illustrations of diagnostic algorithms, treatment, diet, genetics, and resources.

The 1996 gene discovery confirmed that hemochromatosis is real and common; evidence also proved that hemochromatosis could be deadly. This reality helped to shape the late 1990s and launched us into the next period in the history of hemochromatosis: the way it is now.

32

The Way It Is Now

What we know about hemochromatosis today is dramatically changed from the previous decades, when people often received the diagnosis because of an autopsy. From 1996 to date, science has given us a gene and key modifiers such as hepcidin; the media have become aware of hemochromatosis and are beginning to promote it; and government health agencies have set aside funding for protocols, research, and education.

Awareness of hemochromatosis has definitely increased. Patients are being diagnosed earlier. Access to treatment is vastly increased. Through the FDA variance program, blood centers can accept hemochromatosis patients more frequently than every fifty-six days, and they do not have to throw the blood away, so long as it passes the same safety inspection as routinely donated blood. The Internet helped raise awareness and has provided patients with free access to literature and resources.

Overall, the status of hemochromatosis has improved and continues to do so. Still, much work has to be done to reach the unaware and to overcome gaps in knowledge and practice. Among the barriers we face today is reaching the very large at-risk but undiagnosed population and the doctors who will inevitably connect with those patients. When we take all hemochromatosis types into consideration, there are at least 75 million Americans at risk that we need to reach. Presently, there are approximately nine hundred thousand physicians in the United States. Among those in the healthcare profession, we must eliminate knowledge gaps about genetics, liver biopsy, blood chemistry ranges, and best practices. We have to ensure that current funding remains and increases so that our ability to reach, educate, and fund targeted research is expanded.

The previous decade brought some challenges and setbacks, such as the 1998 unbundling of blood chemistries removing serum iron and ferritin, the 2001 controversial Scripps Research Institute report finding that only a small percentage of people with hemochromatosis ever develop disease, and the 2007 U.S. Preventive Task Force report recommending against genetic screening for hemochromatosis. Finally, patient apathy toward the seriousness of hemochromatosis is one barrier we never expected to encounter.

The Scripps study rocked the scientific community when lead investigators Ernest Beutler and Vincent Felitti announced that HFE is not very penetrant; that is, many people may have the gene mutations, but few of them will develop disease—less than 1 percent according to the Beutler et.al. report.

Following this report, scientists began a volley of heated exchanges that remain ongoing today. Beutler and Felitti's findings, they argue, were greatly biased and not representative of the general population. Other large population-based, non-U.S.-based studies that seemed more representative were being ignored.

The National Institutes of Health's $30 million HEIRS project (hemochromatosis iron overload study) of one hundred thousand people in the United States and Canada eventually provided some evidence that supported a greater penetrance. The HEIRS findings correlate more closely with other large population-based studies in Australia and Ireland.

At the core of the argument of the Scripps Institute was ascertainment bias. Participants of the study were enrolled in a major preventive healthcare program, had excellent insurance coverage, and some had given as much as eighteen units of blood but were still accepted as eligible to participate. Forty-two previously diagnosed patients were dropped from the outcome data.

As a result of these more current large-population based studies, approximately half of the patients who are homozygous for classical type 1 hemochromatosis will load iron. Of these, about two-thirds will develop disease. Given this information, penetrance is 35 to 45 percent, significantly higher than the 1 percent reported by Beutler and Felitti.

In 2007, the U.S. Preventive Task Force recommended against genetic screening for hemochromatosis on a population-wide basis. What was not emphasized sufficiently is that the task force was recommending against genetic screening. They went on to say that targeted biochemical screening was appropriate and even encouraged. Unfortunately, this latter recommendation was overlooked by many who simply read the abstract of the paper without focusing on the details of the recommendations.

Discontinuation of funding for targeted iron research at the Iron Disorders Centers of Excellence was another setback. With targeted iron research, we can deliver evidence of a significant cause of disease: HFE and its modifiers. The Iron Disorders Institute, in partnership with Penn State University, established a center of excellence for iron related research. The IDI was fortunate to award and to facilitate awards to Penn State totaling more than $300,000 for a team to investigate iron's role in neurodegenerative diseases. The research directed by IDI Medical and Scientific Advisory Board member James Connor yielded remarkable discoveries about iron's ability to speed the onset and advancement of Alzheimer's or cancer. Because the source of funding for this research center was a congressional earmark, the funding was halted.

The removal of serum iron and ferritin from routine blood chemistry panels closed the window of opportunity for early detection. This low-tech type of screening helped to identify thousands of patients with hemochromatosis. Although this issue is discussed in an earlier chapter, it is worth repeating. With serum iron and TIBC removed from the blood chemistry panels, millions lost the added benefit of discovering elevated iron early enough to intervene with preventive and treatment measures, with relatively simple adjustments like regular blood donation, diet, modest behavioral changes, or a combination of those. Removal of these tests also resulted in skyrocketing lab costs. For patients with insurance, this consequence remained relatively obscure. Most insurance companies, and even Medicare, will not reimburse the cost of these tests without a prior diagnosis of iron deficiency or iron overload. The unintended results of this mean that, for the millions of people who lack insurance coverage adequate to cover the costs of the tests, and for millions more without any insurance at all, the impact was—and continues to be—devastating. Before the unbundling, a blood chemistry panel that included serum iron, TIBC and serum ferritin, and the complete blood count ran about $100; after the unbundling, the same set of tests cost patients more than $400 out of pocket!

In 2005 the Iron Disorders Institute board of directors voted to focus its efforts to restore at least serum iron to routine biochemical panels and to make every effort to also restore serum iron, serum ferritin, and TIBC or UIBC to these panels.

In the CDC survey of patients with hemochromatosis, when asked what led to their diagnosis, 45 percent reported that their diagnosis resulted from a routine or ancillary blood test such as serum iron.

Finally, a barrier to early detection that no one expected was patient apathy. High-risk patients expressed lack of concern about early detection, compliance with therapy, or taking any measures to prevent hemochromatosis-related disease. In 2004, the Iron Disorders Institute reported to CDC that the issue of apathy was emerging and that we could not fathom how such attitudes could be possible. The CDC conducted a study of siblings and blood relatives of people with hemochromatosis and reached the same conclusion as IDI.

The areas of apathy seem to center on two key issues. First, siblings or family members do not believe that hemochromatosis offers any threat to their health. Second, once hemochromatosis patients who undergo therapeutic phlebotomy reach normal iron levels, they behave as though they are cured. They skip treatment appointments or drop out of maintenance entirely.

One blood-bank special collections coordinator remarked to IDI, "Many hemochromatosis patients take their condition for granted. They act like they just had a cold and with a few blood donations they are cured."

We often hear from patients two to three years after their diagnosis and successful iron balance. Of those who stopped listening and learning about hemochromatosis following this period, many report that symptoms have come back and in some cases are even worse. Sadly, for some, the damage is too far gone to reverse. The opportunity for disease prevention and inexpensive therapy has passed for these patients.

When HHC is diagnosed in a blood relative, all other blood relatives are at risk of disease or premature death. In the CDC family-based detection survey, a disturbing number of siblings of diagnosed HHC patients reported that they were not concerned. They stated reasons including absence of symptoms, that they felt their doctors would inform them, or that they thought the condition was rare (their chances of inheritance low).

At a family workshop, the twenty-six-year-old son of a man diagnosed and receiving phlebotomies remarked without hesitation that he wasn't going to give blood. At the time, this young man's serum ferritin was higher than 600 ng/mL and his TS percentage was greater than 70 percent. He went on to say that his dad looked OK, discounting the fact that his dad was receiving therapy. The son announced that he would be just fine; after all, he had no symptoms, which also discounts the fact that his iron levels were very high.

Society has changed dramatically in its attitudes and approaches to health. People are much more proactive. Physicians, too, have changed the way they practice medicine—adapting to the demands of an Internet era and soaring healthcare costs.

Hemochromatosis is the good-news disease; it is the only health condition that gives back. When hemochromatosis is detected, the patient becomes a blood donor for life. If these patients donate blood and take care of themselves, they reduce their risk for all the major chronic diseases (heart failure, diabetes, arthritis, liver disease) and premature death. They also lower their risk of needing a new liver, thus shortening the list of people on the transplant waiting list. By staying well, they remain on the job, need fewer sick days, and enjoy a longer and higher-quality life.

33

How It Must Be

To combat unnecessary pain, suffering, and premature death caused by hemochromatosis, and some of the stigmas associated with this disorder, we need to continue what we are doing but on a grander scale. We must have the ability to ensure adequate epidemiology and surveillance for the CDC; funding from the NIH for targeted and iron expert–led research; funding for screening, outreach, and education; policies that protect patients; consensus by proven experts on best practices; and standardized laboratory ranges.

Funding for screening, outreach, and education are key if we are going to detect disease in its early stages, help patients, and educate physicians.

Experts with a proven record of clinical experience should be developing best practices for hemochromatosis. Regular summits for discussion should include a wide variety of stakeholders, such as clinicians, policy makers, and patients, so that best practices consider all perspectives.

Standardized laboratory ranges would eliminate the confusion about what is normal and what is not. Take, for example, normal serum ferritin ranges, which are as low as 8 ng/mL for some laboratories and as high as 328 ng/mL for others.

Patients with hypothyroidism, a consequence of hemochromatosis, even if they have symptoms, can be told that their thyroid function is normal. This occurs because of the wide range for normal thyroid-stimulating hormone (TSH), a routinely used test to determine thyroid function. When the thyroid is underactive (i.e., hypothyroidism), TSH is elevated. IDI's upper range for normal TSH is 3.5, and most physicians use laboratories for which the range for normal TSH is 5.0 or higher.

Laboratory ranges must be standardized so that all reference ranges are the same. Once this is accomplished, disease or the risk of disease will be detected earlier and therapy will be more uniform.

At a 2009 Iron Disorders Institute Regional Hemochromatosis Conference, twenty-nine medical professionals attended. Of these, 90 percent were seeing patients and stated that they would make changes to their practice as a result of what they learned at this seminar.

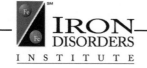

PART SIX

Taking Care of Yourself

34

Finding a Doctor and Treatment Center

A knowledgeable physician who recognizes that hemochromatosis is common, inherited, and often the cause of multiple symptoms will likely order the correct tests, provide good therapy, and begin to screen patients who are in high-risk categories.

Dr. Sharon McDonnell, of the CDC, when asked what kind of doctor IDI should suggest to hemochromatosis patients, responded, "Find one who will listen."

A frequent request made by individuals who contact IDI Patient Services for information is the names of physicians who are knowledgeable about hemochromatosis.

The IDI maintains a database that includes names of physicians who are treating HHC patients and who are using the IDI's Hemochromatosis Reference Guides. As part of its long-range goals for educating physicians about hemochromatosis, the IDI encourages each individual to return literature published by the IDI about hemochromatosis to his or her family doctor. In this way, a physician can learn more about hemochromatosis through his or her patient, while the patient maintains a familiar routine and preserves an already-established relationship.

In cases where the person declines to revisit a particular doctor, the Iron Disorders Institute's Patient Services will provide the individual with a physician's name if available. A package of information about hereditary hemochromatosis is then sent to the person. Another is sent to the former physician.

A physician who diagnoses one case of HHC is equipped to diagnose an entire family.

There are a number of U.S. healthcare providers who follow IDI's advisory board guidelines for diagnosis, treatment, liver biopsy, diet, and genetic testing. These physicians are in the IDI national registry and can be accessed online on at our website, or by calling IDI Patient Services.

On the occasion when a physician may not be aware of the IDI guidelines, a patient can introduce the doctor to the standards by delivering a copy of the IDI Hemochromatosis Physician Reference Chart. The IDI provides these free of charge to patients who wish to have these guidelines followed. The charts are also available online.

Clinicians find the IDI reference charts very helpful. Information in the charts can protect the patient against over-bleeding and underbleeding, and can offer noninvasive options to liver biopsy. Quick reference to information about symptoms, normal ranges, diagnostics, treatment options, diet, and genetics makes the charts unique and appreciated. The sample order for therapeutic phlebotomy calls for a pretreatment hemoglobin of 12.5 g/dL (or 38 percent hematocrit), which protects a patient from being overbled but also allows for his or her blood to be used rather than discarded.

Patients can now have phlebotomy treatments at blood centers with an FDA variance to use hemochromatosis blood for transfusion purpose. Prior to 1999 hemochromatosis patients had to pay out of pocket for phlebotomies; their blood was labeled "biohazard" and thrown away. This was discouraging for patients who knew that their blood was being wasted. Efforts were made to persuade the FDA to investigate the safety of hemochromatosis blood.

In April 1999, the Advisory Committee on Blood Safety and Availability unanimously concluded that blood obtained from people with hemochromatosis posed no greater risk than blood obtained from routine donors. Patients with HHC across the United States cheered. Many patients with HHC were already donating regularly, but they had to watch helplessly as their blood was discarded as unfit for use. When the committee made its recommendation, everyone thought that a long and wasteful practice had been stopped. Those of us present when the recommendation was made applauded the FDA for its decisiveness.

Today, not all eligible blood centers offer a hemochromatosis program. According to Dr. Mary Townsend, medical director of Coffee Memorial Blood Center and chair of the Scientific, Medical, and Technical Committee on blood availability for America's Blood Centers, "Many private blood centers want the blood, but they can't just begin taking it without going through major operational changes."

First, a center must apply for an FDA variance-21 (according to the regulations at C.F.R. 640.3 (d) and 21 C.F.R. 640.3 (f)). The variance does not come without conditions. Although at present the FDA considers HHC blood safe for use, the FDA must be accountable to members of the public who receive this blood. Therefore, it is only prudent for the FDA to ask for additional data as a condition of any center permitted an FDA variance. It is important to keep in mind that blood-banking systems were designed to manage a public commodity that, above all, must be safe for use. The FDA's recommendation could have included that HHC blood be labeled—a deterrent for use by anyone who knows little about iron. Extra data gathering seemed a small price to pay to gain access to such a rich resource of blood; centers are willing to comply, but it takes a lot of work and time to do the extra record keeping.

"That's not the only problem," Dr. Townsend adds. "Let's say a center applies for and receives a variance. That is the easy part; now they are tasked with rewriting standard operating procedures for donor qualification. Medical history, reasons for deferral, and testing procedures need to be changed. Therapeutic phlebotomy algorithms (process and order of procedures) have to be written and included; blood center employees have to be trained," she continues. "Further, some HHC donors need to donate as often as twice a week. Computer systems are not set up to track this level of frequency."

"It's not just a matter of hiring someone to rewrite the software," commented Gregory Hart, director of the Blood Connection in Greenville, South Carolina. "Computer software programs that blood centers use must be approved by the FDA."

In 2002 IDI began calling blood centers to survey them about the variance; comments ranged across the board. Some centers felt that they were too small and did not have the funds to restructure themselves or to hire additional workers to handle the added workload. Some local hospitals continue to refuse to use HHC blood, so why go through the expense and time to restructure when the local demand for this blood is nonexistent? Also, some centers don't draw therapeutics, and some just want to wait for more information based on experience. Their well-entrenched concern for safety in the blood supply seems the key drawback to application for a variance and use of HHC blood. A person with HHC is perceived as having a potentially life-threatening disorder that requires blood extraction.

"Education is key," says Dr. Townsend. "Without significant education, it will never be understood that HHC is not a blood disease but a disorder of metabolism."

What many do not know about hemochromatosis blood is that there is essentially no more iron in a unit of blood drawn from someone with HHC than there is in a unit of blood drawn from a non-HHC donor. Iron in individuals with HHC remains in their tissues (stored in ferritin or hemosiderin) and can be removed only by special means (phlebotomy or iron chelation). Every standard unit of blood contains about 250 milligrams of iron, the same as blood from anyone else who is donating.

It is clear that individuals with HHC have a valid complaint when they see their blood discarded. It is also clear that the Department of Health and Human Services and many blood centers see this as a waste of a precious resource and wish to see the blood used. With adequate time, education, and appreciation on the part of both sides, the blood issue will likely correct itself.

35

Treatment Routine: Phlebotomy and Blood Donation

Therapeutic Phlebotomy Treatment for Iron Overload

Your physician has determined that therapeutic phlebotomies are the preferred medical treatment for your diagnosis of iron overload.

The advantage of this treatment is that therapeutic phlebotomies are inexpensive, are relatively simple to perform, and have increasingly demonstrated an increased survival rate for patients that have a condition warranting their use, such as hemochromatosis. There is mounting evidence that many, but not all, of the medical conditions caused by excess iron are reversible as a result of therapeutic phlebotomies.

The initial goal of your treatment is to remove excess iron from you as quickly as possible without compromising your health and to prevent irreparable damage to your vital organs. Thereafter, less frequent phlebotomies will usually be required to maintain a minimally acceptable level of iron to satisfy your body requirements. The frequency and duration of treatment will vary for each individual.

It is vitally important that you convey your reactions to treatment along with your observations to your physician. These symptoms may include heart irregularities, severe abdominal pain, fatigue, or shortness of breath. Your phlebotomist, under your physician's guidance, will strive to keep you as comfortable as possible, with little inconvenience to you and without affecting your medical treatment or your health. Remember, you are ultimately responsible for your health; therefore, it is advisable that you become knowledgeable about your disease and treatment.

The Iron Disorders Institute strongly advises you to discuss your specific treatment with your physician so that you do not place your health at risk.

Frequently Asked Questions (FAQs)

The following FAQs have been asked by patients when they were first diagnosed. IDI can provide a Patient's Phlebotomy Activity Checklist of procedures that patients being treated for iron overload have found helpful in the past.

What is therapeutic phlebotomy?

A therapeutic phlebotomy is simply the process of collecting blood as a medical treatment, similar to blood donation at a blood bank. The only difference is that therapeutic phlebotomy requires a doctor's order (prescription). Therapeutic phlebotomy is another tool available to doctors to combat unhealthy or dangerous levels of iron in your body. An example is in the treatment of

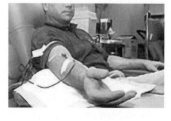

hemochromatosis, which is a condition with an overabundance or high concentration of body iron for which therapeutic phlebotomies are performed to remove the excess iron.

How is a phlebotomy performed?

A tourniquet is applied above the penetration site before a needle is inserted into a vein. Usually, your blood will be collected from one of your arms into a sterile container, similar to donating blood. The penetration site is the front elbow area, or cubital region, where two commonly used superficial veins are located. The median cubital vein is preferred by most phlebotomists. The median vein is often used as an alternate site.

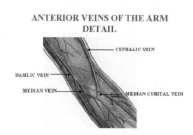

ANTERIOR VEINS OF THE ARM
DETAIL

CEPHALIC VEIN

BASILIC VEIN

MEDIAN VEIN

MEDIAN CUBITAL VEIN

How much blood is removed with each phlebotomy?
Generally, one unit of blood is withdrawn. A unit is 450 to 500 milliliters, or approximately 1 pint. However, your diagnosis, physical condition, or body mass may warrant a lesser or greater volume under strict parameters established by your physician. Also, your intolerance to blood extraction may warrant extracting a lesser volume on a more frequent schedule.

How much iron is removed with each single phlebotomy?
Approximately 200 to 250 milligrams of iron are removed per unit of blood.

How long does a phlebotomy take?
The length of time for a phlebotomy is generally twenty to thirty minutes, but you should expect to spend at least one to two hours at your blood-drawing facility. The medical staff will use the remaining time to ensure that you are healthy enough to undergo a phlebotomy by reviewing your blood test results and measuring your vital statistics, such as blood pressure, respiration, and temperature. Afterward, the staff will remeasure your vital statistics to ascertain that your blood pressure has returned to normal for you. During this period you should rehydrate by consuming liquids.

Why is a tourniquet used?
A tourniquet, or constrictive band, is used to distend your veins. For patients who will have frequent or indefinite phlebotomies, 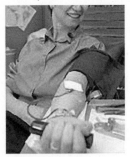 a blood pressure cuff provides considerably more comfort because the cuff is wider and pressure can be controlled much easier than with tourniquets, which are made of rubber, latex, or other synthetic elastic material and are much narrower and more restrictive.

The narrower tourniquets must be removed entirely to release pressure on the selected vein, whereas the blood pressure cuff can be decreased to relieve discomfort without impeding blood flow or pressure can be reapplied if the flow slows. Elastic tourniquets may also cause bruising in some patients.

Are there different kinds of sterile containers?

Yes—there are two types of sterile containers used for therapeutic phlebotomies: standard containers, also referred to as blood bags or gravity bags, and vacuum bottles. Both have advantages and disadvantages. The vacuum bottle is preferred for frequent or long-term therapeutic phlebotomy treatments. The type of container determines the needle size.

How are the needles used for phlebotomy sized?

Needles are measured by gauge; the smaller the gauge, the larger the needle is. For example, a 16-gauge needle is larger in bore size than a 20-gauge needle.

What are the advantages and disadvantages of blood bags?

Blood banks prefer to use blood bags because red blood cells are not damaged in the extraction process because of the associated large-bore, 16-gauge needles. There is also less chance of clots forming in the large needle bore. The blood bag can also be used for a therapeutic phlebotomy. The disadvantage is that, over time, scarring, or sclerosis, will form with frequent venesections at the same penetration site.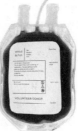

Why is the vacuum bottle preferred over blood bags?

The vacuum bottle can be used for therapeutic phlebotomies for patients who have difficulty with the larger needles. The needles associated with vacuum bottles, called butterfly needles, are both smaller and interchangeable, and range in gauge size from 20 to 24. Thus, patients experience less pain with minimum sclerosis from repeated needle penetrations. The vacuum bottles are more adaptable to a patient's tolerance. However, the incidence of clotting is increased because of the smaller bore.

Butterfly needle

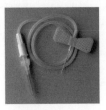

The smaller guage needle makes insertion into the vein easier. Wings are pinched together to allow the phlebotomist a secure grip.

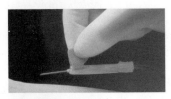

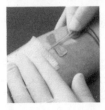

The needle is inserted into a vein in the arm and a connecting tube is attached to a blood bag.

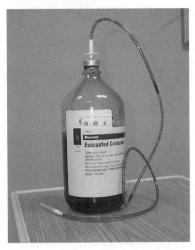

Standard vacuum bottle with attached needle and tube.

How long will it take to reduce my stored iron levels?

How long it takes to reduce your stored iron to acceptable levels may be as quick as several weeks to several months, or indefinitely, depending on the type of iron overload and your physician's guidance. There are generally two phases or stages for therapeutic phlebotomy treatment: a de-ironing or induction phase and a maintenance phase. Each phase has a different frequency rate of phlebotomies.

What is the purpose of my de-ironing phase?

The goal is to remove the excess iron as rapidly as you can tolerate frequent phlebotomies, or blood extractions. This phase is sometimes referred to as the induction phase in the treatment of iron-overload disorders.

What is the phlebotomy frequency for my de-ironing phase?

The frequency may be once every other week, once a week, or several times a week, depending on your ferritin, or stored iron levels; body mass; and tolerance to phlebotomy. Your physician establishes the frequency and the length of time on the basis of relevant blood test results and your physical condition.

What is the purpose of my maintenance phase?

The objective of the maintenance phase is to manage iron levels to prevent toxicity or organ damage, yet retain adequate iron to satisfy your body's requirements in the manufacture of red blood cells.

What is the phlebotomy frequency for my maintenance phase?

The frequency is considerably less than that of the de-ironing phase. Your need to be phlebotomized is determined by factors such as your blood test results and body mass. Important among the blood tests are your level of ferritin (stored iron) and your TS percentage. There are wide variations because of each individual's physical attributes; consequently, some patients have phlebotomies as often as every month, while others may have as few as one or two phlebotomies per year.

How long will my treatment last?

The length of your treatment will depend on your iron-overload diagnosis. For example, you will need to have phlebotomies indefinitely if you have been diagnosed with hereditary hemochromatosis (HHC). However, if your diagnosis was acquired iron overload, then your physician may cease the therapeutic phlebotomies when your ferritin level reaches an acceptable level and is maintained without subsequent phlebotomization.

Your physician will order periodic blood tests to monitor your iron levels as the treatment phase dictates. These tests include, but are not limited to, an iron panel, which includes serum ferritin, total iron-binding capacity (TIBC), fasting serum iron (Fe), and a complete blood count (CBC), which includes hematocrit (Hct), hemoglobin concentration (Hgb), and mean cell volume (MCV).

How rapidly will my iron levels fall?

Serum ferritin drops approximately 30 ng/mL per full unit. If it falls more rapidly, there may be other reasons for elevated ferritin. Use of nicotine products, alcohol consumption, or inflammation due to a chronic illness—such as infection, arthropathy, and diabetes—can affect serum ferritin levels.

How will my de-ironing phase be monitored?

Prior to each phlebotomy, your hemoglobin or hematocrit will be checked. Periodically, a TS percentage and serum ferritin should be performed. Extremely high ferritin levels suggest that frequent monitoring of the test result would serve very little purpose. However, if your blood tests indicate only marginally high stored iron levels, then common sense suggests that your ferritin levels should be watched more closely. Monitoring stored iron levels is a judgment call by your physician.

How will my maintenance phase be monitored?

During the maintenance phase, your physician will monitor your hematocrit or hemoglobin prior to each phlebotomy to ensure that you have not become anemic or have begun to load iron. Your iron panel blood tests will also be monitored during this stage, more than likely every three to six months, or possibly only yearly.

What role does mean cell volume have in monitoring my iron levels?

The use of MCV is a relatively new development showing great promise in avoiding iron deficiency anemia in patients who are aggressively bled. Monitoring MCV values, after establishing a base value at the beginning of the de-ironing phase, will preclude developing iron anemia. The MCV will drop by about 3 percent of baseline when excess iron is removed.

Are alternate treatments available?

Yes, iron-chelation therapy is available but is generally reserved for patients with severe iron overload and anemia. Also available is double red-blood-cell apheresis (DRCA). These and other alternatives are discussed in the next chapter.

Should I modify my diet?

Yes. At a minimum, you should limit foods that contain large amounts of iron, such as red meat and iron fortified cereals. Also avoid supplements that contain iron. The key to iron reduction in your diet is moderation. The Iron Disorders Institute's *Hemochromatosis Cookbook* provides easy-to-prepare, old-fashioned recipes and menus with tips on how to absorb less iron from the diet.

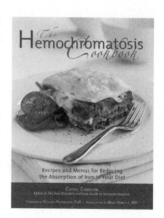

Should I keep a record of my phlebotomies?

Yes, it is highly recommended that you keep a journal of your phlebotomies, including such information as dates, amount of blood withdrawn, penetration site, and so on. In addition, your journal should contain blood test results. Your journal will be invaluable in helping you to understand your specific treatment and, more important, in discussing your treatment with your physician. A spiral notebook, electronic spreadsheet, and the Personal Health Profile offered by IDI are several techniques that you can use to record your treatments.

Are there any methods to prevent my blood from clotting during the phlebotomy?

The use of a pillow under the upper part of the arm will reduce the natural tendency of your arm to bend at the elbow, which can restrict blood flow during a phlebotomy. Your blood flow will also have the additional benefit of increased gravity.

Some patients advocate taking a single 81-milligram aspirin (baby aspirin) the evening before a scheduled phlebotomy to aid in blood flow. However, aspirin is considered an anticoagu-

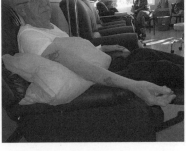

lant and should not be taken without consulting with your physician.

How can I overcome anxiety about the pain associated with needles?

A prescription topical antiseptic, like Emla cream, can be applied to the penetration site an hour before a scheduled phlebotomy to reduce the pain associated with needle penetration. To prevent unnecessary evaporation of a topical anesthetic, cover the affected area with a piece of clear plastic wrap. Caution: Some medical conditions, such as liver disease and glucose-6-phosphate dehydrogenase deficiency (G6PD) may interact with topical anesthetics. Discuss this with physician or pharmacist.

Also, once your phlebotomy needle is in place, ensure that your phlebotomist places a gauze pad under the needle and then tapes the needle in place. The gauze pad keeps the needle's bevel off the roof of the vessel, thus reducing the possibility of restricted blood flow, while the tape needle leaves your phlebotomist's hands free, preventing even the slightest movement by your phlebotomist from being telegraphed to the penetration site.

What is iron avidity, and how is it addressed?

Iron avidity is a condition in which the body is loading iron rapidly. Serum ferritin may be on the low to normal side while TS percentage is elevated. This is believed to be a natural response by the body to the repeated blood loss. The body will compensate in an effort to survive. In the same way that the body's defense mechanisms are activated when a harmful invader gets into the system, the body may also perceive the chronic blood loss as a threat to life.

There are two approaches to addressing iron avidity. Both approaches include discontinuation of blood removal until stores are greater than 50 ng/mL and TS percentage has returned to a normal range, below 45 percent. In addition to discontinuing blood removal, depending on how iron deficient a person has become, it may be necessary to take iron supplements. An alternative to oral iron is to increase lean red meat consumption. A combination of red meat and iron supplements is also another possibility. The Iron Disorders Institute favors the approach of consuming lean red meat because meat contains so many other nutrients, such as B12 and zinc—which are important to blood-cell production. Iron pills will replenish iron stores faster, but there may be side effects such as intestinal upset. Whichever approach you use to replenish iron stores, it is up to you and your physician to decide. Providing that there is no other problem present, both of these approaches will eventually bring iron stores back into balance, which is the goal.

36

Specialized Treatment

Phlebotomy is the most efficient known therapy for most individuals with hemochromatosis or iron overload. The procedure is straightforward and inexpensive, and most people tolerate the procedure well. In exceptional cases, the physician may consider options to standard phlebotomy such as apheresis, also known as double red-cell apheresis (DRCA), chest port, partial phlebotomy, and iron-chelation therapy.

Apheresis

The procedure of apheresis (known as red-blood-cell and plasma apheresis [RBCP] or double red-cell apheresis [DRCA]) is similar to blood donation, except that blood components such as platelets, white blood cells, red blood cells, and plasma are separated during the donation process. Also, this procedure takes a little longer than routine blood donation. Apheresis utilizes a computerized cell separator, which safely and automatically removes a specific component and returns the remaining components to the donor. A patient's hemoglobin is checked prior to apheresis just as it is in routine blood donation. Afterward, the donor reclines on a contour chair where a needle is inserted into a vein in the arm.

The DRCA donation is used as an option to routine phlebotomy. The volume of red cells is not actually quite double the amount of red cells removed in standard phlebotomy. Apheresis allows donors to give full transfusion doses of red cells and plasma through the same process used to donate one component such as platelets. After the red cells and plasma are removed, the remaining fluids are returned to the donor. Donors lose a smaller amount of fluids through the DRCA process than through a regular whole blood donation. A saline solution is added to components that are returned to the donor.

According to Dr. James Smith of the Oklahoma Blood Institute, "The advantage to apheresis over standard phlebotomy is that a standard unit of blood contains about 40 percent red blood cells. A unit removed by apheresis contains nearly 80 percent RBC." If one does the math, it becomes apparent that one apheresis treatment removes approximately double the iron, or an impressive 500 milligrams per treatment, compared with 250 milligrams in a standard phlebotomy. Though apheresis is more efficient than phlebotomy for iron removal, it is expensive and may not be affordable for many people. Centers with a variance to accept hemochromatosis blood may also be able to offer apheresis. This is left to the individual blood center system and depends on their variance and standard operation procedures.

Dr. Mary Townsend, medical director of the Coffee Memorial Blood Center, agrees that individuals with iron overload can consider apheresis. Dr. Townsend points out that apheresis can be helpful for people who live in rural areas and must travel long distances for treatment. These individuals can get the equivalent of two phlebotomies with one apheresis treatment.

For John, "apheresis can't be beat." After two years of repeated elevated levels of serum iron and eventually finding a physician who knew to test TS percentage and ferritin, John was properly diagnosed with hemochromatosis. His TS percentage was 91 percent, and his ferritin level was higher than 1,000 ng/mL. Nearly two years earlier, a previous physician had seemed unimpressed by John's ferritin level of 690. A second test by the same physician didn't alarm him either; by this time, John's ferritin was 1,092 with a TS percentage of 58 percent. However, by this time, the physician had heard of hemochromatosis and referred John to a hematologist, where he received his diagnosis and began phlebotomy treatments. Fifteen phlebotomies spread over nineteen months were not aggressive enough to reduce ferritin to a safe range. John began to look for alternatives. After reading about apheresis, he decided this was the therapy approach for him.

His physician wasn't certain John was correct, but he took care to measure John's hematocrit prior to each treatment, which resulted in successful de-ironing. John's prescription read: "Two unit apheresis every two weeks until serum ferritin is lowered to ~20 ng/mL as long as hematocrit remains greater than 35 percent and hemoglobin remains within range of 14 to 18 g/dL." In addition, for this critical period of time for John's therapy, the physician ordered tests of monthly serum iron, ferritin, and liver enzyme levels.

Three years later, and upon being successfully de-ironed, John obtained genetic analysis and was found to be homozygous for C282Y. He concludes that his parents had to be carriers, as they never had symptoms of any disease. Afterward, John's brother Patrick was diagnosed with hemochromatosis by liver biopsy.

Apheresis is available in any blood center; however, it is not routinely offered as a treatment option for those with hereditary hemochromatosis. A blood center must have a provision in its FDA variance to include apheresis for HHC. Visit our website (www.irondisorders.org) for a list of centers offering apheresis as part of their HHC program.

Chest Port

Patients with exceptionally high amounts of iron, usually confirmed by liver biopsy, might benefit from an implant or chest port. Chest port or central venous catheters are tubes threaded through the vein in the upper chest under the collarbone. Two types are commonly used: internal, which is surgically implanted under the skin, or external, where the entry site portion is visible outside the skin.

A phlebotomist who performs therapeutic phlebotomy is also qualified to remove blood through a port. Hemoglobin and/or hematocrit levels are measured prior to extraction just as with other types of blood extraction. Blood is extracted from the port through a tube leading into a vacuum bag or bottle. This type of bag or bottle is needed to suction the blood through the needle into a tube and then into a blood bag.

Vacuum bags or bottles hold the same amount of blood, one unit, or 450 to 500 cubic centimeters of blood, the same as a standard blood bag.

A saline solution is used to clean the port and is followed by a heparin flush. Heparin is a blood thinner used to prevent clotting, one of the problems of using this device. Another problem with ports is that they can work their way out of the body and have to be replanted.

Ports are not considered a routine method for therapeutic phlebotomy. These devices are generally used to give medication in cases where a patient requires large amounts of medicine that must be given often, such as with AIDS and cancer. However, this device can work well for some patients for whom iron levels are extremely high, especially when access to veins is impaired or difficult.

After complications caused by phlebotomy, Jim, diagnosed with hemochromatosis, needed an alternative. His arms were bruised and painful; he was not going to be able to tolerate the twice-weekly blood extractions that his high iron levels required. With a ferritin level more than 1,800 ng/mL and TS percentage greater than 60 percent, Jim's attending physician felt that de-ironing had to be aggressive.

An ultrasound-guided liver biopsy confirmed Jim's hemochromatosis. Fortunately, there was no cirrhosis, and cancer was ruled out, so the thought of repeated phlebotomy and anemia didn't sound too bad to him. After five extractions, however, Jim couldn't tolerate therapeutic phlebotomy; his doctor recommended a chest port.

Jim's overall experience with the port was very good. He found the port convenient and efficient, commenting that approximately 600 cubic centimeters of blood were removed each time rather than the standard 450 cubic centimeters. He had a unique problem in that his port worked its way out of his body and had to be removed. This was not painful as much as it was uncomfortable. Jim's physician removed the port, bandaged the area, and decided that Jim was sufficiently de-ironed. So he did not insert a new port.

Itching and burning at the site were among Jim's complaints, in addition to two other problems. One, a false drop in platelets, was traced to a heparin flush done before blood work rather than after. Blood for complete blood count (CBC) is drawn from the port; because it had been flushed with heparin prior to drawing blood needed to run the CBC, his platelet level readings were misleadingly low. Jim's second problem was that he had to deal with moderately severe anemia. His physician inappropriately extracted blood until hemoglobin was at 9.5 g/dL, which left Jim with uncomfortable symptoms: fatigue, sensitivity to cold, leg cramps, dizziness, heart arrhythmia, headache, and muscle weakness. He missed more work than usual, and he was not very good company to his family.

"I don't think I needed to be bled so aggressively toward the end," remarks Jim. "This was not so much because of the port," he adds, "but a belief my doctor held that anemia was a necessary part of the therapy. I'm not so sure I agree."

Chest ports require surgical implantation. This is a serious procedure and should be discussed at length with one's physician. Most people with iron overload are not candidates for this treatment option.

Minimal Extraction

Individuals who are frail, elderly, weigh less than 110 pounds, or whose veins are scarred and not accessible might benefit from a smaller needle such as the butterfly needle. This type of needle is usually a 20- to 22-gauge needle rather than the 16- to 18-gauge needle used for standard phlebotomy. Because the needle is smaller, removal of a standard unit of blood will take longer. Some individuals, such as those with heart conditions, especially arrhythmia, might not need a full unit removed, in which case minimal extraction or half-unit (250 cubic centimeters) can be considered.

Iron-Chelation Therapy

The type of chelation therapy used to de-iron patients who have iron overload should not be confused with ethylenediaminetetraacetic acid (EDTA), a method used by some alternative medicine practitioners: EDTA is a broad-spectrum chelator, meaning that it binds with and removes a wide number of minerals.

Therefore, it is not specific. In contrast, deferoxamine (brand name Desferal), deferasirox (brand name Exjade), and deferiprone (brand name Ferriprox) are highly specific for iron. The latter two are iron chelators that can be taken orally.

Iron-chelation therapy is the removal of iron pharmacologically with an iron-chelating agent such as the products mentioned earlier. Individuals who are transfusion dependent or who have conditions in which anemia is present at the same time as iron overload require iron-chelation therapy to remove excess iron.

Desferal is not absorbed in the gut (intestinal tract); therefore, this drug must be administered intravenously or given by subcutaneous injection, using a portable battery-operated infusion pump.

Generally, the pump is worn at night, where slow infusion of the iron-chelating agent is administered over a period of about eight hours for a duration of four to six nightly infusions per week. Patients might be given an additional 2 grams of Desferal intravenously for each unit of blood transfused. Desferal is injected separately from blood transfusions.

Desferal is administered subcutaneously (under the skin) slowly at first, beginning with 1 gram three to four times per week, with monitoring of iron excretion in a cumulative twenty-four-hour urine sample. If effective, the dose can then be adjusted upward, 1 gram at a time, up to four times per week, until the patient reaches a tolerable dose level. The dose should not exceed 50 milligrams per kilogram of weight, or about 3 grams per day. Periodic examination of the patient is necessary until positive response to treatment is confirmed.

In the United States, Desferal and Exjade are presently the only drugs approved for removal of iron by chelation. These drugs are very efficient at removing iron, but the process takes longer since chelation removes only about 6 to 10 milligrams of iron per treatment—compared with phlebotomy, which removes 250 milligrams per treatment. For this reason, iron chelation is not appropriate for most patients with hemochromatosis or iron overload. It is, however, currently the only treatment available for those who are transfusion dependent. People with conditions such as thalassemia, some forms of leukemia, sideroblastic or aplastic anemia, or myelodysplasia (MDS) may need whole red-blood-cell transfusion to survive.

With every unit of blood received by transfusion, these patients are receiving approximately 250 milligrams of iron. With repeated transfusions, accumulation of iron occurs within one to one and a half years, and if a patient has complications such as leukemia, a complex treatment scenario is created.

Attending physicians will likely address the underlying cause of anemia first, before addressing iron overload. Iron-chelation therapy can then be administered to reduce iron levels after the primary condition causing anemia has been stabilized. For those with thalassemia major and who have been transfusion dependent for a lifetime, chelation therapy should begin at the same time as transfusions or very early in the onset of using transfusion.

Some physicians use a combination of iron chelators and therapeutic phlebotomy, especially for patients with diabetic neuropathy and arthropathy. Dr. Paul Cutler, of Buffalo, New York, reports that this combination therapy results in 50 percent increased improvement over standard phlebotomy alone. Individuals with cardiac involvement might benefit from the combination of Desferal and phlebotomy.

However, anyone with severe kidney damage is not a candidate for this type of treatment, as Desferal is excreted not only via bile and feces but also via urine. Women who are pregnant or nursing, and children younger than three have restrictions on the use of iron-chelation drugs. It is not known how much of the drug gets into breast milk; thus, a mother who is receiving this type of treatment might consider low-iron soy-formula substitutes.

Immediate symptoms of adverse reaction to iron-chelation therapy with Desferal might include visual disturbances, blurred vision, rash or hives, itching, vomiting, diarrhea, stomach or leg cramps, fever, rapid heartbeat, hypotension (low blood pressure), dizziness, anaphylactic shock, and pain or swelling at the site of intravenous entry. Long-term problems might include kidney or liver damage, loss of hearing, or cataracts. Some side effects have been reported with Exjade but can be addressed by adjusting the dose.

Patients should report such symptoms immediately to their physician, who can adjust dosage. Further, physicians might examine a patient's visual status with slit-lamp fundoscopy (means of examining the eye) and hearing status with audiometry or a hearing test. Liver enzymes (ALT, AST, GGT, and ALP), a kidney function test such as blood urea nitrogen (BUN), serum ferritin, and TS percentage might also be measured by the attending physician.

In Conclusion

As with any drug or therapeutic approach, patients should be proactive and learn as much as they can about any medications or procedures recommended to them.

Patients should especially read about side effects and risks so that they can have an informed conversation with their healthcare providers. Some hemochromatosis patients may seek an approach to therapy that is less tedious than routine phlebotomy. They may turn to herbal remedies and use concentrated forms of mixtures that claim to get rid of excess iron. This can be dangerous, especially because of the damage that can be done to the liver. Individuals with iron overload who are considering therapy options are encouraged to seek information about therapy from reliable sources such as respected scientific journals and organizations. Patients should read as much about a new therapy as possible, make no hasty decisions about the therapeutic course of action, and discuss therapy options in detail with a qualified physician and perhaps other patients who may offer details of their experiences.

37

Diet, Supplements, and Behavior

> "Among 2,851 participants, following diagnosis of HHC, 65 percent were told to avoid iron supplements, 38 percent were told to eat less iron-rich foods, [and] 27 percent were given no diet advice."
> —*1996 Centers for Disease Control and Prevention HHC Patient Survey*

When Harry Kieffer was diagnosed there was no Internet, no genetic testing, and information about a hemochromatosis diet was nearly not existent. Chris Kieffer, one of the founding directors of Iron Disorders Institute, got the idea that if a diet for iron-deficiency anemia would help build up iron stores, it made sense that doing just the opposite should help people like Harry who did not need the iron. For several years, Chris limited Harry's diet of red meat including venison, a favorite of Harry's. She read labels watching every milligram of iron regardless of the source. In time, we have learned a great deal about foods and substances that impair or increase iron absorption. Questions about diet are among the most frequently asked by patients.

Food Choices, Supplements, and Behavior Can Dramatically Influence Iron Balance

Some hemochromatosis patients believe that by following a strict diet, phlebotomy may not be needed. Although there are documented cases of hemochromatosis patients having success with this approach, high levels of iron cannot be managed in this way. For a person with serious iron overload, blood loss is the most expedient way to lower iron levels. A diet plan can significantly reduce absorption of iron from the diet and therefore affect levels of stored iron in ferritin. However, no food or supplement can pull iron out of ferritin. These substances can only impair absorption of iron, and therefore reduce the amount of iron that is stored in ferritin. As a result, a patient may need fewer therapeutic phlebotomies.

No single food or substance is a cure-all and no beneficial food need to be eliminated from the diet. A person can develop iron-deficiency anemia with a specialized diet, such as a strict vegetarian diet. These individuals usually do not have excessive iron stores to begin with.

For hemochromatosis patients, as with anyone, a balanced diet is the key. A good diet plan needs to be easy to follow and adhere to, and it needs to be dynamic, changing, as the individual's needs change. All foods, including those rich in vitamin C, should remain in the diet of a person with hemochromatosis. Women with hemochromatosis can safely breast-feed their newborns and infants and are encouraged to do so. Those who enjoy an alcoholic beverage can do so once excess iron levels are addressed and as long as the liver is healthy.

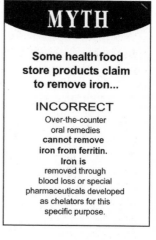

MYTH

Some health food store products claim to remove iron...

INCORRECT

Over-the-counter oral remedies **cannot remove iron from ferritin.** Iron is removed through blood loss or special pharmaceuticals developed as chelators for this specific purpose.

Hemochromatosis patients can generally eat normally by observing a few easy-to-remember practices. As with anyone, intake of sugars, fats, and processed foods should be limited; but in particular, hemochromatosis patients should avoid eating organ meats, raw shellfish, and animal fat.

The Hemochromatosis Cookbook is a great resource for planning menus. The book contains helpful menu-planning forms, iron content in foods, grocery checklists, charts, and an eating plan that allows for flexibility.

Controlling the amount of iron a person absorbs depends on the bioavailability of iron in the diet. Bioavailability is the degree to which a nutrient is available to the body for its intended use. Although most people think spinach is high in iron, possibly because of growing up with the cartoon antics of Popeye the Sailor, the iron from spinach is actually not well absorbed. Spinach contains oxalates, which impede iron from being absorbed, making the bioavailability of iron contained in spinach almost nonexistent. According to the nutrient bioavailability expert Dr. Raymond Glahn, of the U.S. Department of Agriculture's U.S. Plant, Soil, and Nutrition Laboratory at Cornell University, "What little iron one gets from eating spinach comes mostly from soil that clings to the leaves."

Types of Iron

People consume two types of iron: heme iron and nonheme iron. Heme iron is derived from organic sources such as the blood proteins, hemoglobin, and myoglobin contained in meat. This type of iron is in a form that is more easily absorbed by the body. About 10 percent or less of dietary iron consumed in American diets is heme iron, even though meat consumption in the United States is high. For people with normal iron metabolism, only 20 to 25 percent of the heme iron consumed is actually absorbed. For example, a four-ounce hamburger contains about 3 milligrams of iron; about 1.2 milligrams are heme and about 1.8 milligrams are nonheme. The amount of heme iron absorbed from that hamburger would be approximately a third of a milligram. People with HHC who have abnormal iron metabolism can absorb up to four times the iron as a person with normal iron metabolism. Therefore, 80 to 100 percent of heme iron can be absorbed, or approximately 1.2 milligrams from the same hamburger. Calcium is the only substance that has been found so far that inhibits heme iron absorption, whereas numerous substances can inhibit the absorption of nonheme iron. Although there are many food and supplement substances that impede or enhance absorption of nonheme iron, the absorption of heme iron is little affected by these foods or products.

About 40 to 45 percent of the iron contained in meat is heme; the other 55 to 60 percent is nonheme. Iron contained in plants is almost entirely nonheme iron, though plants can contain minute traces of heme iron. Nonheme iron represents the majority of dietary iron that humans consume. Nonheme iron is inorganic and is derived from grains, nuts, fruits, vegetables, fortifiers, or contaminant iron such as from water, soil, or cooking utensils. Unlike heme iron, the iron from all these sources must be changed before absorption can take place.

When nonheme iron is ingested, it is in a form called ferric iron. Humans cannot absorb ferric iron; it must be united with oxygen to become ferric oxide. The body cannot absorb ferric oxide either, but when ferric oxide reaches the stomach, it mixes with stomach acid (hydrochloric acid) and is changed into ferrous iron. Ferrous iron is the form of iron that can be absorbed; it moves out of the stomach into the first part of the intestine, called the duodenum. This is the point at which scientists believe that the majority of absorption takes place. There may be another absorption site further down in the intestinal tract where minute amounts of iron can absorbed.

Certain substances can interfere with the absorption of iron; knowing what these are and avoiding or including these substances with main meals can help individuals control dietary iron absorption.

There are foods and substances that increase or decrease iron's bioavailability. These should be taken into consideration for balancing body iron in any adult.

For infants, breast milk contains the most highly bioavailable form of iron and should be the first choice of nourishment for a baby, unless circumstances such as health of the mother are in question. Women with hemochromatosis who are not on medications that can get into their milk can breast-feed their newborn or infant and are encouraged to do so.

The excess iron in a female with hemochromatosis is contained in the tissues of her body stored in ferritin. These excesses do not get into her milk. The content of breast milk is carefully regulated by the body's natural mechanisms. As part of these mechanisms, breast milk contains lactoferrin, a protective iron-binding protein that guards against harmful pathogen infiltration. Lactoferrin also helps in the delivery of just the right amount of bioavailable iron to the child. Note in the chart on the next page of infant formulas and milks that breast milk is low in iron but bioavailable iron is high.

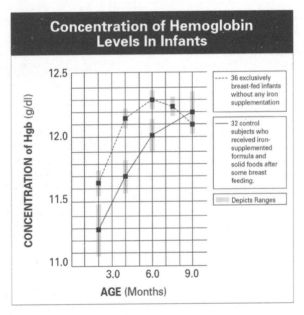

Iron Absorption — Breastmilk • Formulas • Cow's Milk			
Substance	Iron Content (mg/L)	Bioavailable iron (%)	Absorbed iron (mg/L)
Nonfortified formula	1.5–4.8	about 10%	0.15–0.48
Iron-fortified formula*	10.0–12.8	about 4%	0.40–0.51
Whole cow's milk	0.5	about 10%	0.05
Breastmilk	0.5	about 50%	0.25

* The average iron content is 6.8 milligrams of iron per liter of formula.

Iron Disorders Institute image file

Concentration of Hemoglobin Levels In Infants

CONCENTRATION of Hgb (g/dl)

AGE (Months)

- - - - 36 exclusively breast-fed infants without any iron supplementation

—— 32 control subjects who received iron-supplemented formula and solid foods after some breast feeding.

Depicts Ranges

Adapted from M. A. Siimes, "Hematopoeisis and Storage of Iron in Infants," in *Iron Metabolism in Infants*, ed. B. Lonnerdal (Boca Raton, FL: CRC Press, 1990), 34–62.

Note also in the chart the hemoglobin values of children who are breast-fed: their values are stronger, one assurance that a child will get the iron needed for rapid growth and development. It should again be mentioned that newborns and infants have exceedingly high iron levels as compared to adult levels. Ferritin in newborns can be well up to 600 ng/mL and TS percentage can be 100 percent; these values are temporary but vital to a child's normal development. A child, even one who is homozygous for HFE mutations, is not at risk for iron overload in these circumstances.

For adults, among the substances that increase the bioavailability of iron and therefore its absorption are ascorbic acid or vitamin C, alcoholic beverages, beta-carotene, super iron additives (Ferrochel or FeEDTA), and meat, especially red meat and hydrochloric acid (stomach acid).

Ascorbic acid or vitamin C occurs naturally in vegetables and fruits, especially citrus; it can also be synthesized for use in supplements. Ascorbic acid enhances the absorption of nutrients such as iron. One glass of orange juice (about 100 milligrams of vitamin C) can counteract the inhibiting effect of a cup of tea. Studies suggest that greater than or equal to 50 milligrams of ascorbic acid would be required to overcome the inhibitory effects on iron absorption of any meal containing more than 100 milligrams of tannic acid. In studies about the effects of ascorbic acid on iron absorption, 100 milligrams of ascorbic acid increased iron absorption from a specific meal by 4.14 times. In a standard meal of meat, potatoes, and milk, 100 milligrams of ascorbic acid increased absorption of iron by 67 percent. The addition of 100 milligrams of ascorbic acid to a specially formulated liquid meal containing 85 milligrams of phytate increased absorption by 3.14. Grapefruit juice is one source of vitamin C that you should not take if you have liver damage or are on medication.

WARNING!!!

Grapefruit juice can cause serious and dangerous side effects, including fatalities, when taken with certain medications. Something in the fruit causes drug potency to be increased up to twelve fold.

Iron Disorders Institute image file

Alcohol enhances iron absorption. Moderate consumption of alcohol has known health benefits, but heavy or abusive drinking, especially when in combination with high body iron levels, increases the risk of liver damage and liver cancer. Studies show that heavy drinkers have high iron levels. Approximately 20 to 30 percent of those who are heavy consumers of alcohol acquire up to twice the amount of dietary iron as do moderate or light drinkers. Alcohol will hasten liver disease such as cirrhosis. Excess alcohol consumption can impair the body's natural antioxidant defenses, establishing an environment conducive for oxidative damage, which affects tissue, cell, and DNA health. Patients who have developed cirrhosis increase their chance of developing liver cancer by 20- to 200-fold. Alcohol in the presence of high iron can also cause brain damage. Alcohol-induced lab rats were found to have an alarming amount of free iron in the cells of their brains. A standard drink is defined as 13.5 grams of alcohol, or 12 ounces of beer, 5 ounces of wine, or 1.5 ounces of distilled spirits. Moderate consumption is defined as two drinks per day for an adult male and one drink per day for females or those older than sixty-five, regardless of sex. Options to consider might be nonalcoholic or low-alcohol-content beer and wine. Although red wine is reported to be healthy for the heart, it is likely that the polyphenol content in red wine provides the greater benefit. Except for the sedating quality of alcohol, a handful of red grapes will provide equal, if not greater, health benefit.

Well water can contain high levels of nonheme iron. For most people this iron is not a concern. Individuals with hemochromatosis who have very high body iron can consider using a water-filter system or switching to bottled water. The iron content in the water is a warning sign that other containments are present in the groundwater. Having the well water tested for contaminants is encouraged. In general, high levels of iron in well water is an indication that the underground water source is being contaminated. Often, the cause can be traced to a nearby landfill where cars or metals are dumped.

Beta-carotene is one of more than a hundred carotenoids that occur naturally in plants and animals. Carotenoids are yellow to red pigments contained in foods such as apricots, beets and beet greens, carrots, collard greens, corn, red grapes, oranges, peaches, prunes, red peppers, spinach, sweet potatoes, tomatoes, turnip greens, and yellow squash. Beta-carotene enables the body to produce vitamin A. In studies of the effects of vitamin A and beta-carotene on absorption of iron, vitamin A did not significantly increase iron absorption under the experimental conditions employed. However, beta-carotene alone significantly increased absorption of iron. Moreover, in the presence of phytates or tannic acid, beta-carotene generally overcame the inhibitory effects of both compounds, depending on their concentrations.

Both FeEDTA and Ferrochel are additive iron compounds that are emerging as candidates for fortification among major food manufacturers. Individuals with conditions such as hemochromatosis who are at high risk for iron overload will need to avoid food products fortified with those two compounds. Both additives were found to exceed absorption capabilities of the commonly used fortifier ferrous sulfate.

Iron Absorption in Humans from Four Different Breakfasts When Fortified

Basal	Basal + 3mgs Ferrous Sulfate	Basal + 3mgs Ferrochel	Basal + 3mgs Fe-EDTA
3.0%	5.3%	10.8%	14.9%

Iron Absorption in Humans from Four Different Breakfasts When Fortified *Plus Phytase*

Basal	Basal + Ferrochel	Basal + Ferrous Sulfate + Phytase	Basal + Ferrochel + Phytase
5.1%	7.9%	10.1%	13.2%

Hydrochloric acid (HCl) is the acid found in the stomach that breaks down food and makes it available for absorption. We all need some HCl for normal digestion. Several acid-reduction medications such as proton-pump inhibitors or antacids can reduce the production of stomach acid and affect iron absorption. These medications should not be taken to lower stomach acid levels unless under the direction of a healthcare provider.

Meat, especially red meat, increases the absorption of nonheme iron. Beef, lamb, and venison contain the highest amounts of heme, compared with pork or chicken, which contains low amounts of heme. Meat also contains animal fats, which can increase absorption of nonheme iron. It has been calculated that 1 gram of meat (about 20 percent protein) has an enhancing effect on nonheme iron absorption equivalent to that of 1 milligram of ascorbic acid. A Latin American–style meal (corn, rice, and black beans) with a low iron bio avail-ability had the same improved bioavailability when either 75 grams of meat or 50 milligrams of ascorbic acid was added. Meat contains about 40 to 50 percent heme iron; the balance is nonheme.

IRON	per 3.2 oz serving MEAT		
	total iron MILLIGRAMS	heme iron percentage of total iron	heme iron MILLIGRAMS
VENISON	4.5	51	2.3
LAMB	3.1	55	1.7
BEEF			
RUMP STEAK	2.9	52	1.5
SIRLOIN STEAK	2.5	52	1.3
ROUND STEAK	3.2	50	1.6
TOP ROUND	2.5	48	1.2
GROUND	2.5	40	1.0
BRISKET	2.0	25	0.5
VEAL	1.9	40*	0.7*
PORK	1.3	23	0.3
PROCESSED MEATS			
SAUSAGE (VEAL)	0.7	40*	0.2*
BOILED HAM	0.7	40*	0.2*
LIVER PATE	5.0	16	0.8
CHICKEN	0.6	40*	0.2*
FISH			
COD	0.2	0.0	0.0
MACKEREL	0.7	0.0	0.0
SALMON	0.6	17	0.1
MUSSELS	4.6	48	2.2
LOBSTER	1.6	40*	0.6*
SHRIMP	2.6	40*	1.0*

* resources vary

Iron Disorders Institute image file

Substances that inhibit absorption of iron include phenolic compounds, phytates, phosphates, oxalates, eggs, and calcium.

Polyphenols are phenolic compounds, including chlorogenic acid, found in cocoa, coffee, and some herbs; phenolic acid, found in apples, peppermint, and some herbal teas; tannins, found in black tea, coffee, cocoa, spices, and walnuts; and polyphenols, found in fruits such as apples, blackberries, raspberries, and blueberries. One must remember, however, that some of these foods also contain vitamin C and beta-carotene. Of the polyphenols, Marabou (Swedish), Dutch, or Swiss cocoa and certain teas demonstrate the most powerful iron-absorption-inhibiting capabilities, in some cases up to 90 percent. Coffee is high in tannin and chlorogenic acid; one cup of certain types of coffee can inhibit iron absorption by as much as 60 percent. Dr. Ray Glahn of the USDA center at Cornell University tasked one of his research fellows with testing some of the recipes in our *Hemochromatosis Cookbook*. His research student reported that the techniques in the book do in fact work and that the marinating approach used in the red meat recipes reduced nonheme iron absorption by as much as 40 percent!

Iron Absorption in Humans from Four Different Breakfasts Containing Coffee/Tea			
Basal	Basal + American Coffee	Basal + Espresso	Basal + Tea
7.5%	6.7%	3.9%	3.9%

Iron Disorders Institute image file

Green tea in concentrated capsule form is one particular supplement that should be taken with caution. Green tea is very high in tannin, but taken in high, concentrated doses, the liver could be damaged.

Excessive consumption of tannin is not recommended for people with liver damage. Make sure that you do not have liver damage, as assessed by a qualified physician, before consuming tannins more than once daily. One glass of tea, a cup of coffee, or a small amount of red wine with a meal will probably be allowed, but do not take a chance without consulting with your doctor about your liver health.

Phytate is a compound contained in soy protein and in fiber found in walnuts, almonds, sesame, dried beans, lentils and peas, cereals, and whole grains. Recent absorption studies in humans have demonstrated that even low levels of phytate (about 5 percent of the amounts in whole-cereal flours) have a strong inhibitory effect on iron absorption. Phytate levels are reduced during yeast fermentation in rye, white, and whole wheat breads, and sourdough leavening results in an almost-complete degradation of phytate. Oatmeal is a food that is rich in iron, but because of the high phytate (fiber) content, almost none of this iron is absorbed.

LUNCH, DINNER, and SNACKS

PHYTATE-RICH FOODS	Phytic acid content percentage of dry weight
Excellent	
Lima beans	0.9-2.5%
Wild rice	2.2%
Red kidney beans	1.2-2.1%
Pinto beans	0.6-2.0%
Navy beans	1.8%
Good	
Rye bread	0.8-1.5%
Corn bread	1.4%
Soybeans	1.4%
Peas	0.9-1.2%
Whole wheat bread	0.6-1.0%
Barley	1.0%
Brown rice	0.9%
Corn	0.9%
SNACKS OR CONDIMENTS (SEEDS AND NUTS)	
Excellent choices	
Sesame seeds	5.3%
Pumpkin seeds	4.3%
Sunflower seeds	1.9%
Peanuts	1.9%

Iron Disorders Institute image file

BREAKFAST

PHYTATE-RICH FOODS	Phytic acid content percentage of dry weight
Excellent	
Wheat bran cereals like All-Bran	3.0–5.0%
Oatmeal	2.4%
Raisin bran	1.8%
Good	
Shredded wheat	1.5%
Rye bread	0.8–1.5%
Whole wheat bread	0.6–1.0%
Special K	0.7%
Product 19	0.5%
Poor	
Rice Krispies	0.24%
Pumpernickel bread	0.16%
White bread or French bread	0.03–0.13%
Cornflakes	0.05%
Raisin bread	0.09%

Iron Disorders Institute image file

Phosphates are compounds used to whiten food products and are found in modified tapioca starch, bacon, toothpaste, certain medications, and some dairy products. The ability of phosphates to inhibit the absorption of iron is not completely understood.

Oxalates are compounds derived from oxalic acid, found in foods such as spinach, kale, beets, nuts, chocolate, tea, wheat bran, rhubarb, and strawberries, and in herbs such as oregano, basil, and parsley. Oxalates impair the absorption of nonheme iron. The presence of oxalates in spinach explains why the iron in spinach is not absorbed. In fact, it is reported that the iron from spinach that does get absorbed is probably from the minute particles of sand or dirt clinging to the plant rather than from the iron contained in the plant.

Eggs contain phosphoprotein called phosvitin, which is believed to be the substance in eggs that impairs the absorption of iron. The binding capacity of this protein with iron may be responsible for the low bioavailability of iron from eggs and possibly the iron-inhibiting ability of eggs, called the egg factor. The egg factor has been observed in several separate studies. One boiled egg can reduce absorption of iron in a meal by as much as 28 percent.

Calcium is an essential mineral; it is found in foods such as milk, yogurt, cheese, sardines, canned salmon, tofu, broccoli, almonds, figs, turnip greens, and rhubarb. The iron-inhibiting capability of calcium has long been a debated issue. Reports that calcium can impair the absorption of both heme and nonheme iron have been supported by the USDA Agricultural Research Department. Where 50 milligrams or less of calcium had no effect on absorption, calcium in amounts of 300 to 600 milligrams inhibited the absorption of heme iron similarly to nonheme iron. One cup of skim milk contains about 300 milligrams of calcium.

Fats, especially animal fats, can trigger free-radical activity. Hemochromatosis patients should sparingly eat animal fats, contained in fatty meats, butter, and whole milk dairy products. Fats derived from plant sources and cold-water fish are among the best choices.

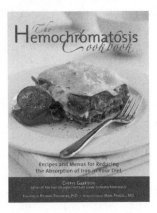

Everyone is different: not all hemochromatosis patients have the same iron levels, eat the same foods, or have the same habits. Patients with very high iron levels—serum ferritin greater than 1,000 ng/mL—will need to take greater precautions. Once iron levels are lowered to a serum ferritin of less than 1,000 ng/mL, some liberties can be taken.

We highly recommend *The Hemochromatosis Cookbook* for eating plans, such as those on the following page.

- *Calculate the nonheme and heme iron content in foods.* Use the food composition charts and the blank worksheets provided in *The Hemochromatosis Cookbook* to calculate the amount of iron in foods you intend to use in your weekly meal plan. Visit www.hemochromatosis.org or www.irondisorders.org and click on the links for diet and iron content in foods.

- *Incorporate foods and substances that impair absorption of iron such as tea, coffee, dairy, and fiber.* These substances, when consumed within two hours of a meal, will reduce the absorption of non-heme iron. The calcium contained in dairy products will inhibit the absorption of both non-heme and heme iron.

- *Do not eat raw shellfish, and take precautions while walking barefoot on beaches.* Oysters especially can be contaminated with *V. vulnificus*; when consumed by a person with high iron, the result may be death by septicemia if emergency medical attention is not received.

- *Eat freely of low-sugar fruits and high-fiber vegetables.* Fruits such as berries, apples, and kiwi versus ripe or high-sugar fruits are the best choices when iron levels are high. Eventually, you can begin to mix in some of the riper, higher-sugar fruits (bananas, pineapple) once iron levels are closer to normal. Do not be concerned about vitamin C or beta-carotene content of these antioxidant-rich foods. Enjoy them between meals or in cooked form; heat destroys vitamin C but not antioxidants.

- *Limit supplemental vitamin C to 200 milligrams per dose.*

- *Limit the amount of alcohol consumed.*

- *Consume good fats.* Use olive oil for cooking and salad dressings. Enjoy avocados and coconuts, which are rich in nutrients and fats known to lower the risk of some cancers.

- *Avoid cooking in cast-iron skillets or on grills.* Cook in glassware when possible, but you do not have to be a fanatic about it. Cornbread cooked in an iron skillet is a real treat that should not be denied to someone with hemochromatosis. The real issue with cast-iron skillets is to not let foods simmer for long periods or to eat high-acid foods (tomatoes) cooked in an iron skillet. Grilled foods at restaurants fall into this category also. Although it is a good idea to reduce the amount of cast-iron cooking for hemochromatosis patients, it is during the times of very high iron levels that these practices need to be tempered. Once iron levels are back down to normal, there is no reason not to enjoy an occasional cast-iron skillet meal.

- *Be compliant with therapeutic phlebotomies.* No diet can replace this important aspect of therapy for those with iron overload.

- *Keep hydrated.* Your body can get some water from foods, but most people tend not to eat adequate amounts of foods with high water content, such as fruits and vegetables. Sports drinks are not the best source of hydration. Adequate hydration reduces the time it takes to remove a pint of blood.

- *Don't smoke or chew tobacco, and limit nicotine consumption.* Chewing tobacco increases the risk of gum, throat, and esophageal cancer. Nicotine-containing gum will elevate iron levels.

- Take a daily iron-free vitamin supplement, especially while undergoing phlebotomy.

Phlebotomy removes other nutrients besides iron. Although a balanced diet might provide sufficient amounts of these nutrients, some people may need supplementation.

The Iron Disorders Institute recommends a daily iron-free multivitamin for patients undergoing therapeutic phlebotomies. Many affordable vitamin supplements are on the market. Phlebotomy removes nutrients other than iron, and substances that inhibit the absorption of iron also inhibit absorption of other nutrients. When a person consumes substances that can inhibit the absorption of iron, those same substances inhibit the absorption of other nutrients such as zinc and copper. Taking a daily multivitamin is one way to ensure that other nutrients blocked from absorption are replenished through supplementation. A once-a-day multivitamin with minerals excluding iron is likely sufficient for any adult with hemochromatosis. Beware of supplements that require a person to take six to eight pills a day. Not only can this be expensive, but one might actually experience gastrointestinal discomfort or undue stress on the liver as a result of high doses of supplements. When looking for a daily vitamin, find a one-dose vitamin, as is the case with the vitamins recommended previously.

Some supplements can be exceedingly harmful, especially because their potency and interactions are not widely known. Vitamin A daily, for example, should not exceed 4,500 international units (IUs) per day from all sources for hemochromatosis patients, unless patients are advised otherwise by a physician because of therapeutic reasons. Vitamin A taken regularly and in large doses can actually shut down the liver. Beta-carotene is another supplement widely used. Emerging evidence points to concerns about supplemental beta-carotene and certain types of cancers. Supplemental zinc can also influence iron balance. Zinc is an essential mineral found in meat, eggs, seafood, and to some degree, in grains. High doses of supplemental zinc can interfere with copper utilization, which can lead to impaired metabolism of iron.

In Summary

Cut back on red meat, limit alcohol consumption, don't eat raw shellfish, and maintain phlebotomies. Find an advocate who will keep reading on your behalf so that you remain current with information about hemochromatosis. We are learning new things everyday; know what we know. Read our books and visit our websites www.irondisorders.org and www.hemochromatosis.org.

38

Being Prepared for Emergencies

Be prepared. When you move to a new area, update your health and contact information and give a copy to someone who may act on your behalf in an emergency. Become familiar with local facilities before you have need for them. These final two points are illustrated in the story of Eric.

Twenty-year-old Eric did not want to donate blood. He was too busy getting ready to go off to college and just didn't want to take the time to drive across town to the local blood center. Diagnosed with an iron-loading disorder at the age of sixteen and successfully de-ironed, Eric felt that the situation was under control. He had plenty of time to go give blood.

Joint pain had been his biggest problem, and Advil took care of that, so the donation could wait a while—after all, how fast could iron accumulate? His family doctor had just tested his iron levels. Ferritin was not too high, sixty-something, he remembers; TS percentage he couldn't quite recall, but it was high, according to the doctor. Maybe that was the sixty-something number. "Next time," he thought, "I'd better write those numbers down somewhere."

Weeks became months; his concerned mother asked about his blood donation schedule. Eric agreed that it would be taken care of within the week. School was hypnotic: new friends, good grades, and great professors kept Eric distracted from his responsibility to give blood. Realizing that it was Friday, and that he had agreed to donate blood within the week, he rushed out the door to take care of the matter.

There was no blood donation center in the town where

he went to school, so he would have to go to the one in his hometown, which was almost a two-hour drive. Fridays were the only days he could leave school because of classes, so Eric headed for the blood center back home. When he arrived, it was closed. Oh well, next time, thought Eric.

During the next few months, Eric noticed that his hair was thinning. His joint pain seemed a bit worse than usual, and now he was having headaches, something he rarely got. Another problem he was reluctant to mention was sex related. Eric noticed that his desire for sex was waning. Although he was not thinking about marriage, he worried about the lack of desire, which should be normal for his age.

After a lengthy discussion about these symptoms with a friend, Eric felt better; he realized that his symptoms were probably related to his iron metabolism condition. He decided he would be more compliant with therapy, give up cola drinks, and take some supplements. That Friday he gave blood. The following week he got sick. Chills, sweating, fever, headache, dizziness, and muscle aches caused Eric to miss class for the first time that semester.

He had e-mailed his mom that he was sick and told her the symptoms. She e-mailed back for him to get to the health center immediately. Worried about the potentially lethal combination of virus or bacteria and excess iron, she called Eric. He sounded somewhat better, but still she was concerned. Although there are no studies to support death by viral or bacterial infection except in the cases of *Yersinia* and *Vibrio*, she didn't want her son to take any chances.

It was 4:00 p.m. Eric had agreed to check out the school health center, buy a thermometer, and call home by 10:00 a.m. the next morning. Forgetting that Eric was to call her the next morning, she called her son's room at 7 p.m. and got the answering machine. Hopeful that he was just sleeping, she left a message. The next morning her son's usual update and hello was not among her e-mail. At 7:00 a.m. she called her son's room. Again, she got the answering machine.

Reality hit, and panic replaced reason. She realized that she did not know the main number of the campus, her son's room number, the name of the hospital, or the health center on campus. The only thing she could remember about Eric's girlfriend, Julie something, was that she had long brown hair. She didn't know how to reach Eric's father, who was remarried and living elsewhere.

She dialed one more time and, to her relief, she heard the familiar, albeit sleepy voice of her twenty-year-old son through the receiver. He had gone to the pharmacy to buy a thermometer to see if he still had a fever. He had taken an over-the-counter cold and sinus medication and had slept deeply, his fever finally breaking.

The two talked about the lethal combination of iron and certain microorganisms, and about how fortunate it was that Eric had just removed 250 milligrams of iron with the recent blood donation. They discussed writing down contact numbers, knowing the local emergency health services, and being prepared when an emergency arises. Eric visited the college campus health center to learn that, though they don't provide therapeutic phlebotomy, they will provide immunization for hepatitis A and B and for meningitis.

Since Eric had let his hepatitis A booster lapse, he was able to take advantage of the college health services for a very small charge. He then went to the emergency room and met with the director of Emergency Services and wrote out a contact list for the floor counselor, his mom, his dad, and one close friend. He contacted the Iron Disorders Institute Patient Services and asked them to send the ER physician and the hospital health center a letter about his condition. The IDI sent a Patient Relocation Information Package to both the ER physician and the health center.

When a person waits until the crisis hits, panic will likely cause that person to do something that will be regrettable later on. Eric's mom is an educated woman. She has an important and demanding job, two factors that kept her from getting details that would have lessened her anxiety over this experience.

Lesson Learned
Do not let events catch you by surprise: make a complete list of important matters, such as your current address, phone numbers, people's full names, roommates, the name and address of your doctors, medications you are taking, and your treatment facility. If you are planning a trip, ask your doctor for an

extra order for a phlebotomy or medications in case you need them while away from home. It is not necessary to have any personal information on such a list; matters of that type should be handled through wills or kept separate from general health information. Obtain a copy of the Iron Disorders Institute Personal Health Profile form. This form is a great place to record lab work, to journal experiences, and to list important details such as medications and contact details.

One Last Thought

Some patients who have had numerous phlebotomies are encouraged to wear a medical ID bracelet noting hemochromatosis, as their veins will be similar in appearance to someone who abuses drugs.

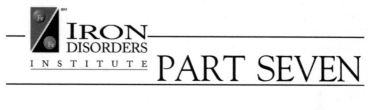

PART SEVEN

Support

39

About the Iron Disorders Institute

The Iron Disorders Institute (IDI) received its nonprofit status in 1998. The IDI exists so that anyone with an iron disorder receives early, accurate (complete) diagnosis and appropriate treatment, and is equipped to live in good health.

Iron Disorders Institute Logo

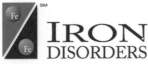

The IDI logo comprises two triangles, one red and the other one black, representing iron excess and insufficiency. Each triangle contains a ball depicting an atom with the letters *Fe*, which is the symbol for iron on the periodic table of the elements, used in chemistry. Together, they symbolize the two atoms of iron that is the limit one molecule of transferrin can hold and the iron contained in ferritin. The triangles, when placed together, create a diagonal slash representing TS percentage. As a whole, the logo symbolizes all things associated with iron balance in health.

Iron Disorders Institute Mascot

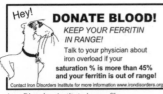

Iron Disorders Institute image file

The cartoon character C. R. Hume is a ferret who is featured on promotional materials used to raise awareness about the importance of periodically checking iron levels. His name is a play on words; when said rapidly, "C. R. Hume" is meant to sound like "serum," and since he is a ferret, he represents serum ferritin. A contest to determine the meaning of C. R.'s name was won by Arthur Callahan, of Memphis, Tennessee.

Products, Services, Programs, and Advocacy

Products

The IDI "Guide To" series is a set of handouts targeting patients and healthcare providers by focusing on one of four categories of iron disorders: iron deficiency anemia, anemia of chronic disease, iron overload with anemia, and hemochromatosis or iron overload. The set includes an introductory pamphlet designed to capture the attention of a person who may be at risk but is not yet diagnosed. A physician reference guide with diagnosis algorithm and other helpful charts is available for the physician and often delivered by the patient. Full-length books on the topic, such as *The Guide to Hemochromatosis, The Hemochromatosis Cookbook, The Guide to Anemia,* and *Exposing the Hidden Dangers of Iron,* are provided for patients and healthcare professionals. Record keeping—with journal forms such as the Personal Health Profile Form—helps patients consolidate data and information. Newsletters (*Nanograms)* and periodic reports (idInsight) detail iron health status and news. Websites keep information current with daily, weekly, and monthly updates.

Services

The IDI provides assistance connecting patients with healthcare providers, healthcare professionals with experts, and physicians with the most current best practices. The IDI offers online discussion and forums for both patients and healthcare providers and a toll-free number to request information.

Programs

The IDI carries out education programs in partnership with the U.S. Centers for Disease Control and Prevention, as well as numerous global healthcare organizations and establishments, with emphasis on the United States.

Advocacy

The IDI advocates for patients by ensuring that hemochromatosis remains a health priority among healthcare policy makers. The IDI organizes efforts to reach delegates and keep them apprised of our critical issues and needs. The IDI's efforts resulted in the first congressional budget line item to educate healthcare professionals about hemochromatosis.

Infrastructure

The IDI uses generally accepted accounting practices and relies on guidance and oversight from three boards. These include a governing board of directors, a medical and scientific advisory board, and an institutional review board.

The board of directors is the governing board for the organization. Members on this board assure that the executive director has both the means and the limitations to ensure that IDI will operate under the best possible environment. Members are a combination of businesspeople and medical professionals who develop policies that dictate limitations, goals, and objectives in terms of "ends" statements. Presently, the board members are Tim Roberson, chairman, of Greenville South Carolina; George Whittenburg, vice chairman, of Amarillo, Texas; Cheryl Garrison, of Greenville, South Carolina; Laura Main, of Newark, Ohio; Chad Bortle, of Newark, Ohio; Tom Gallagher, of Albany, New York; Aran Gordon, of London, England; Gerry Koenig, of Austin, Texas; Prad Phatak, MD, of Rochester, New York; and Herbert Bonkovsky, MD, of Charlotte, North Carolina.

The IDI Medical and Scientific Advisory Board comprises a group of experts who have extensive clinical experience with iron disorders such as hemochromatosis. Each expert represents a key area of importance, such as genetics, diagnosis, management, and body systems (heart, lungs, brain, bones and joints, hormone-producing organs, metabolism, infection, cancer, epidemiology, and surveillance). Members of this board ensure that the content of IDI's publications and programs is medically accurate, scientifically current, and recommends the best practices for patient care.

Members appear in alphabetical order here, except for

emeritus members at the end of the list. Their titles and a brief description of their area of expertise and interests is included. Since all of these individuals have published extensively, have served on multiple boards and panels, and are leaders in their field, we provide only a glimpse of their profile. To request a copy of their CVs or to invite them to presentations, contact the Iron Disorders Institute.

Iron Disorders Institute Medical and Scientific Advisory Board Members

Ann Aust, PhD, Department of Chemistry and Biochemistry, Utah State University

Dr. Aust is an expert in inhaled carcinogenic materials such as iron-containing asbestos and other particulates prominent in some U.S. environments.

Bruce R. Bacon, MD, Director, Division of Gastroenterology and Hepatology, Saint Louis University School of Medicine

Dr. Bacon is a gastroenterologist; he is an expert in liver diseases and is the cofounder and co–medical director of the Saint Louis University Liver Center.

George Bartzokis, MD, Brain Research Institute, David Geffen School of Medicine at UCLA Department of Neurology

Dr. Bartzokis is a psychiatrist and an expert in brain iron; his interests include investigating iron's role in aging and in neurodegenerative diseases such as Alzheimer's, Parkinson's, and multiple sclerosis. Dr. Bartzokis is the inventor of the MRI technique used to detect abnormal iron clusters in the brain.

Herbert L. Bonkovsky, MD, Chairman, Iron Disorders Institute Medical and Scientific Advisory Board

Dr. Bonkovsky is a gastroenterologist; he is an expert in iron metabolism and hepatic (liver) imaging techniques. He is the inventor of the MRI technique used to qualify and quantify hepatic (liver) iron. His areas of interest include porphyrin metabolism and imaging techniques such as MRI.

Arthur Caplan, PhD, director of bioethics University of Pennsylvania; and Chairman, Iron Disorders Institute Institutional Review Board

Dr. Caplan is a bioethicist; he is the Emanuel and Robert Hart Professor of Bioethics, chair of the Department of Medical Ethics, and director of the Center for Bioethics at the University of Pennsylvania in Philadelphia. His areas of interest include transplantation research ethics, genetics, reproductive technologies, health policy, and general bioethics. Dr. Caplan writes a regular column on bioethics for MSNBC.com.

James Connor, PhD, Professor and Vice Chair, Department of Neuroscience and Anatomy; Director, G. M. Leader Alzheimer's Disease Research Laboratory

Dr. Connor is a neuroscientist; he is an expert in the relationship between iron and neurodegenerative disease. He was one of the first to suspect an association between hemochromatosis or iron overload and depression. In his current work, he has identified an antibody to the divalent metal transporter DMT1, believed to play a significant role in iron absorption. Dr. Connor is also the director of the IDI–Pennsylvania State University Centers of Excellence at Hershey, Pennsylvania, which produced unique evidence of iron's role in Alzheimer's disease onset and the progress of some cancers.

James Cook, MD, University of Kansas Medical Center

Dr. Cook is a hematologist and oncologist, and an expert in iron balance. His area of interest is in iron-deficiency anemia, anemia of chronic disease, and iron-overload states. Dr. Cook participated in the early stages of discovery and use of the serum transferrin receptor (sTfR), a test that is not affected by inflammation in the way serum ferritin is affected.

Joanne M. Jordan, MD, MPH, Associate Professor, Medicine and Orthopaedics, University of North Carolina School of Medicine, Chapel Hill, North Carolina

Dr. Jordan is an expert in osteoarthritis, genetics of osteoarthritis, ethnic health disparities, biomarkers, heavy metal exposures, disability, and hemochromatosis arthropathy.

Kris Kowdley, MD, Virginia Mason Healthcare System, Seattle

Dr. Kowdley is a hepatologist; he is an expert in liver diseases and organ transplantation. He established one of the first hemochromatosis and iron disorders patient clinics in Seattle. His areas of interest include liver transplantation and hepatic scanning techniques.

John Longshore, PhD, Carolinas HealthCare System

Dr. Longshore is a laboratory scientist and an expert in molecular analysis. His findings in progress include possibility of higher prevalence of HFE mutation for hemochromatosis in the U.S. South and occurrence of C282Y in nonwhites.

Patrick MacPhail, MD, PhD, Department of Medicine, University of Witwatersrand

Dr. MacPhail is a hematologist and oncologist; he is an expert in African siderosis. His work includes research on the relationship between iron overload and genetics in Africans.

Arch Mainous III, PhD, Medical University of South Carolina, Charleston

Dr. Mainous is biostatistician; he is an expert in epidemiology and surveillance. He has synthesized decades of National Health and Nutrition Examination Survey (NHANES) data, providing some of the first consolidated evidence of excess iron and premature death.

Gordon McLaren, MD, University of California, Irvine, and VA Long Beach Healthcare System

Dr. McLaren is a hematologist and oncologist; he is professor in the Division of Hematology and Oncology at University of California Irvine Medical Center (UCIMC), Physician at the VA Long Beach Healthcare Center, and Medical Director of the UCI field center of the NIH-sponsored Hemochromatosis and Iron Overload Screening (HEIRS) Study.

Robert T. Means Jr., MD, University of Kentucky and Veteran's Administration Medical Center, Lexington, KY

Dr. Means is a professor of Internal Medicine, Division of Hematology, Oncology and Blood & Marrow Transplantation at the University of Kentucky Medical Center. He is also senior associate chair, Department of Internal Medicine, University of Kentucky College of Medicine. Dr. Mean's interest in iron includes iron's role in cancer and the inflammatory response.

David Meyers, MD, MPH, Department of Medicine, Division of Cardiovascular Disease, University of Kansas Hospital

Dr. Meyers is a cardiologist and an expert in cardiovascular disease. His more than two decades of work include writing the Kansas Primary Care Physicians Preventive Health Guidelines. He provides scientific substantiation of a connection to reduced incidence of cardiac arrest and frequency of blood donation.

P. D. Phatak, MD, Head of Hematology and Medical

Oncology, Rochester General Hospital; Vice Chairman, IDI Medical and Scientific Advisory Board

Dr. Phatak is a hematologist and oncologist; he is an expert in iron balance in blood and blood-forming organs, including cancers of those systems. He has led or participated in many large population-based studies of hemochromatosis prevalence, cost to treat, and genetic penetrance.

Mark Princell, MD, Spartanburg Regional Health Systems, South Carolina

Dr. Princell is a family practice physician; he is an expert in emergency services.

Barry Skikne, MD, University of Kansas Medical Center

Dr. Skikne is a hematologist and oncologist; he is an expert in iron balance, both excess and insufficiency. His years in the field include pioneer work on the serum transferrin receptor (sTfR)—a test that is not affected by inflammation in the way serum ferritin is affected.

Gene Weinberg, PhD, Professor of Microbiology, Indiana University

Dr. Weinberg is an expert in iron, infectious disease, and cancer. His work focuses on the prevention of chronic disease by lowering iron levels. He promotes reducing the amount of dietary iron and discontinuation of contributive factors to excess body iron, such as tobacco and alcohol use. His more than forty years of work in the field of iron's relationship to cancer has earned him prestige and recognition worldwide. His book *Exposing the Hidden Dangers of Iron* discusses iron's role in each of the body's systems.

Lewis Wesselius, MD, Mayo Clinic, Scottsdale, Arizona

Dr. Wesselius is a pulmonologist and associate professor of medicine at Mayo Clinic, and expert in iron in the lungs. His areas of interest include airways disease, lung cancer, occupational lung disease, and interstitial lung disease.

Mark Wurster, MD, Ohio State University

Dr. Wurster is a doctor of internal medicine and an expert in diagnostics. He established the first hemochromatosis patient centers in Ohio, at Ohio State University.

Leo R. Zacharski, MD, Dartmouth College, New Hampshire

Dr. Zacharski is a hematologist and oncologist, and professor of medicine at Norris Cotton Cancer Center, Dartmouth-Hitchcock Medical Center. Dr. Zacharski's areas of interest include iron's role in cancer and iron surveillance research.

Emeritus Medical and Scientific Advisory Board Members

The following esteemed scientists have served on the advisory board; their contributions continue to be acknowledged in IDI's materials.

Nancy Andrews, MD, PhD, Duke University School of Medicine

Dr. Andrews is a professor of pediatrics and of pharmacology and cancer biology. She led the team that cloned the HFE knockout mouse, which is used extensively in research. Her early contributions to IDI's reference charts include pediatric ranges for serum ferritin, TS percentages, and inputs to the normal ranges of serum ferritin for adults.

John Beard, PhD, formerly professor of Nutrition, Pennsylvania State University

Dr. Beard was a nutritionist and an expert of the effects of iron deficiency on cognitive and behavioral performance, thyroid metabolism, and thermoregulation. His work includes investigating the benefits of iron supplementation in youths, women of childbearing age, and the elderly. He was one of the first to serve on the Iron Disorders Institute Sceintific Board. John died suddenly in early 2009.

David Brandhagen, MD, formerly with the Department of Gastroenterology and Hepatology, Mayo Clinic

Dr. Brandhagen died tragically in an automobile accident in 2004; his work as a hepatologist specializing in diseases of the liver and liver transplantation continues to be cited and expanded on. In his practice, he treated more than two hundred hemochromatosis and iron-overload patients. His important clinical experience in HHC is accented by numerous awards and honors, including the 1998 American Federation of Medical Research Award.

Alan Buchanan, PhD, University of Arizona

Dr. Buchanan is a medical ethicist. The focus of his work is on the ethical, legal, moral, and social implications of genetic testing.

John Feder, PhD, Bristol-Meyers Squibb Pharmaceutical Research

Dr. Feder was a key participant on the HFE gene discovery team. Two prevalent mutations, C282Y and H63D, are now known to contribute to abnormal iron metabolism. His current work focuses on novel gene therapies, and he is an adviser to those pursuing genetic research.

Nancy Olivieri, MD, FRCP (C), Hemoglobinopathy Program, Hospital for Sick Children, Toronto

Dr. Olivieri is internationally known for her research and expertise in thalassemia. Over the past fifteen years, her work has included contributions to development of new approaches to therapy for those with thalassemia and sickle-cell anemia.

Jukka Salonen, MD, PhD, MSc, PH, Department of Medicine, University of Kuopio

Dr. Salonen, a leading epidemiologist, conducted the first major study of incidence of cardiac attack in men relative to ferritin levels. His ongoing work includes incidence of cardiac attack in heterozygotes.

40

Support across the United States and around the World

When people are first diagnosed with hemochromatosis, they experience an immediate heightened concern about the future of their health. This reality sensitizes them to their own mortality and to how hemochromatosis might affect their families. Unanswered questions about therapy, missed diagnoses, efforts to bring about awareness, research, and physician education can be overwhelming.

Reason can sometimes give way to emotion, especially when these individuals meet disinterest about hemochromatosis from their physicians. People can feel that they are waging war against an unseen adversary and that they are completely alone. The idea of being alone can frighten anyone, especially when a person's health is concerned. We all want to believe that, no matter how our health is today, there are groups of people working on behalf of such important matters as our health and well-being for the future and that support is available.

Outreach, Patient Advocacy, and Support
The Iron Disorders Institute has several alliances with other patient groups, governmental health agencies, policy makers, and industry leaders who are in a position to create or amend policies so that patients are protected and receive the best health care possible.

The IDI Network of Charitable Health Alliances is made up of a group of national and international voluntary health agencies that address various disease consequences of iron imbalances. The IDI often serves as the first contact for patients with questions about their health. Given our iron expertise, we educate patients about iron imbalances and then refer them to the appropriate alliance expert or support group that can address a specific need. An example of this type of partnership is exemplified in the IDI's relationship with the Arthritis Foundation. Excess iron is a risk factor for osteoarthritis and osteoporosis, two bone and joint diseases that the Arthritis Foundation addresses. Patients with hemochromatosis often have these two diseases as a consequence of HHC. Working together with IDI, the Arthritis Foundation publishes articles about iron imbalances in its magazine *Arthritis Today*. Also, IDI refers patients to the Arthritis Foundation for help with therapies and support. Moreover, IDI has on its advisory board a hemochromatosis arthritis expert who addresses questions or issues from the Arthritis Foundation. In this type of relationship, the patient receives the best access to care.

Ambassadors
Ambassadors are individuals who volunteer time to write, attend conferences, and distribute information about breaking news and events within their community.

Influential Health-Related Contributors
Health-related contributors include medical universities, treatment centers, genetic laboratories, the insurance industry, manufacturers of diagnostic aids and treatment equipment, publishers of health-related materials and media health resources, and organizations such as the American Medical Association, the American Clinical Laboratories Association, the American Society of Hematology, American Advancement for the Study of Liver Diseases, the American Academy of Family Physicians, etc.

Government Health Alliances
These include any government agency associated with health. The major agency is the U.S. Department of Health and Human Services, which encompasses the Centers for Disease Control and Prevention and the National Institutes of Health.

Other U.S. government health agencies include the Veterans Administration, the Food and Drug Administration, and the U.S. Department of Agriculture, for example.

Support Groups

The IDI offers different venues for support; in addition to its toll-free information line, patients can participate in local workshops and the IDI online discussion group Excess Iron List, which has been active for more than a decade and is a place where hundreds of patients register comments, ask questions, and learn about important issues pertaining to iron. From these dialogues, the IDI can identify education opportunities for patients and healthcare providers. Besides the online discussions, IDI works with a national network of treatment centers at blood donation facilities, universities, hospitals, and clinics. Periodic offerings of family workshops are made available at these centers. Another activity gaining popularity are educational web seminars offered by special invitation and hosted by IDI. In these seminars, topics of interest such as diet, genetics, and therapy are well received by patients and healthcare providers.

Community-Based Support Groups

One of the most successful patient support groups was created and maintained by Mardi Brick, of Santa Cruz, California. Mardi was motivated to help others because of her personal experience with hemochromatosis. Several family members died without a diagnosis. Mardi suspects hemochromatosis in most of these deaths because she is a C282Y homozygote. Her support group is called the Ironic Family, inspired by Roberta Crawford's book *Ironic Elephant*. The book is based on the Chinese parable about three blind men who come upon an elephant. Because they encounter different aspects of the elephant, their descriptions are totally different, which is not unlike the way hemochromatosis patients describe their experiences. In a book called *Hemochromatosis Adventures*, Mardi uses the theme of an African safari and highlights some of the adventures that she and patients in her group have embarked on in their journey with HHC. Her book is available through IDI Patient Services, which you can reach toll-free at (888) 565-4766.

The IDI's network of support-group coordinators is ever expanding. Coordinators are credentialed professionals such as registered nurses, physician's assistants, genetics counselors, physicians, teachers, and licensed nutritionists. Our concern is that the public receives answers to their questions from trained professionals rather than individuals who are not medically qualified to address questions. Foremost is the health and well-being of individuals with iron disorders. We encourage people to take charge of their health but to approach matters well informed and not to take action based on an emotionally charged event.

Other Organizations in the United States and around the World

The Iron Disorders Institute commends everyone who has worked to bring awareness to this most important health issue known as hemochromatosis or iron-overload disease. In an effort to strengthen an alliance between U.S. and international hemochromatosis organizations, Chris Kieffer, a founding director of IDI, contacted groups to participate. Organizations such as Iron Overload Diseases and the American Hemochromatosis Society were contacted to obtain permission to publish their mission statement or website information. Readers can visit their websites (www.ironoverload.org and www.americanshs.org) to learn about these two U.S. organizations. The American Hemochromatosis Society promotes IDI publications and provided the following information about the organization.

American Hemochromatosis Society

The American Hemochromatosis Society (AHS) was established in 1998, with headquarters in Del Ray Beach, Florida. Sandra Thomas is the founder and president. The mission of AHS is to educate and support the victims of HHC and their families, as well as to educate the medical community on the latest research on hemochromatosis. The aim of the AHS is to identify through genetic testing the more than 35 million Americans who unknowingly carrying the single- or double-gene mutation for HHC, which puts them at risk for loading excess iron.

The AHS recognizes and envisions that it is possible now and in the future to prevent needless deaths, disability, organ damage, costly joint replacements, and organ transplants caused by HHC or iron overload through the following:

- Routine and universal HHC screening of the American public
- DNA newborn HHC screening for all children in America
- Establishment of universal guidelines for diagnosis and treatment of HHC in children and adults
- Various AHS projects, which involve patient, family, community, and governmental cooperation and support for screening and awareness, including the Children HHelping Children Screening & Awareness Project for pediatric HHC, the Seniors HHelping Seniors Screening & Awareness Project for geriatric hereditary hemochromatosis, the Hereditary Hemochromatosis Congressional Challenge for DNA testing of all members of Congress, and the Hereditary Hemochromatosis Celebrity Challenge for DNA testing of celebrities, including those in the film and music industry.

Pioneers for Awareness, Outreach, and Education

Until the late 1970s, there were no formally organized groups addressing the issue of HHC. Few people at that time had actually been diagnosed. Mayo Clinic, an icon of U.S. health care, had only thirteen confirmed cases of hemochromatosis by the mid-1960s. The condition was thought to be rare, an older male's disease.

As the world grew smaller through television and air travel, and as people moved from city to city or even to different countries, information about hemochromatosis began to emerge. Through the efforts of individuals like Marie Warder, Dr. Margit Krikker, and Roberta Crawford, people with hemochromatosis gradually had a source of information. These pioneering women all shared a common goal: to raise awareness about hemochromatosis and iron overload.

Marie Warder organized an international hemochromatosis network that connected people worldwide on the issue. The Hemochromatosis Research Foundation in Albany, New York, founded by Dr. Margit Krikker, was the first U.S. organization to address hemochromatosis in America. Next was Iron Overload Diseases, of Palm Beach, Florida, founded by Roberta Crawford.

For the following twenty years, Warder, Krikker, and Crawford struggled to get the attention of physicians. They wrote countless letters, worked long hours, and gave generously of their time to speak anywhere in the world when asked to do so. Their stories are part of history and represent the beginnings of service to families with hemochromatosis or iron overload all over the world.

International Network Established

The Canadian Hemochromatosis Society, in Richmond, British Columbia, was founded by Marie Warder as one of the first international hemochromatosis patient groups. Marie's story demonstrates her motivation to reach out and help people with hemochromatosis.

Marie figured out long before her physician did that she was a carrier for hemochromatosis. Her husband, Tom, had been diagnosed in 1975, but not until their daughter Leigh was diagnosed in 1979 did Marie put it all together. Her family was living in Johannesburg, South Africa, at the time of Tom's diagnosis but had moved to Canada by the time Leigh received her diagnosis. For Marie, it was the love of her family that inspired her and drove her to challenge theories that had become entrenched in the minds of many physicians. One theory she was determined to dispel was that premenopausal females do not accumulate iron. She looked at her thirty-two-year-old daughter, who was living proof that menstruating females can indeed become overloaded with iron.

Marie wrote letters to newspapers and magazines but was met with indifference. As she encountered one family after another who seemed to find her regardless of where they lived in the world, Marie decided that an organization had to be established. In 1978 she started the Canadian Hemochromatosis Society (CHS). But it would be in November 1982, after three years of struggle with financial setbacks and government red tape, that the Canadian Hemochromatosis Society would finally be incorporated, with seven members.

By 1985 CHS had more than 450 members, and an international network began in South Africa and stretched around the world to Great Britain, Australia, and France. Marie's family—Leigh, Tom, and Shaun—helped her immeasurably to run the demanding network of societies. Marie appeared on television, in newspaper articles, and was written about in *Reader's Digest*. Her ardor was apparent when she challenged the Canadian Red Cross to take HHC blood, and when she persuaded Consumer and Corporate Affairs to change misleading "reduced iron" labels on food packages. Her drive to raise awareness, designating the month of May as HHC Awareness Month in Canada, resulted in the proper diagnosis of more than five hundred individuals. In June 1991, Marie was awarded the Canada Volunteer Award from the office of the health minister in recognition of her work. Her efforts are known throughout the United Kingdom, Ireland, Holland, Belgium, France, Germany, Australia, the United States, and South Africa.

The Bronze Killer, her book about the Warder family experience with hemochromatosis, is in its third printing. Now retired, Marie knows that her organization is in good hands. Charm Cottingham stepped in to continue a watchful eye over the organization that Marie had started some twenty years earlier. Charm's husband died early as a result of hemochromatosis. His autopsy revealed massive upper gastrointestinal hemorrhage secondary to esophageal varices, or varicose veins in the esophagus. He had hemochromatosis with cirrhosis, pancreatic atrophy, an enlarged heart, testicular atrophy and ascites, aortic valve damage, myocardial degeneration in the left ventricle, old renal infarcts, old right cerebral infarct, and old and recent splenic infarcts. He was only sixty-one. Charm continues to raise awareness on behalf of Canadians with hemochromatosis.

Today there is a growing number of hemochromatosis organizations with an international network, with representation in Australia, the United Kingdom, the Netherlands, Italy, South Africa, Spain, Belgium, Brazil, Ireland, Israel, France, the United States, the Ukraine, and New Zealand.

41
Role of U.S. Government Health Agencies

All governmental health agencies are funded by U.S. tax dollars specifically allocated to the various agencies. Nearly 20 percent of the total U.S. budget is distributed among these entities.

Reimbursement guidelines for physicians, provision of funding for research and development of new therapies or cures, epidemiology, and surveillance are some of the ways that governmental health agencies influence health care. Every U.S. citizen is affected by what these agencies do, whether or not we have private insurance. Knowing about how our governmental health agencies function will help bring about a better understanding of how the agencies contribute to the health and well-being of every U.S. citizen. Ideally, our government health agencies work hand in hand with patient advocacy groups to establish policies and to inform and educate the public.

Reimbursement guidelines are developed by the Health Care Finance Administration (HCFA) for Medicare. Physicians must follow these guidelines to be reimbursed for services, including the cost of laboratory tests for anyone receiving Medicare benefits. Because it is easier to maintain one set of operations policies and procedures, the guidelines also apply to patients not yet on Medicare. For this reason, whatever is enacted in law for Medicare will likely affect the population as a whole.

Research that is funded through the U.S. government is available in the form of grants, which scientists apply for periodically during the year. Grants are awarded on merit. The U.S.

Department of Health and Human Services is by far the largest grant-producing agency in America, sending out more than sixty thousand grants per year.

U.S. Department of Health and Human Services

The guardianship of U.S. health begins with the secretary of health and human services and the U.S. surgeon general. The first public statement about hemochromatosis was made by Dr. David Satcher, former assistant secretary of health and U.S. surgeon general: "Early detection of iron overload disease (such as hemochromatosis) represents a major chronic disease prevention opportunity. Detection and treatment (phlebotomy) for iron overload early in the course of the illness can substantially reduce the severity of the symptoms, organ damage, and death from associated chronic disease."

The U.S. Department of Health and Human Services comprises twelve operating divisions:

1. Office of the Surgeon General (under the Secretary of Health)
2. Agency for Healthcare Research and Quality
3. Agency for Toxic Substances and Disease Registry
4. Administration on Aging
5. Administration for Children and Families
6. Centers for Disease Control and Prevention
7. Food and Drug Administration
8. Health Care Financing Administration
9. Health Resources and Services Administration
10. Indian Health Service
11. National Institutes of Health
12. Substance Abuse and Mental Health Services Administration

Each operating division contributes in some way to the health and well-being of a hemochromatosis patient.

Centers for Disease Control and Prevention's Priorities for Hemochromatosis

- Educating healthcare providers about early diagnosis and treatment of the disorder
- Promoting laboratory standardization and quality assurance for diagnostic tests to provide an evidence-based response to universal screening issues and recommendations for diagnostic test cutoff points
- Improving the estimate of the prevalence of hemochromatosis and its associated morbidity and mortality in the United States
- Estimating the prevalence of iron overload within overload illnesses
- Describing the clinical course of the disorder
- Determining the risks and benefits of universal screening for early detection of hemochromatosis

National Institutes of Health

While many institutes of the NIH are directly or indirectly funding hemochromatosis and iron-related disease research, the following are most prominent in their funding efforts for this disorder:

National Institute of Diabetes and Digestive and Kidney Diseases

"Hereditary hemochromatosis is the most common genetic mutation known in the United States. The excessive iron accumulation in patients with the full-blown disease results in liver and heart failure, as well as diabetes and other ailments. Diagnosis has been a major problem, but the recent discovery of the gene, HFE, responsible for most cases of hereditary hemochromatosis, has revolutionized the opportunity both to understand and diagnose this genetic disorder. Clinical and basic science investigators are engaged in an intensive study of its cause and pathology. As a model genetic disease, hemochromatosis also will help us learn how to apply genetic knowledge to patient care and how to deal with societal implications of genetic diseases."
—David G. Badman, PhD, Hematology Program Director, Deputy Director for Basic Program Administration (retired)

Division of Kidney, Urologic, and Hematologic Diseases (DKUHD), National Institute of Diabetes and Digestive and Kidney Diseases (NIDDK), National Institutes of Health (NIH)

The NIDDK conducts and supports much of the clinical research on the diseases of internal medicine and related subspecialty fields, as well as many basic science disciplines. The institute's Division of Intramural Research encompasses the broad spectrum of metabolic diseases, such as diabetes, inborn errors of metabolism, endocrine disorders, mineral metabolism, digestive diseases, nutrition, urology and renal disease, and hematology. Basic research studies include biochemistry, nutrition, pathology, histochemistry, chemistry, physical biology, chemical biology, molecular biology, pharmacology, and toxicology.

The NIDDK's extramural research is organized into divisions of program areas. One is the Division of Diabetes, Endocrinology, and Metabolic Diseases (DEM). The division provides research funding and support for basic and clinical research in the areas of type 1 and type 2 diabetes and other metabolic disorders, including cystic fibrosis; endocrinology and endocrine disorders; obesity, neuroendocrinology, and energy balance; and development, metabolism, and basic biology of liver, fat, and endocrine tissues. The division also provides funding for the training and career development of individuals committed to academic and clinical research careers in these areas.

Division of Digestive Diseases and Nutrition

The Division of Digestive Diseases and Nutrition (DDN) has responsibility for managing programs in basic and clinical research, as well as training and career development, related to liver and biliary diseases; pancreatic diseases; gastrointestinal disease, including neuroendocrinology, motility, immunology, absorption, and transport in the gastrointestinal tract; nutrient metabolism; obesity; and eating disorders.

Division of Kidney, Urologic, and Hematologic Diseases

The Division of Kidney, Urologic, and Hematologic Diseases (KUH) provides research funding and support for basic and clinical research in areas of kidney disease, including end-stage renal disease, kidney disease of diabetes, IgA nephropathy, hemolytic uremic syndrome, polycystic kidney disease, hypertensive nephrosclerosis, acute renal failure and fluid and electrolyte disorders; urinary tract diseases, including benign prostatic hyperplasia, urinary tract infections, kidney stones, impotence, urinary incontinence, and interstitial cystitis; and disorders of the blood and blood-forming organs.

Past Hemochromatosis Research Funded by the NIDDK

- *Penn State College of Medicine*: To determine how the hemochromatosis protein normally controls iron absorption within the intestine. Humans have an automatic iron-regulation mechanism. In people with normal iron metabolism, this system allows us to take in more iron when needs are great, such as with growth spurts, blood loss, and trauma. This same system can reduce the amount of dietary iron absorbed when chronic illness is present. For those with hemochromatosis, an inborn error of metabolism, this regulatory process may contribute to excessive absorption of iron. This study will contribute to a better understanding of iron regulation in the gut.

The principal investigators are Dr. James R. Connor, of the Department of Neuroscience and Anatomy; Dr. Jing Hu and Dr. Harriet C. Isom, of the Departments of Microbiology and Immunology and Pathology; Dr. Edward E. Cable, research associate; Dr. Michael J. Chorney, of the Departments of Microbiology and Immunology and Pediatrics; Dr. John Beard, of the Nutrition Department; and Dr. Mel Billingsley, of the Department of Pharmacology and director of Hershey's Macromolecular Core Facility.

- *Kaiser Permanente/Scripps Research Institute*: To determine the gene frequency of the three HFE mutations (C282Y, H63D, S65C) and to relate genotypes to various clinical and laboratory values in 10,198 adults.

The principal investigators were Drs. Ernest Beutler, Vincent Felitti, Terri Gelbart, and Ngoc Ho.

The research program was begun in 1997 as a joint project with Dr. E. Beutler, of the Scripps Research Institute, and Dr.

V. Felitti, of Kaiser Permanente. It was funded with two grants from the NIDDK and supplemented with a grant from the CDC and the Stein Endowment Fund. Results of the observational study are published in the September 5, 2000, issue of *Annals of Internal Medicine* ("The Effect of HFE Genotypes on Measurements of Iron Overload in Patients Attending a Health Appraisal Clinic").

The National Heart, Lung, and Blood Institute

The National Heart, Lung, and Blood Institute (NHLBI) provides leadership for a national program in diseases of the heart, blood vessels, lungs, and blood; blood resources; and sleep disorders.

The NHLBI plans, conducts, fosters, and supports an integrated and coordinated program of basic research, clinical investigations and trials, observational studies, and demonstration and education projects. Research is related to the causes, prevention, diagnosis, and treatment of heart, blood vessel, lung, and blood diseases, and sleep disorders. The NHLBI plans and directs research in the development and evaluation of interventions and devices related to prevention, treatment, and rehabilitation of patients suffering from such diseases and disorders. It also supports research on clinical use of blood and all aspects of the management of blood resources. Research is conducted in the institute's own laboratories and by scientific institutions and individuals supported by research grants and contracts. For health professionals and the public, the NHLBI conducts educational activities, including the development and dissemination of materials in the foregoing areas, with an emphasis on prevention.

The NHLBI supports research training and career development of new and established researchers in fundamental sciences and clinical disciplines to enable them to conduct basic and clinical research related to heart, blood vessel, lung, and blood diseases; sleep disorders; and blood resources, through individual and institutional research training awards and career development awards.

The institute coordinates relevant activities in these areas, including the related causes of stroke, with other research institutes and federal health programs. Relationships are maintained with institutions and professional associations, and with international, national, state, and local officials, as well as with voluntary agencies and organizations working in the foregoing areas.

Hemochromatosis Research Funded by the NHLBI

As part of the NHLBI, the Warren G. Magnuson Clinical Center is the setting for the Hemochromatosis Protocol, a long-term study of HHC. Lead investigator Susan Leitman, MD, and her team of specialists accept eligible patients into the program. Therapy approaches such as double red-cell apheresis are available to patients who are candidates for this type of therapy. From the hemochromatosis protocol, we have some of the first solid evidence about reducing excess iron levels without forcing a patient to experience the symptoms and discomfort of iron-deficiency anemia.

The NHLBI and the National Human Genome Research Institute (NHGRI) jointly funded a multicenter, multiethnic, primary care–based sample of one hundred thousand adults in a five-year study to determine the epidemiology of HFE prevalence; the genetic and environmental determinants; and the potential clinical, personal, and social impacts of iron overload and HHC, called HEIRS (Hemochromatosis–Iron Overload Study).

Contributors to the investigation in the field centers include Ronald Acton, MD, University of Alabama; Paul Adams, MD, London Health Sciences Centre, London, Ontario, Canada; Victor Gordeuk, MD, Howard University; Christine McLaren, PhD, University of California, Irvine; and Emily Harris, PhD, Kaiser Permanente Center for Health Research, Portland. Contributors in the central lab include John Eckfeldt, MD, PhD, University of Minnesota, and in the data-coordinating center, David Reboussin, PhD, Wake Forest University.

National Institute of Neurological Disorders and Stroke

The National Institute of Neurological Disorders and Stroke (NINDS) supports the study of stroke, sleep disorders, epilepsy, Alzheimer's, Parkinson's, multiple sclerosis, restless legs syndrome,

ADD/ADHD, and depression, all conditions known to be related to iron imbalances.

The NINDS has provided grants for three different research projects, with principal investigators Drs. James Connor, Department of Neuroscience and Anatomy, and John Beard, Department of Nutrition, Penn State University. There is a known link with iron to such neurological problems as Alzheimer's, early-onset Parkinson's, ADD/ADHD, depression, epilepsy, hypothyroidism, and hypogonadism. These three critically important research projects will be helpful in understanding the mechanisms by which iron influences these illnesses. The three research programs are to study the dynamics of iron transport into the brain to determine the role of iron in the outcome of infants who are hypoxic or ischemic at birth and to determine whether the brain regulates iron uptake, and if so, how.

*   *   *

The Iron Disorders Institute continues to advocate for you. Learn about ways you can help us carry out our mission. The Iron Disorders Institute exists so that any person with an iron disorder receives early, accurate diagnosis and appropriate treatment, and is equipped to live in good health.

Visit our websites: www.irondisorders.org and www. hemochromatosis.org.

Appendix A:
QUICK Checklist for Physicians

This checklist provides the necessary basics such as the routine blood tests and a sample order for phlebotomy. This would be a good checklist to cut out and post on your refrigerator so you can take a look before visiting the doctor or to keep in your pocket as a handy reference.

QUICK Checklist for Physicians

A. Tests to Determine Iron Status
  1. Serum iron (fasting)
  2. Total iron-binding capacity (TIBC)
  3. Serum ferritin
  4. SI divided by TIBC × 100 = transferrin-iron saturation percentage (TS%)
  5. Complete blood count

B. Begin Therapy Promptly
Patients with serum ferritin greater than 1,000 ng/mL at the time of diagnosis are at increased risk for liver damage.

C. Avoid Overbleeding
Sample phlebotomy order:
Phlebotomize 500 cc once a week [the period should reflect frequency] if Hgb ≥ 12.5g/dL (approximate hematocrit of 38%)

D. MCV will drop by ~3% when iron levels are in a healthy range

This checklist is based on a large body of evidence and clinical expert opinion. A bibliography or citations for the basis of these recommendations is available by request from **info@irondisorders.org.**

Download a PDF copy of the Iron Disorders Institute Hemochromatosis Reference Chart, which includes reference ranges, a diagnostic algorithm, treatment options and frequency guidelines, genetics and diet information. Also see QUICK Checklist for Patients.

Appendix B:
QUICK Checklist for Patients

This checklist sums up the important things to remember as a patient. Once you get familiar with your condition, this checklist can serve as a reminder of the basics.

QUICK Checklist for Patients

A. Keep records of your iron-profile test results
1. Serum iron (fasting)
2. Total iron-binding capacity (TIBC)
3. Serum ferritin (SF)
4. SI divided by TIBC × 100 = transferrin-iron saturation percentage (TS%)
5. Complete blood count

B. Cut back on or avoid alcohol, red meat, and supplemental vitamin C, and do not eat raw shellfish.

C. Keep iron in a healthy range: TS% 25–35; SF 25–75 ng/mL

D. Keep learning: hemochromatosis is with you for the rest of your life.

See Physician's QUICK Checklist.

Glossary

absolute neutrophil count: a measure of the actual number of neutrophils present in the blood per unit volume.

aceruloplasminemia: lack of ceruloplasmin, a copper-containing serum protein essential for normal function of transferrin-iron transport

acidosis: a condition resulting from accumulation of too much acid in the body as a result of excess carbon dioxide. Acidic individuals may sigh frequently, have insomnia, or suffer from migraines. Neutral pH is 7.0—greater than 7.0 is alkaline, less than 7.0 is acidic. Ideal body pH is around 7.4.

acquired immune deficiency syndrome (AIDS): a usually fatal condition whereby the immune system loses the ability to fight infection because of the human immunodeficiency virus (HIV), which can be contracted from sexual contact with an infected person, use of a syringe also used by an infected person, or from an infected mother who passes the virus to a fetus.

acquired nonreversible sideroblastic anemias: forms of sideroblastic anemia that occur later in life and for which the cause cannot be reversed. Also called acquired idiopathic SA.

acquired reversible sideroblastic anemias: forms of sideroblastic anemia that can be reversed by eliminating the cause, such as nutritional deficiencies or use of certain drugs.

activated partial thromboplastin time (APTT): (or partial thromboplastin time) a test that measures the intrinsic clotting time in plasma.

acute: occurring suddenly and severely but of short duration; can define "sharp" pain.

Addison's disease or syndrome (adrenal insufficiency): inactive or underactive adrenal function.

adhesions: bands of fibrous tissue that cause organs to abnormally bind together, most commonly found in the abdomen, frequently following surgery. Can cause abdominal pain.

adrenal cortex: the outer layer of the adrenal gland where various hormones, including cortisone, estrogen, testosterone, cortisol, androgen, aldosterone, and progesterone are secreted

adrenal gland: a pair of triangle-shaped ductless hormone glands that rest above the kidneys; part of the endocrine system. They secrete hormones, including adrenaline (from the adrenal medulla) and cortisol, aldosterone, and adrenal androgens (from the adrenal cortex).

adrenal insufficiency: see *Addison's disease.*

adrenal medulla: the middle part of the adrenal gland that secretes epinephrine (same as adrenaline) and the neurotransmitter norepinephrine.

adrenocorticotropic hormone (ACTH): hormone secreted by the anterior pituitary gland that stimulates adrenal glands to secrete hormones such as cortisone, the body's natural pain-reliever. ACTH is secreted during moments of stress, trauma, major surgery, and fever.

adrenocorticotropic hormone (ACTH) deficiency: a condition in which the pituitary produces too little ACTH.

advanced directive: written instructions, as in a living will, whereby all hospitalized patients have a form on file indicating their desires.

alanine aminotransferase (ALT): an enzyme (see also *SGPT*) that can concentrate in muscles, liver, and brain. Increased levels indicate cell death or disease in these tissues.

aldosterone: a hormone excreted by the adrenal cortex; indirectly regulates blood levels of potassium and chloride, bicarbonate, as well as pH, blood volume, and blood pressure.

alkaline phosphatase (ALP): an enzyme that is concentrated in developing bone, plasma, and kidney and is excreted by the liver. Increased levels may indicate biliary obstruction or diseases of the pancreas, lung, liver, or bone. ALP can also be naturally elevated in youths who are experiencing bone growth.

alkalosis: abnormal condition in which body fluids are more alkaline than normal.

allele: any one of a series of two or more different genes that occupy the same position (locus) on a chromosome. Since autosomal chromosomes are paired, each autosomal locus is represented twice. If both chromosomes have the same allele occupying the same locus, the condition is referred to as homozygote for that allele. If the alleles at the two loci are different, the individual or cell is referred to as heterozygous for both alleles.

allergen: a substance that causes an allergic reaction.

allogeneic bone marrow transplantation: process in which bone marrow cells from a donor are infused into a patient.

alpha-fetoprotein (AFP): an oncofetal protein produced by the fetal liver and yolk sac during the first trimester. Increased maternal serum levels may indicate neural tube or abdominal wall defects in the fetus. Increased nonmaternal AFP may indicate tumor development in the breast, ovaries or testes, kidney, or liver.

alveolus (alveoli, pl.): tiny air sacs in the lungs where the exchange of carbon dioxide and oxygen occurs.

Alzheimer's disease: Named for the neurologist Alois Alzheimer (1864–1915). A chronic, progressive disorder that accounts for more than 50 percent of all cases of dementia.

amenorrhea: cessation of menstruation for at least three months in a woman who has previously menstruated. Causes include pregnancy, breast-feeding, eating disorders, endocrine disorders, psychological disorders, menopause (usually thirty-five years of age or older), surgical removal of the uterus or ovaries, or very strenuous athletic activities.

amino acids: organic compounds mostly made of proteins. The body contains at least twenty amino acids. Ten are essential, which means that the body does not make or form these, so they must be acquired through diet.

aminoglycosides: a class of antibacterial antibiotics that includes amikacin, gentamicin, kanamycin, neomycin, netilomycin, streptomycin, and tobramycin. Can combine with iron to cause damage to kidneys and hearing.

amosite: a form of carcinogenic asbestos with a high content of iron.

amylase: a type of enzyme that splits starches; classed as either alpha (found in animals) or beta (found in plants).

amyloidosis: disorder in which starchlike glycoproteins (amyloids) accumulate in tissues, impairing function.

anaphylaxis: also called anaphylactic shock, a severe allergic reaction to a foreign substance that the patient has had contact with. Infused or injected iron can cause anaphylaxis in some patients.

androgens: hormones that stimulate pubic and underarm hair growth in both males and females but that are produced in much greater quantities (especially testosterone from the testes) and are more important in stimulating and maintaining secondary sexual characteristics in males.

androstenedione: hormone; precursor of testosterone and estrogen. Increased levels may indicate adrenal tumor or congenital adrenal hyperplasia.

anemia: reduced red blood cell mass; condition in which the iron needs exceed the supply of iron in the body. See *anemia of chronic disease, aplastic, Cooley's, Falconi's, hemolytic, iron deficiency, pernicious, pyridoxine-responsive, sickle cell, sideroblastic, thalassemia.*

anemia, aplastic: serious disease caused by a failure of the bone marrow to produce blood cells. Symptoms may include paleness; weakness; bleeding from the nose, mouth, rectum, or internally; frequent infection; and unexplained bruising. May be caused by neoplasm (tumor) or destruction of the bone marrow by exposure to certain chemicals, anticancer drugs, immunosuppressive drugs, or antibiotics. Cause is sometimes unknown. Curable if cause can be identified and treated successfully.

anemia, Cooley's: (also known as thalassemia) inherited disorder in which a recessive trait is responsible for interference with hemoglobin synthesis.

anemia of chronic disease: mild anemia that accompanies the body's inflammatory defense mechanisms during episodes of infection, cancer, and other specific disorders.

anemia, hemolytic: inherited disorder in which premature destruction of mature red blood cells occurs.

anemia, hypoplastic: failure of the bone marrow to produce one or several blood cells or an overall reduction of all blood cells. In hypoplastic anemias, one or more types of blood cells are affected, compared with aplastic anemia, in which all types of cells are affected.

anemia, iron-deficiency: anemia caused by blood loss, dietary insufficiencies, or rapid growth in which iron demands exceed intake and stores.

anemia, megaloblastic: a type of anemia in which red blood cells that are larger than normal, usually resulting from a deficiency of folic acid or vitamin B12.

anemia, pernicious: anemia caused by inadequate absorption of vitamin B12 due to the absence of intrinsic factor, a chemical secreted by mucous membranes of stomach anemia, pyridoxine-responsive; corrected by treatment with pyridoxine (B6)

anemia, pyridoxine-responsive: an anemia that responds to pyridoxine (B6) treatment.

anemia, renal disease: anemia associated with acute and chronic renal failure.

anemia, sickle-cell: severe, incurable anemia that occurs in people who have an abnormal form of hemoglobin in their blood cells. It is an inherited disease and derives its name from the sickle-shaped cells that are present with the disorder.

anemia, sideroblastic: type of anemia in which the bone marrow deposits iron prematurely into red blood cells. The cells do not transport oxygen to the body as efficiently as normal cells.

anemia, thalassemia major: see *anemia, Cooley's.*

anesthesiologist: see *physicians, types of.*

angina: chest pain or pressure usually beneath the sternum (breastbone). Caused by inadequate blood supply to the heart. Often brought on by exercise, emotional upset, or heavy meals in someone who has heart disease.

angiocardiography: cardiac catheterization used to visualize the heart chambers, arteries, and veins.

angiography: (or arteriography) an X-ray technique used to determine blood-flow abnormalities and some tumors, and to pinpoint internal bleeding. Radiopaque contrast material is injected into the desired artery during X-ray. Blood-flow abnormalities and tumors can be easily seen using this procedure.

angiomas: benign tumors, usually congenital, made up of mostly blood vessels or lymph vessels.

angioplasty: the use of surgery to make a damaged blood vessel function properly again; may involve widening or reconstructing the blood vessel.

angiotension-converting enzyme (ACE) inhibitor: a drug used to treat high blood pressure that decreases pressure inside blood vessels.

anisocytosis: excessive variation in red cell size; presence of red blood cells with increased variability as measured by red-cell distribution width (RDW).

anterior pituitary: master endocrine gland at base of brain; its hormone-producing cells are very sensitive to iron toxicity.

antibody: a protein made by white blood cells that reacts with a specific foreign protein as part of the immune response; fights infection or harmful foreign substances (antigens).

antidiuretic: substance that controls the amount of water reabsorbed by the kidney.

antigen: a marker on the surface of cells that identifies what type of cell it is. A substance that stimulates the formation of a specific antibody and that will combine with that antibody.

antinuclear antibody (ANA): used to diagnose various autoimmune diseases, such as rheumatoid arthritis, scleroderma, or systemic lupus erythematosus.

antioxidant: a chemical that can neutralize or destroy oxygen radicals that have been formed by the catalytic action of iron.

apheresis: a therapeutic procedure in which whole blood is removed from the patient or donor and blood components such as red cells, leukocytes, and plasma are separated. Can be used to treat conditions such as iron overload or sickle-cell anemia.

aplastic: failure of an organ or tissue to develop normally.

apoptosis: programmed cell death; the body's normal method of disposing of damaged, unwanted or unneeded cells.

arrhythmia: an irregular heartbeat. May be rapid or seem to skip beats. May be due to iron loading of cardiac cells

arthralgia: pain in a joint.

arthritis: inflammatory condition of the joints, characterized by pain, stiffness, and swelling. See *rheumatoid* and *seronegative rheumatoid arthritis.*

arthrography/arthrogram: X-ray of a joint with contrast dye.

arthropathy: disease of a joint.

arthroscopy: a procedure that allows direct examination of the interior of a joint using an endoscope.

ascites: accumulation of fluid in the abdomen; may be a complication of cirrhosis, congestive heart failure, kidney malfunction, cancer, peritonitis, or various fungal and parasitic diseases.

aspartate aminotransferase (AST): a liver enzyme concentrated in the muscles, liver, and brain. Increased levels may indicate liver diseases such as hepatitis, cirrhosis, or tumors.

aspiration: withdrawal by suction of fluids, air, or foreign bodies.

ataxia: defective muscular coordination, as in an unsteady gait.

atherosclerosis: common disorder of the arteries characterized by thickening, loss of elasticity, and calcification of artery walls. Results in decreased blood supply to the brain and lower extremities. Typical signs include pain on walking, poor circulation in feet and legs, headache, dizziness, and memory defects.

atransferrinemia: congenital disorder in which little or no transferrin is produced.

atrophy: the wasting away of a tissue or organ.

autoantibody: an antibody made by a person's body that reacts with his or her own tissues.

autoimmune disease: a disorder in which the body's immune system attacks itself; sometimes referred to as autoimmune response.

autoimmune hemolytic anemia: a condition in which antibodies attack the red blood cells, causing them to be prematurely destroyed.

autoimmune thyroiditis: chronic inflammation that can lead to Graves' disease (hyperthyroidism) or hypothyroidism if the thyroid gland diminishes in size. See *Hashimoto's thyroiditis, hypothyroidism.*

autosomal dominant: a pattern of inheritance in which the dominant gene on any non–sex chromosome carries the defect.

autosomal gene: located on a non–sex chromosome.

autosomal recessive: non–sex chromosome in which two defective gene copies must be inherited, one from each parent, for a disease to manifest itself.

bacteria: plural of *bacterium*; tiny, single-celled microorganisms. Some are naturally present in the intestinal tract; some are pathogenic and can cause disease.

bacteriuria: the presence of bacteria in the urine.

basal ganglia: collection of nerve cell bodies.

basophils: a type of white blood cell responsible for controlling inflammation and damage of tissues in the body.

benign: noncancerous tumor or growth that does not interfere with normal function.

beta-blocker: a drug used to treat hypertension (high blood pressure), heart arrhythmia, circulation, and sometimes angina or migraine. Drug slows the heart rate and reduces pressure inside blood vessels. Beta-blockers can also regulate heart rhythm.

bile duct: passages that convey bile from the liver to the hepatic duct, which joins the duct from the gallbladder to form the common bile duct, which enters the duodenum.

biliary disease cirrhosis: a form of liver cirrhosis marked by enlargement of the liver and jaundice.

bilirubin: red-blood-cell waste product in bile; blood carries it to the liver. Orange-yellow in color, it contributes to the yellow color of urine. Abnormal accumulation of bilirubin in the blood and skin results in jaundice. Increased bilirubin level may also be involved in extensive liver damage.

biopsy: removal of a small amount of tissue or fluid, usually by needle, for laboratory examination; aids in diagnosis.

blast cells: immature cells that mature into various blood cells.

bleeding, gastrointestinal: condition of internal blood loss occurring somewhere in the digestive system: esophagus, stomach, small and large intestine.

bleeding time: lab test performed to determine the time for blood flow to cease (normally two to eight minutes).

blood: liquid pumped by the heart through arteries, veins, and capillaries. Blood consists of a pale yellow fluid called plasma, red blood cells (erythrocytes), white blood cells (leukocytes), platelets (thrombocyte-essential blood-clotting element), and suspended chemicals, hormones, proteins, fats, and carbohydrates. Men have about 70 ml/kg of body weight and women about 65 ml/kg. See *plasma*.

blood pressure: measure of tension caused by blood pressing against the walls of the arteries as it flows through the body.

blood sugar: measure of glucose in the blood.

276

blood test: a lab procedure in which blood is drawn from the arm, a port, or obtained by finger prick to examine for specific values such as blood cell size, shape, color, and volume, or the presence of specific abnormalities or disease.

blood urea nitrogen (BUN): a blood test that measures the amount of urea nitrogen in the blood; used to determine liver and kidney function.

bone marrow: specialized soft tissue that fills the core of bones, especially the sternum and long bones. Yellow marrow consists primarily of fats and does not participate in hematopoiesis (blood cell production). Red marrow produces all the types of blood cells. Most of the body's red and white blood cells are produced in bone marrow.

bone marrow aspiration: removal of a portion of the soft organic material filling the cavities of the bone. Used to evaluate and diagnose many blood diseases such as anemia, leukemia, iron storage deficiency, bone marrow deficiencies, or identification of tumors.

bone marrow transplant: procedure in which bone marrow filled with disease is destroyed by radiation or chemotherapy and then replaced with healthy cells from a donor. Therapeutic use of bone marrow from healthy, antigen-matched donor in patients who have a variety of neoplastic or metabolic diseases.

brain infarctions: localized area of brain tissue death resulting from lack of oxygen to that area because of an interruption in blood supply. Severity of symptoms following brain infarction depends on the location of the infarct and the extent of damage. See *infarction*.

breast cancer: a malignancy of the breast.

cachexia: weakness, loss of appetite, or emaciation associated with serious infection or cancer.

calcification: a process in which organic tissue becomes hardened by the deposition of minerals such as calcium when the mineral calcium contained in the blood is deposited into tissues from injury, infection, or aging. Often it is part of healing and not a sign of active disease, but it can lead to impaired organ function such as in kidneys and arteries.

calcitonin: a hormone produced by the parathyroid glands that affects levels of calcium in the blood.

calcium: mineral contained in the blood that helps regulate the heartbeat, transmit nerve impulses, contract muscles, and form bones and teeth.

calcium channel blocker (CCB): a drug used to relax the blood vessels and heart muscle, causing pressure inside blood vessels to drop. CCB drugs can be used to regulate heart rhythm.

cancer: abnormal and malignant growth of cells that invade nearby tissues, often spreading (metastasizing); also called carcinoma.

***Candida* (*C. albicans*):** a genus of yeasts (fungi) that is part of the normal body flora found in the mouth, skin, intestinal tract, and vagina. Abnormal growth of *Candida* results in a yeast infection called candidiasis.

carcinogen: a chemical or radioactive agent that induces normal cells to become malignant.

cardiac arrest: a sudden stop of heart function; "sudden death."

cardiac catheterization: a procedure in which a thin hollow tube is inserted into a blood vessel. The tube is then advanced through the vessel into the heart, enabling a physician to study the heart and its pumping activity.

cardiac enzymes: various enzymes that are indicative of injury to the heart, such as creatine kinase (CK), aspartate aminotransferase (AST), and lactate dehydrogenase (LDH), which are of variable specificity to cardiac muscle.

cardiologist: see *physicians, types of.*

cardiomyopathy: disease that weakens the heart muscle so that the heart cannot efficiently pump blood. May be curable if the underlying cause is curable, such as quitting smoking or drinking.

cardiotoxicity: damage to heart muscle cells as by certain anticancer drugs (e.g., adriamycin) that combine with iron; an iron-trapping agent (dexrazoxane) may be employed with the anticancer drug

case-control study: comparison of cases with healthy controls matched for such factors as age and sex.

catabolize: to break down complex chemical compounds into simpler ones.

celiac disease: (also called celiac sprue) a malabsorption disease caused by an intolerance for gluten, a protein present in most grains, which affects the jejunal portion of the small intestine.

cerebellum: the portion of the brain lying below the cerebrum and above the pons and medulla.

cerebrospinal fluid (CSF): a clear, normally colorless, and blood-free fluid that cushions and nourishes the brain and spinal cord.

ceruloplasmin (Cp): a blood glycoprotein that binds with copper but is also essential to the transport of iron; most of the copper in the blood is attached to it. An increased Cp level may indicate biliary cirrhosis or infection, while decreased Cp level are present in Wilson's disease or hemochromatosis.

chelator: chemical agents that can tightly bind one or more transition series metals such as iron, manganese, zinc, or copper; pharmaceutical strengths are specially formulated to bind with iron and might on rare occasions be prescribed for hemochromatosis patients with exceptional complications and very high levels of iron.

chemotherapy: treatment of cancer with medication intended to kill cancer cells without harming healthy tissue. Used to treat cancers that cannot be completely cured or treated with surgery or radiation.

cholelithiasis: gallstones.

cholesterol: complex chemical produced by the liver and contained in dietary fats that is transported through the bloodstream attached to lipoproteins. Low-density lipoproteins (LDLs) carry cholesterol that builds up plaque; high-density lipoproteins (HDLs) carry cholesterol to the liver where the body can get rid of it.

chondrosarcoma: a cancer arising in cartilage cells.

chromosome: structures inside the nucleus of living cells that contain hereditary information (DNA).

chronic: long-term, or continuing. Chronic illnesses are usually not curable, but they can often be prevented from worsening by controlling symptoms.

chrysotile: form of asbestos that comprises mainly magnesium (rather than iron) silicate and that is much less carcinogenic than forms that contain high iron.

cirrhosis: a chronic disease of the liver in which scar tissue replaces normal, healthy tissue, causing loss of function of liver cells and decreased blood flow through the liver.

coagulation, blood: the process of lumping together blood cells to form a clot.

colitis: inflammatory condition of the large intestine. It can occur in episodes, such as irritable bowel syndrome, or it can be one of the more serious, chronic, progressive, inflammatory bowel diseases, such as ulcerative colitis. Irritable bowel syndrome is characterized by bouts of colicky abdominal pain, bloating, diarrhea or constipation, and fatigue, often due to emotional stress. Treatment includes stress reduction, diet changes, and sometimes medication.

collagen: albuminoid substance of the white fibers of connective tissue, cartilage, and bone.

colonoscopy: investigation of the inside of the colon using a long, flexible fiber-optic tube called an endoscope.

colony-stimulating factors: cytokines (hormones) that stimulate the formation of various kinds of blood cells.

colostrum: the first milk secreted after the birth of the child; has an unusually high content of lactoferrin, which is instrumental in suppressing potential pathogenic bacteria in the infant's intestine.

complement: a system of serum proteins that work to help antibodies destroy antigens.

complete blood count (CBC): usually includes hemoglobin, hematocrit, the number of red and white cells, mean corpuscular volume (MCV), mean corpuscular hemoglobin (MCH), and the mean corpuscular hemoglobin concentration (MCHC).

compound heterozygote: in hereditary hemochromatosis, a patient who has inherited a single CY mutation and a single HD mutation.

computed tomography (CT): sometimes called a CAT scan. A technique used in radiology in which a three-dimensional image of a body structure is constructed by computer. Beams pass through the body and are detected by sensors. Information from sensors is computer processed and then displayed as an image on a televisionlike screen. Sometimes contrast agents are used to block certain tissues. Tumors, primary and metastatic, show up as bright white spots on the film.

congenital: present at, and existing from, the time of birth.

congestion: abnormal fluid accumulation in the body, especially the lungs.

congestive heart failure: life-threatening condition in which the heart loses its full pumping capacity and fluid accumulates in the lungs, causing shortness of breath. Usually accompanied by fatigue and edema (abnormal accumulation of fluid in body tissues) in the extremities.

connective-tissue disease (collagen disease): any one of many abnormal conditions characterized by inflammatory changes in small blood vessels and connective tissue. Some collagen diseases include systemic lupus erythematosus (chronic inflammation resulting in arthritis), scleroderma (autoimmune disease resulting in hardening of the skin), polymyositis (muscle inflammation), and rheumatic fever (resulting in heart valve damage).

Coombs' (direct): test used to identify hemolysis due to autoimmune reaction.

Coombs' (indirect): test used to detect circulating antibodies to red blood cells.

coronary: encircling, as the blood vessels that supply blood directly to the heart muscle; loosely used to refer to the heart and to coronary artery disease.

coronary thrombosis: presence of blood clot obstructing the coronary artery and flow of blood to the heart.

corticosteroids: hormones produced by the adrenal cortex that regulate sexual function, salt and water balance, the body's response to stress, metabolism, and immune system function.

corticotropin: a hormone released by the pituitary gland that stimulates the adrenal glands' production of hormones.

cortisol: (also called hydrocortisone) a hormone released by the adrenal cortex that affects the metabolism of fats, carbohydrates, and proteins.

creatine phosphokinase (CPK, CP, or CK): an enzyme found predominantly in the heart muscle, skeletal muscle, and the brain. Elevated levels indicate damage to these organs.

creatinine: compound found in the blood, urine, and muscle tissue. Elevated creatinine in the blood usually indicates the presence of kidney disease.

crocidolite: highly carcinogenic form of asbestos with very high content of iron silicate.

Crohn's disease: chronic inflammatory condition primarily involving the colon and the terminal portion of the small intestines, but can be present in the mouth, esophagus, stomach, duodenum, appendix, rectum, and anus.

cross-match: type and cross; test in which the blood cells of a donor and a recipient are mixed together to determine whether they are compatible.

culture: procedure used to identify the source of infection; specimen of blood, urine, sputum, or stool is taken and tested to determine the type of infection and the appropriate antibiotic.

cytokines: chemicals made by the cells that act on other cells to stimulate or inhibit their function; hormonelike proteins secreted by many different cell types that regulate cell proliferation and function; for example, cytokines that stimulate growth are called growth factors.

cytopenia: a deficiency of cells in the blood.

cytotoxic: destructive to cells.

DCT1: divalent cation transporter No. 1; enables enterocytes to accumulate various essential metal ions from diet.

deferasirox: (marketed as Exjade), oral iron chelator.

deferiprone: oral iron-chelating drug used by thalassemic patients in India and Europe; not yet available in the United States.

deferoxamine: a drug used in iron-chelation therapy.

Delaney amendment: passed by U.S. Congress in 1970s to prevent adulteration of U.S. foods by carcinogens. Unfortunately, iron (a well-known carcinogen) was exempted because its addition to foods in the U.S. had begun in earlier decades.

deoxyribonucleic acid (DNA): the chemical in the cell nucleus that carries the genetic instructions for producing new cells.

depression: a condition accompanied by feelings of hopelessness, sadness, and discouragement, often with inability to function or participate in activities. A depressed person can have dramatic weight changes and sleep disturbances.

dermatitis herpetiformis: a chronic disease of the skin marked by a symmetric itching eruption of vesicles and papules that occur in groups; relapses are common; associated with gluten-sensitive enteropathy and IgA immune complexes beneath the epidermis of lesioned and normal-appearing skin.

Desferal: injectable iron-chelating drug used by patients with iron overload and anemia.

desmopressin (DDAVP): synthetic drug that resembles vasopressin. It is used in nonreplacement treatment for von Willebrand's disease.

diabetes: either of two disorders, diabetes insipidus or diabetes mellitus. Diabetes insipidus is a metabolic disorder of the hormone system caused by a deficiency of antidiuretic hormone (ADH) normally secreted by the pituitary gland and is usually a temporary condition. Diabetes mellitus is a chronic metabolic disorder due to insufficient or ineffective insulin. Two forms of diabetes mellitus are type 1 (or juvenile-onset diabetes) and type 2 (or adult-onset diabetes). Insulin-dependent people are those with an inability to produce enough insulin to process carbohydrates, fat, and protein efficiently and so require insulin injections. Non-insulin-dependent people are most prevalent among obese adults. Often controlled with weight loss, exercise, and diet.

diabetic coma: result of not taking insulin properly or from the presence of stress from surgery, infection, or improper diet. Warning signs include increased thirst, vomiting, nausea, and headache.

diabetic ketoacidosis: serious complication of diabetes mellitus in which the body produces acids that cause fluid and electrolyte disorders, dehydration, and sometimes coma.

diabetic retinopathy: vision disorder seen most frequently in people who have had poorly controlled insulin-dependent diabetes mellitus for several years; can lead to loss of vision.

dialysis: medical procedure for filtering waste products from the blood of some patients with kidney disease.

differential: percentage of different types of blood cells in the blood. In diagnosis, a particular test or procedure that helps to narrow the possible causes of an illness.

digitalis: a drug used to increase the force of the heart's contraction and to regulate specific irregularities of heart rhythm.

dilated cardiomyopathy: enlargement of the heart's chambers, causing the heart to lose its pumping ability.

diuretic: a drug that helps eliminate excess body fluid; usually used in the treatment of high blood pressure and heart failure.

diverticulosis: refers to a condition in which the inner lining of the large intestine (colon) bulges out (herniates) through the outer, muscular layer.

Doppler studies: named after the Austrian scientist Johann Christian Doppler (1803–1853); measurements of systolic blood pressure using sound waves. Doppler studies are also used to measure fetal heart rate in expectant mothers.

doxorubicin: an antibiotic used to treat several forms of cancer (e.g., adriamycin).

dyserythropoiesis: abnormal red-blood-cell synthesis, characterized by nuclear abnormalities, including abnormal chromatin pattern, bizarre shapes, and nuclear fragmentation.

dyspnea: shortness of breath.

echocardiogram: the record of a procedure (echocardiography) using ultrasound waves to depict internal heart structure.

echocardiography (EEG or EKG): a test that bounces sound waves off the heart to produce pictures of its internal structures.

edema: abnormal accumulation of fluid in body tissues.

effusion cardiac: fluid in the sac (pericardium) around the heart.

electrocardiogram (EKG or ECG): the most common test used to diagnose a heart attack, it measures electrical activity during heartbeats.

electrophoresis: separation of molecules by size and electrical charge; electric current in the molecules can be forced through a gel with pores of a size that will separate specific molecules.

embolism: sudden blockage of a blood vessel by a embolus (blood clot).

embolotherapy: a procedure to occlude (plug in) abnormal blood vessels; used to treat pulmonary arteriovenous malformation (PAVM) and brain telangiectasias.

endocarditis: serious bacterial infection of the membrane lining of the heart and valves or heart muscle. Symptoms include fever and heart arrhythmia and can result in valve damage that requires surgery. Those with mitral valve prolapse may be more susceptible to this condition and may have to be premedicated with antibiotic prior to dental work or surgical procedure.

endocrine disorders: any disorder involving the endocrine system. The endocrine system is made up of organs that secrete hormones into the blood to regulate basic functions of cells and tissues. Endocrine organs are pituitary, thyroid, parathyroid, adrenal glands, pancreas, ovaries (in women), and testicles (in men).

endocrine gland: an organ containing a group of cells that produce and secrete hormones into the bloodstream.

endocrinologist: physician specializing in care and treatment of all types of disorders of the ductless glands.

endoscope/endoscopy: an endoscope as used in the field of gastroenterology is a thin flexible tube that uses a lens or miniature camera to view various areas of the gastrointestinal tract.

endothelial cells: cells in the tissue layer that line blood vessels.

endothelium: cells that form the inner lining of the heart, blood vessels, lymph channels, and various body cavities.

enema: introduction of a solution into the rectum and colon to stimulate bowel activity and empty the lower intestine for either feeding or therapeutic purposes, to give anesthesia, or to aid in X-ray studies.

enterocytes: cells in the lining of the small intestine that function in absorption of specific nutrients from diet.

enteroscopy: a visual examination of the inside of the intestine using a device called an enteroscope.

enzyme: a chemical (protein) originating in a cell that can act outside the cell and regulate reactions in the body; acts as a catalyst to induce chemical changes in other substances.

enzymopathy: disease that results from inability by the patient's cells to form a specific enzyme.

enzyme erythrocyte: red blood cell.

eosinophils: a type of white blood cell that reacts to allergies and can destroy parasites.

epinephrine: the principal hormone that raises blood pressure and heart rate, and is secreted by the adrenal medulla; also called adrenaline.

epistaxis: nosebleed.

erythrocyte: a mature red blood cell.

erythropoiesis: synthesis (creation) of red blood cells.

erythropoietin (EPO): a hormone produced in the kidneys that stimulates the production of red blood cells in the bone marrow.

Escherichia coli (E. coli): bacteria that normally live in the digestive tract of humans and animals that are passed on to others when infected feces contaminate food, water, or any other substance that people or animals might ingest.

esophageal varices: enlarged veins on the lining of the esophagus subject to severe bleeding; often they appear in patients with chronic alcoholism and other forms of liver disease. Symptoms include severe pain. May be caused by infection, irritation, or most commonly, from the backflow of stomach acid.

esophagitis: inflammation of the mucous-membrane lining of the esophagus.

esophagus: hollow tube that provides passage from the back of the throat to the stomach.

erythrocyte sedimentation rate (ESR): test for evidence of inflammatory activity.

estrogen: the female sex hormone; a hormone produced primarily by the ovaries in women that stimulates breast development, menstruation, and other secondary sexual changes.

ethanol: a form of alcohol contained in beverages.

Exjade: brand name for deferasirox, an oral iron chelator.

exocrine gland: a gland (like a salivary gland or the digestive enzyme-producing part of the pancreas) that releases a secretion external to or at the surface of an organ, often through a canal or duct.

fasting: going without food for a period of time, such as twelve-hour fasting before blood work.

Fe: symbol for the element iron.

febrile: an elevated body temperature.

fecal: pertaining to body waste, matter discharged from the bowel.

fecal occult blood test: test in which a stool sample is chemically tested for hidden blood.

ferritin: a complex protein formed in the intestine, containing about 23 percent iron. The amount found in serum is directly related to iron storage in the body. Increased ferritin levels may indicate iron loading and conditions such as hemochromatosis; when low, iron deficiency anemia exists.

ferroportin: an iron-export protein; a mutation in the ferroportin gene may lead to high macrophage iron and is associated with African siderosis fibrosis, or abnormal formation of connective or scar tissue.

ferrous sulfate, gluconate: common forms of oral iron.

fertility: ability to reproduce.

fetal: pertaining to the fetus.

fibroids: abnormal growth of cells in the muscular wall of the uterus; uterine fibroids are composed of abnormal muscle cells and are almost always benign. Cause is unknown. They usually decrease in size without treatment after menopause.

fibrosis: abnormal formation of connective or scar tissue.

fluids: nonsolid, liquid, or gaseous substances; secretions.

folate (folic acid): folate and folic acid are forms of water-soluble B-complex vitamins and needed for normal function of red and white blood cells. Folate is found in foods, and folic acid is the synthetic form found in supplements and fortified foods.

folic acid anemia: a shortage of red blood cells due to lack of folic acid in the diet.

FT3 (triiodothyronine): free T3; one form of thyroid hormone that occurs when T4 is converted.

FT4 (free thyroxine): one form of thyroid hormone in response to thyroid-stimulating hormone.

fulminating infection: infection that occurs suddenly and with great intensity.

fungi: a yeast, mold, or mushroom.

gallbladder disease: any disease involving the gallbladder or biliary tract. The gallbladder is a reservoir for bile; the biliary tract is the passageway that transports bile to the small intestine. Gallbladder disease is a common, often-painful condition requiring surgery. It is commonly associated with gallstones and inflammation.

gallstones: calculi or stones formed in the gallbladder.

gamma glutamyl transpeptidase (GGT): an enzyme found mainly in the liver but also in many other parts of the body. Increased GGT levels are involved in hepatitis, cirrhosis, jaundice, and other chronic diseases.

gastritis: irritation, inflammation, or infection of the stomach lining. Cause is sometimes unknown but may be due to excess stomach acid, food allergy, viral infection, or adverse reaction to alcohol, caffeine, or some drug. Symptoms may include nausea, diarrhea, abdominal pain, cramps, fever, weakness, belching, bloating, and loss of appetite. Usually curable in one week if cause is eliminated.

gastroenteritis: inflammation of the stomach and intestines accompanying many digestive-tract disorders. Causes may include bacterial, viral, or parasitic infections; food poisoning; food allergy; excess alcohol consumption; and emotional upset. Symptoms are the same as gastritis. Recovery usually occurs within one week. See *gastritis.*

gastroenterologist: see *physicians, types of.*

gastrointestinal disease: any disorder of the gastrointestinal tract, which includes the mouth, esophagus, stomach, duodenum, small intestine, cecum, appendix, ascending colon, transverse colon, descending colon, sigmoid colon, rectum, and anus.

gastrointestinal disorders: any condition or disease relating to any part of the digestive system, including the mouth, esophagus, stomach, small intestine, large intestine, and rectum. May also include some conditions relating to the liver, gallbladder, and pancreas.

gastrointestinal (GI) symptoms: any symptoms relating to the stomach or intestine, such as vomiting, diarrhea, constipation, bloating, flatulence, ascites, abdominal pain, or heartburn.

gastrointestinal tract: the entire length of the digestive system,

running from the stomach through the small intestine, large intestine, and out the rectum and anus.

gene expression: the process by which proteins are made from the instruction coded by DNA gene transfer, or insertion of unrelated DNA into the cells of an organism.

genetic code: adenine (A), thymine (T), guanine (G), and cytosine (C) are the amino acid letters of the DNA code; each gene's code combines the four bases in various ways to spell three-letter words that specify the sequence of amino acids that will constitute proteins.

genetic mutation: (genetic variation) any abnormal change in the makeup of a gene. A substitution of one of the DNA bases to result in an altered amino acid insertion in the gene product.

germ line: inherited material that is passed on to the offspring.

globin: one of the six proteins associated with the hemoglobin molecule.

glucagon: a hormone that works with insulin to regulate glucose levels in the blood.

glucose: simple sugar that is the body's major source of energy.

glucose-6-phosphate dehydrogenase (G6PD): an enzyme; G6PD deficiency is an inherited X-linked autosomal recessive disorder that can result in hemolytic anemia when an individual consumes fava beans or alcoholic beverages or is given certain drugs such as antimalarial or sulfa drugs. The constant hemolysis (destruction of red blood cells) leads to siderosis or iron overload.

glucose tolerance test: useful in the diagnosis of diabetes or hypoglycemia.

gluten: the insoluble protein (prolamin) constituent of wheat and other grains; a mixture of gliadin, glutenin, and other proteins; the presence of gluten makes dough cohesive or stretchy.

glycogen: substance formed from glucose, stored chiefly in the liver.

When blood sugar is too low, glycogen is converted back to glucose for the body to use as energy.

gonadotropin: hormone that stimulates function of the gonads produced by the anterior pituitary.

gonads: parts of the reproductive system that produce and release eggs (ovaries in the female) or sperm (testes in the male).

granulomas: nodule of firm tissue formed as a reaction to chronic inflammation, such as from foreign bodies or bacteria.

growth hormone (GH): a hormone regulating cell division and protein synthesis needed for normal growth.

Hashimoto's thyroiditis: a form of autoimmune thyroiditis that results in inflammation of the thyroid gland and hypothyroidism.

HbA1c: a monitor of the rise and fall of blood sugar over a period of time. If the blood glucose level has been carefully controlled and regulated over a period of five to six weeks, the HbA1c level will be normal; if it is elevated, it is an indication that the blood glucose level has not been controlled and has also been elevated.

HBV: hepatitis B virus, commonly known as serum hepatitis.

HCV: hepatitis C virus, commonly known as serum hepatitis. Contracted from infected blood as a result of transfusion prior to July 1991 or from contaminated personal items such as razors, nail clippers, toothbrushes, syringes, tattoo needles, and so on.

heart attack: See *myocardial infarction.*

heart failure: loss of pumping ability by the heart, often accompanied by fatigue, breathlessness, and excess fluid accumulation in body tissues.

Helicobacter pylori: a bacterium found in the cells of the stomach lining that can be a risk factor for some gastric diseases; gram-negative bacterium that grows in stomach mucosae and derives nutritional iron from human lactoferrin; associated in some, but not all, people with gastritis, ulcers, and stomach cancer.

hematocrit (Hct): the percentage of total blood volume consisting of red blood cells, found by centrifuging the whole blood and measuring the volume of red cells in a given volume of blood. Decreased hematocrit levels are associated with anemia, hyperthyroidism, cirrhosis, bone marrow failure, and numerous other pathogenic conditions.

hematologist: a physician specializing in the study of blood and in the diagnosis and treatment of disorders of the blood and blood-forming tissues, including bleeding disorders and blood diseases.

heme: the iron-containing portion of the hemoglobin molecule.

heme synthesis: a process by which iron accumulates in the mitochondria (the functional portion of the cell) and waits to be inserted into the heme ring of a red blood cell. The enzymatic process of heme production is complicated but essential before iron can be inserted into the heme ring to form hemoglobin. If any of these enzymes are abnormal, iron accumulates, resulting in iron-overload condition.

hemochromatosis: inherited metabolic disorder in which excessive iron may accumulate in the liver, pancreas, heart, brain, joints, and skin, resulting in liver disease, diabetes mellitus, heart attack, hormonal imbalances, depression, impotence, and a bronze or ashen gray-green skin color.

hemoglobin (Hgb, Hb, or Hbg): the red-blood-cell protein-iron compound responsible for transporting oxygen from the lungs to the cells and transporting carbon dioxide from the cells to the lungs.

hemoglobinopathy: diseases associated with abnormal hemoglobin.

hemolysis: process by which red blood cells break down and hemoglobin is released. Occurs normally at the end of the life span of a red blood cell. It may also occur abnormally with certain diseases or conditions such as hemolytic anemia.

hemolytic anemia: a disorder characterized by chronic premature destruction of red blood cells.

hemolytic disorder: characterized by the premature destruction of red blood cells. May or may not result in anemia, depending on the ability of the bone marrow to increase production of red blood cells.

hemolytic episode: separation of hemoglobin from red blood cells.

hemoptysis: coughing up blood.

hemorrhage: severe internal or external bleeding.

hemosiderin: an iron-containing compound that is not contained in ferritin. Hemosiderin collects in vital organs such as the heart, joints, liver, lungs, brain, gonads, and pancreas, impairing function.

hemosiderosis: a condition marked by excessive iron in the tissues, especially in the liver and spleen; also called siderosis.

hepatic coma: stupor or coma caused by buildup of waste products in the blood that are toxic to the brain. Normally, the liver neutralizes waste products, but because of extensive liver damage they continue to circulate in the blood.

hepatic disease: any disease involving the liver, including many types of hepatitis and cirrhosis.

hepatic dysfunction: poor liver function.

hepatitis: an inflammatory liver condition.

hepatitis A: form of viral hepatitis caused by the hepatitis A virus that is contracted through contaminated food or water, usually because of unsanitary conditions (improper hand washing after restroom use) or contaminated shellfish. Hepatitis A is usually mild, though it can be severe; the acute stage lasts about two weeks. There is a hepatitis A vaccination.

hepatitis, acute viral: characterized by rapid onset of symptoms, loss of appetite, vomiting, fever, joint pain, itchy skin (with some forms of hepatitis), jaundice, flulike symptoms, enlarged liver, loss of appetite, upper-right-quadrant abdominal pain, abnormal liver function, dark urine, and clay-colored stool.

hepatitis-associated antigen (HAA): a protein used to detect hepatitis A and/or B virus.

hepatitis B: form of viral hepatitis caused by the hepatitis B virus that can enter the body through blood transfusions contaminated with the virus or from the use of contaminated needles or instruments. Infection may be very severe and result in prolonged illness, cirrhosis, or death. There is a hepatitis B vaccination. See *cirrhosis*.

hepatitis C: form of viral hepatitis caused by the hepatitis C virus, spread through blood or sexual contact; there is no vaccine.

hepatitis, chronic: inflammation of the liver lasting more than six months; can be due to hepatitis B or C, alcohol, drugs, medications, toxic chemicals, or autoimmune conditions.

hepatocellular injury: injury of liver cells.

hepatologist: see *physicians, types of.*

hepatoma: malignant tumor that begins in the liver (primary site of cancer), as opposed to liver cancer that has spread from another site.

hepatotoxicity: destructive effect on the liver usually caused by a medication or alcohol.

hepcidin: liver hormone that inhibits intestinal absorption of excessive iron and, during inflammatory episodes, suppresses macrophage release of iron.

hereditary: inherited, transmitted genetically from generation to generation.

heterozygote: an individual who has two dissimilar members of a gene; a carrier of a gene mutation.

HFE: first identified in 1996, the first hemochromatosis-associated gene, located on chromosome 6. Two mutations were reported Cys282Tyr (C282Y) and His63Asp (H63D). Of these, the C282Y mutation is considered a major cause of iron loading.

high-density lipoprotein (HDL): a lipoprotein produced mainly in the liver but also in the intestine; carries cholesterol to the sites where it is needed. Also called good cholesterol.

histocompatibility antigens: see *human lymphocyte antigen.*

homozygote: an individual who has two identical members of a mutated gene.

hormone: a chemical produced by a specific gland or tissue that is released into the bloodstream to a target organ. Controls body functions such as growth and sexual development. For example, insulin is a pancreatic hormone.

human growth hormone (HGH): hormone needed for normal growth and sexual maturity from birth until the end of puberty; secreted by cells in the pituitary gland.

human lymphocyte antigen (HLA): a genetic "fingerprint" existing on the surface of a specific type of white blood cell, this antigen is determined genetically and is therefore useful in paternity investigation and compatibility with tissue transplantation.

hyper-: a prefix; excessive, above, or beyond.

hyperglycemia: too much sugar in the blood, as in diabetes.

hyperinsulinemia: an excessive amount of insulin in the blood.

hypersplenism: a type of disorder that causes the spleen to rapidly and prematurely destroy blood cells.

hypertension (high blood pressure): increase in the force of blood against the arteries as blood circulates through them. Often has no symptoms. Essential or primary hypertension, the most common kind, has no single identifiable cause. Secondary hypertension is caused by an underlying disease.

GLOSSARY

hyperthyroidism: overactivity of the thyroid, the endocrine gland that regulates many body functions.

hypertrophic cardiomyopathy: heart muscle disease that leads to thickening of the heart walls, interfering with the heart's ability to fill with and pump blood.

hyperviscosity: blood that is too thick.

hypo-: a prefix; deficient, beneath, or under.

hypochromic: refers to a red blood cell with a decreased concentration of hemoglobin.

hypochromic erythrocytes: pale red blood cells due to subnormal content of hemoglobin.

hypoferremia: subnormal content of iron in the blood.

hypoglycemia: a condition of low blood sugar.

hypogonadism: gonads with deficient secretion and that are small in size.

hypothalamus: a centrally located structure of the brain that regulates the pituitary gland.

hypothyroidism: underactive thyroid gland.

hypoxia: oxygen deficiency.

hysterectomy: surgical removal of total or partial uterus; may be followed by onset of iron loading.

ichthyosis: dry, itchy skin with adherent scales idiopathic; condition for which no cause is yet known.

idiopathic: refers to a disease or condition of unknown cause.

Ig or immunoglobulin, IgG, IgA, IgM: antibodies. Tests that measure immune status.

IgA: increases in chronic non-alcoholic disease, primary biliary cirrhosis.

IgG: increases in infections of all types, liver disease, myeloma, and rheumatoid arthritis.

IgM: increases in malaria, infectious mononucleosis, and rheumatoid arthritis.

ileostomy: a surgical procedure in which the lower part of the small intestine (the ileum) is cut and brought to an opening in the abdominal wall, where feces can be passed out of the body.

infarction: an infarct or area of tissue that undergoes necrosis (cell death) as a result of loss of blood supply due to an occlusion (blockage) or stenosis (narrowing or constriction of blood vessels).

infection: presence and growth of a microorganism that produces tissue damage.

infectious mononucleosis: infectious viral disease that affects the liver, respiratory system, and lymphatic system.

infertility: the inability or diminished ability to produce offspring.

inflammation/inflammatory: a nonspecific immune response that occurs in reaction to any type of bodily injury. Common symptoms are pain, redness, swelling, and warmth at the injured area. Fever commonly occurs with extensive inflammation as well.

inflammatory bowel disease: a group of disorders that cause the intestines to become inflamed (red and swollen). These disorders usually last a long time and reoccur frequently. Symptoms include abdominal cramps and pain, diarrhea, weight loss, and bleeding from the intestines. Crohn's disease is one type of inflammatory bowel disease.

insulin: a hormone secreted by the beta cells of the islet of Langerhans of the pancreas that regulates blood glucose levels; works with glucagon to regulate glucose levels in the blood and to supply fuel to the body's cells for the production of energy.

insulin resistance: reduced sensitivity to insulin by the body's insulin-dependent processes (as glucose uptake, lipolysis, and inhibition of glucose production by the liver) that results in lowered activity of these processes, an increase in insulin production, or both. It is typical of type 2 diabetes but often occurs in the absence of diabetes.

internist: see *physicians, types of.*

interstitial: occupying space between tissues, such as interstitial fluid.

interstitial fibrosis: formation of fibrous tissue between normal tissues.

intestines: (also known as the bowels) divided into the large and small intestines.

intrinsic factor: a hormone produced in the stomach; essential for the absorption of vitamin B12.

iron: an essential micronutrient and a metallic element widely distributed in nature. As part of hemoglobin, iron is essential for the transport of oxygen in the blood and is part of some of the enzymes needed for cell respiration.

iron avidity: an affinity for iron. Often seen in hemochromatosis patients, where the TS percentage is elevated but the serum ferritin is normal or low. See *overbleeding.*

iron-chelation therapy: the removal of iron from the tissues using a drug formulated to specifically bind with iron.

iron-deficiency anemia: a type of anemia due to blood loss, insufficient iron in the diet, or demands for iron that exceed stores, such as during a growth spurt.

iron overload: a potentially fatal condition in which iron accumulates in tissues of the body, seen in some hemolytic anemias and hemochromatosis; a common side effect of numerous blood transfusions.

iron panel: series of tests that measure levels of iron and iron actively in the body, such as serum iron, transferrin, total iron-binding capacity (TIBC), transferrin-iron saturation percentage, serum transferrin receptor, unbound or unsaturated iron-binding capacity (UIBC), hemoglobin, and hematocrit.

ischemia: decreased blood supply to a body organ or part.

islet of Langerhans: collection of cells in the pancreas that produce insulin.

IV: intravenous.

jaundice: condition of yellow skin, yellow whites of the eyes, dark urine, and light-colored stools. It is a symptom of diseases of the liver and blood caused by abnormally elevated amounts of bilirubin in the blood.

joint aspiration: the drawing off of excess fluid from around a joint by the means of suction.

juvenile hemochromatosis: onset of iron loading prior to age thirty.

ketoacidosis: serious disorder that results from a deficiency or inadequate use of carbohydrates. Characterized by fluid and electrolyte disorders, dehydration, and mental confusion. If left untreated, coma and death may occur. It is usually a complication of diabetes mellitus but may also be seen in starvation and rarely in pregnancy if diet is inadequate. See *diabetes mellitus*.

knockout: inactivation of specific genes in yeast or mice to determine identity of specific function coded by the gene.

koilonychia: (also known as spoon nails) a malformation of the nails in which the outer surface is concave; often associated with iron deficiency or softening by occupational contact with oils.

Kupffer cell: a type of cell found in the liver and a part of the reticuloendothelial system (RES).

lactoferrin: a protein found in human secretions such as tears, seminal and vaginal fluids, saliva, and mother's milk that binds with iron to withhold the iron from harmful germs.

lamina: a thin, flat layer or membrane.

left ventricular assist device (LVAD): a mechanical device used to increase the heart's pumping ability.

libido: sexual drive or urge.

lipase: a fat-splitting enzyme found in the blood, pancreatic secretion, and tissues.

liver biopsy: procedure in which a tiny sample of the liver is removed using a needle inserted into the liver so that a tissue sample can be examined for liver damage or malignancy (liver cancer). This procedure helps determine what is occurring in the liver and the extent of liver damage.

liver function tests: include alanine aminotransferase (ALT), also known as serum glutamic pyruvic transminase (SGPT); aspartate aminotransferase (AST), also known as serum glutamic-oxaloacetic transaminase (SGOT); gamma-glutamine transferase (GGT); and alkaline phosphatase (ALP).

locus: the place on a chromosome where a specific gene is located.

low-density lipoprotein (LDL): see *cholesterol.*

lung: organ of respiration. The primary purpose of the lung is to bring air and blood together so that oxygen can be added to the blood and carbon dioxide removed from it. The lungs are composed of lobes (three in the right lung and two in the left lung). Lobes are divided into lobules that contain blood vessels, lymphatic nerves, and ducts that connect the alveolar air space where oxygen and carbon dioxide exchange takes place. It is in this space that alveolar macrophages can become loaded with iron when iron is inhaled.

lymph: a clear, transparent filtrate of plasma that is collected from tissues throughout the body and eventually flows to the lymphatic system.

lymphatic system: an important aspect of the body's immune system, consisting of vessels that carry lymph fluid from tissues throughout the body through the lymph nodes to the venous blood circulation.

lymphocyte: one of three types of white blood cells (the others being granulocytes and monocytes), and the primary cell of the immune response, responsible for attacking antigens; divided into two forms, B cells and T cells.

lymphoma: cancer of the lymph glands.

lysozyme: enzyme in body fluids that digests bacterial cell walls.

macro-: prefix; combining form meaning large or long.

macrocytic: descriptive term applied to a larger-than-normal red blood cell.

macrocytosis: a condition in which cells are abnormally large.

macrophage: a monocyte (a type of white blood cell) that has left the bloodstream and settled in a tissue. Macrophages are found in large quantities in the spleen, lymph nodes, alveoli, and tonsils, and are one of the major cells of the immune system.

magnetic resonance imaging (MRI): a diagnostic procedure in which a large magnet surrounds a person; radio frequencies interact with the magnet to provide information to a computer.

malabsorption: inadequate absorption of nutrients from the intestinal tract, especially the duodenal portion of the small intestine.

malaise: vague feeling of body discomfort generally prior to onset of illness.

GLOSSARY

malignant: able to destroy normal tissue; may lead to death. Usually refers to cancer growth.

maternal: pertaining to, or inherited from, the mother.

mean corpuscular hemoglobin (MCH): the measure of the amount or weight of hemoglobin within a red blood cell. Part of complete blood count and helps determine types of anemia.

mean corpuscular hemoglobin concentration (MCHC): the measure of the average concentration or percentage of hemoglobin within a single red blood cell; MCHC is part of a complete blood count and helps determine types of anemia.

mean corpuscular volume (MCV): the average volume or size of a single red blood cell. Used to determine types of anemia, liver disease, vitamin B deficiencies, alcoholism, and thalassemia.

mean platelet volume (MPV): the average volume (size) of platelets.

megaloblastic anemia: a type of anemia in which red blood cells are larger than normal, usually resulting from a deficiency of folic acid or vitamin B12.

melanoma: any of a group of malignant tumors, primarily of the skin. The most severe form of skin cancer.

Mendelian inheritance: manner in which genes are passed to offspring; examples include autosomal

dominant, autosomal recessive, and sex-linked genes.

menorrhagia: excessive or prolonged menstrual bleeding with blood loss exceeding 80 milliliters per cycle.

metabolism: combined chemical and physical processes that take place in the body. Involves distribution of nutrients, growth, energy production, elimination of wastes, and other body functions. There are two phases of metabolism: anabolism, the constructive phase formation of tissues and organs, and catabolism, the breaking-down phase during which molecules are broken down.

metacarpals: bones of the hand to which finger bones are attached.

metastasis: process by which cancerous cells or infectious germs spread from their original location to other parts of the body.

micro-: prefix; denotes small size or extent.

microbes: microorganisms (small, living organism); many are capable of producing disease.

microcytic: red blood cells that are abnormally small.

microcytosis: blood disorder characterized by abnormally small (microcytic) red blood cells often associated with iron deficiency anemia, lead poisoning, or thalassemia.

mitochondria: self-replicating portion of the cell where metabolic and respiratory functions provide a cell's energy source.

mitral valve: valve located in the heart between the left atrium and left ventricle.

mitral valve prolapse: condition in which the mitral valve becomes floppy, resulting in mitral regurgitation.

monocyte: one of three types of white blood cells (the others being granulocytes and lymphocytes), normally constituting 3 to 7 percent of the blood-circulating macrophages.

morphism: in blood production, the structure and formation of a blood cell.

myelodysplastic syndromes (MDS): Myelodysplastic syndromes (MDS) are disorders of bone marrow characterized by increased cell production with dysplastic (abnormal) maturation. A high percentage of MDS cases progress to acute myeloid leukemia and for this reason, MDS is referred to as a preleukemic condition.

myeloid: pertaining to, derived from, or resembling bone marrow.

myocardial infarction (MI): heart attack; death of an area of heart muscle due to interruption of its blood supply. Arteries narrowed by atherosclerosis may be occluded (blocked) by blood clot (coronary thrombus). Symptoms include crushing, viselike chest pain that may radiate especially to the left arm, neck, or jaw; shortness of breath; faintness; anxiety; ashen color; perspiration; and arrhythmia.

myoglobin: iron-containing pigment that provides the red color in muscles; it also contains oxygen needed by the muscles for proper function.

necrotizing enterocolitis: severe infectious bacterial invasion of intestinal lining in non-breast-fed infants who lack maternal lactoferrin.

neoplasm/neoplastic: a new and abnormal formation of tissue, as a tumor or growth. It serves no useful function but grows at the expense of the healthy organism.

nephrosis: conditions in which there are degenerative changes in the kidneys or kidney disease.

nephrotoxicity: damage to kidneys.

neurological: pertaining to the nervous system.

neuropathy: damage to nerve tissue.

neutropenia: low neutrophil (poly) count; a deficiency of neutrophils in the blood.

neutrophil: the most numerous of the white blood cells, important for helping the body fight infections.

nonalcoholic steatohepatitis (NASH): fatty liver not caused by alcohol consumption; can be associated with C282Y mutation; patients have elevated serum ferritin and insulin resistance.

nonspecific liver disease: poor liver function in the absence of a known cause.

normo-: prefix; denotes normal or usual.

normochromic: refers to a red blood cell with a normal concentration of hemoglobin.

normocytic: refers to a red blood cell of normal size.

nuclear medicine scanning test: any test involving the use of radioactive substances to diagnose a number of certain conditions. The substances are either injected into the body or inhaled, the dose of radiation is minimal, and the substances used either lose their radioactivity in a short time or are excreted.

obstruction: a blockage.

oncology: study of cancer.

orthopedist: see *physicians, types of.*

osteoarthritis: degenerate joint disease; can be an early sign of iron loading.

osteoporosis: a general term describing any disease process that results in reduced bone mass.

ovaries: female reproductive organs (gonads) that release eggs and female sex hormones.

overbleeding: lowering iron levels too low, resulting in unnecessary iron deficiency anemia.

ovulation: the periodic ripening and discharge of the ovum from the ovary. Ovulation occurs approximately fourteen days before the next menstrual period.

packed cells: red blood cells that have been separated from the plasma and used for conditions that require red blood cells but not the liquid components of whole blood.

pancreas: an exocrine and endocrine organ. The exocrine portion secretes digestive enzymes into the duodenum; the endocrine portion secretes insulin, which regulates blood sugar; glucagon, which stimulates the liver to convert glycogen to glucose; and somatostatin, which inhibits the release of insulin, glucagon, growth hormone, and gastrin so that levels of these hormones do not exceed normal (negative feedback system).

pancreatitis: inflammation of the pancreas. Chronic pancreatitis usually follows recurrent attacks of acute pancreatitis. Pancreas gradually becomes unable to supply digestive juices and hormones necessary for good health.

parathyroids: four glands located on the corners of the thyroid gland that release parathyroid hormone and calcitonin, which affects fluid balance and the levels of calcium in the blood.

parenchyma: cells in an organ that are responsible for specific function(s) of the organ; for example, the hepatocytes in the liver.

parenteral: subcutaneous, intramuscular, or intravenous injection of drugs or nutrients to bypass the intestinal route.

Parkinson's disease: a neuropathy involving a rhythmic tremor and rigidity of muscle action; associated with accumulation of iron in the substantia nigra portion of brain

paroxysmal nocturnal hemoglobinuria (PNH): a rare, acquired bleeding disorder where the hemolysis is intermittent, occurring during sleep.

paternal: pertaining to, or inherited from, the father.

pediatric: concerning the treatment of children (younger than age eighteen).

percutaneous: refers to the skin; medication by application of an ointment or removal or injection of a fluid by a needle.

pericardial: pertaining to membranes surrounding the heart.

pericarditis: an inflammation of the two layers of the thin, saclike membrane that surrounds the heart.

peripheral blood smear test: a blood test; the examination of the edge, sometimes called the feather edge, of a blood sample in which most of the red cells are almost touching.

pernicious anemia: chronic anemia that occurs as a result of vitamin B12 deficiency due to the lack of intrinsic factor, a substance secreted by the mucous membranes of the stomach that is essential for absorption of B12.

petechiae: tiny red dots on the skin due to bleeding under the skin.

phagocyte: see *macrophage.*

phagocytize: to engulf and destroy microorganisms or cells, a function performed by certain white blood cells.

phenotype: an observed trait or characteristic; for example, the increased intestinal absorption of iron in hemochromatosis.

phlebotomy: therapeutic withdrawal of blood from the vein.

phosphates: form of inorganic phosphorus found in the body.

physicians, types of:
    anesthesiologist: specialist in administering an anesthetic agent, usually for surgical procedures.
    cardiologist: specialist in care of disorders of the heart.
    emergency care physician: treats conditions requiring immediate care.
    endocrinologist: specialist in care and treatment of all types of disorders of the ductless glands.
    family practitioner: one who cares for the entire range of diseases affecting persons of all ages and sexes and not limited to a particular organ system or disease; a general practitioner.
    gastroenterologist: physician whose practice covers disorders

of the stomach, intestines, and related structures, such as the esophagus, liver, gallbladder, and pancreas.

general practitioner: see *family practitioner*.

hematologist: specialist in the study of blood and in the diagnosis and treatment of disorders of the blood and blood-forming tissues, including bleeding disorders and blood diseases.

hepatologist: specialist in diseases of the liver.

internist: specialist in the treatment of diseases of the internal organs by nonsurgical means.

nephrologist: one who is concerned with the structure and function of the kidneys.

neurologist: specialist in diseases of the nervous system and the brain.

ob-gyn: specialist in pregnancy, childbirth, and gynecology (female reproductive system).

oncologist: specialist in cancer; often hematologists are oncologists.

orthopedist: specialist in prevention and correction of musculoskeletal disorders.

pathologist: specialist in analyzing tissue for disease.

pediatrician: physician treating children and children's diseases.

psychiatrist: specialist in the study, treatment, and prevention of mental disorders.

psychologist: specialist in the study and treatment of disorders of the mental processes that affect behavior.

pulmonologist: physician whose practice is concerned or involved with the lungs.

radiologist: physician trained in the diagnostic and/or therapeutic use of X-rays, CT scans, MRIs, and ultrasounds.

rheumatologist: specialist in rheumatic diseases of the joints.

surgeon: specialist who does surgery; general or specific, such as a head-neck surgeon, cancer surgeon, heart surgeon, and so on.

urologist: physician whose practice is concerned with disorders of the urinary tract.

phytates: natural compounds found in whole grains that suppress intestinal absorption of excessive nonheme iron.

pica: an appetite or craving for substances not fit as food or of no nutritional value, such as clay, dried paint, ice, hair, coins, dirt, paper, starch.

plasma: the liquid part of the blood and of the lymph; the fluid (noncellular) portion of the circulating blood.

platelet: nonnucleated cells essential for blood clotting.

platonychia: thickened spots in center of fingernails.

polycythemia: increase in red blood cells in the body. The disease has three forms. Polycythemia vera involves overproduction of red blood cells, white blood cells, and platelets. Secondary polycythemia is a complication of diseases or factors other than blood cell disorders. Stress polycythemia involves decreased blood plasma.

polycythemia vera: (also called my-eloproliferative disorder) abnormal increased production of red blood cells and hemoglobin concentration, white blood cells, and platelets. Cause is unknown. Treatment may include withdrawing blood at certain intervals, radioisotope therapy, and drug therapy. Treatment is needed to prevent blood clots from forming that could cause a stroke, heart attack, or blockage in a vein or artery.

polydipsia: excessive thirst.

polyp: an abnormal growth that develops on the inside of a hollow organ such as the colon, stomach, or nose.

polyuria: excessive production of urine.

porphyria: excretion of porphyrins into the urine.

porphyria, acute intermittent (AIP): rare, inherited disorder characterized by excessive formation and excretion of porphyrins (see *porphyrins*). Symptoms include recurrent abdominal pain, often accompanied by nausea, vomiting, constipation, and dark urine.

porphyria cutanea tarda: inherited metabolic disorder involving the synthesis of red pigment (heme) in blood cells due to a defective enzyme (uroporphyrinogen decarboxylase) in the liver, which results in an increase in porphyrins in the skin. Increased porphyrins lead to photosensitivity where the skin is damaged by sunlight. This type of porphyria

usually associated with chronic alcoholism marked by skin lesions and enlarged liver. See *porphyria, acute intermittent.*

porphyrins: any number of pigments widely distributed in hemoglobin, myoglobin, and cytochromes.

portal shunt: transjugular intra-hepatic portosystemic shunt (TIPS). A flexible stent composed of an expandable stainless-steel mesh inserted through the jugular vein and fed down through the portal vein. Helps maintain pressure in the portal vein in those with esophageal varices, a life-threatening condition of bleeding varices.

posthemorrhagic anemia: loss of red blood cells due to massive or prolonged bleeding.

preeclampsia: toxic complication of pregnancy involving increased blood pressure and serum iron, kidney damage, and edema.

progesterone: a female hormone involved in the menstrual cycle.

prolactin: a hormone that stimulates milk production in women who are breast-feeding.

proliferation: growth by reproduction of similar cells.

prostate-specific antigen (PSA): an antigen found in all men that is greatly increased in cases of prostate cancer.

protein: one of a class or kind of complex compounds synthesized by all living things, which provide the amino acids essential for growth and repair of tissue.

protein metabolism: process by which protein foods are used by the body to make tissue proteins, together with breaking down tissue proteins to produce energy. Food proteins are first broken down into amino acids, then absorbed into the blood, and finally used in body cells to form new proteins.

pruritus: itching.

pulmonary: concerning or involving the lungs.

pulmonary congestion (or edema): fluid accumulation in the lungs.

pulmonary edema: fluid accumulation in lungs.

pulmonologist: see *physicians, types of.*

pulse oximeter: a clip placed on the tip of the ear, finger, or toe and connected to a machine that measures the oxygen in the blood.

pyelonephritis: infection of the kidney.

pyridoxine: vitamin B6.

pyruvate kinase deficiency (PK): an inherited hemolytic anemia due to a deficiency of the enzyme pyruvate kinase (PK).

Q wave: the downward or negative wave of an electrocardiogram (EKG) that follows the P wave. Abnormal or elongated Q wave is an indication of problems with the conduction system of the heart.

Q-T wave: an electrocardiogram measure; in an iron-loaded heart (and in congestive heart failure), the Q-T wave is lengthened.

quantitative phlebotomy: removal of a certain amount of blood as advised by the physician.

recessive trait: an inherited trait that is outwardly obvious only when two copies of the gene for that trait are present, as opposed to a dominant trait where one copy of the gene for the dominant trait is sufficient to display the trait.

red-blood-cell distribution width (RDW): an indication of the variation in red blood cell size.

red cell indices: aids in the classification of anemias. Indices include mean corpuscular volume (MCV), mean corpuscular hemoglobin (MCH), and mean corpuscular hemoglobin concentration (MCHC).

reductase: an enzyme that accelerates the reduction process of chemical compounds.

renal: pertaining to the kidneys.

restless legs syndrome: uncontrollable jumpiness or twitching in the legs.

restrictive cardiomyopathy: heart muscle disease in which the muscle walls become stiff and lose their flexibility; typically results from another disease elsewhere in the body such as amyloidosis (abnormal protein fibers accumulate in the heart muscle), sarcoidosis (inflammatory diseases that causes the formation of small lumps in organs), and hemochromatosis or iron overload.

reticulocyte count: the number of reticulocytes, usually expressed as the percentage of red blood cells.

reticulocytes: young, immature red blood cells. The normal reticulocyte count in the peripheral blood is 1 percent. The reticulocyte count is a measure of effective erythropoiesis.

reticulocytosis: excess amount of reticulocytes in the blood.

reticuloendothelial system (RES): the system of the body that includes the function of defense against infection and disposal of the products resulting from the breakdown of cells. Includes the macrophages, Kupffer cells of the liver, the bone marrow, spleen, and lymph system.

retina: the light-receptive layer and terminal expansion of the optic nerve in the eye.

rheumatic fever: inflammatory disease occurring primarily in children as a result of delayed reaction to streptococcal throat; may result in rheumatic heart disease, heart muscle, and valve damage.

rheumatoid arthritis: inflammatory condition characterized by joint disease that involves muscles, cartilage, and membrane linings of the joints. Three times more common in women than men. Symptoms include red, warm, painful joints and are usually symmetrical (i.e., affect both sides). Sometimes accompanied by weakness and fatigue. If disease is severe, permanent deformity and crippling may result.

rheumatologist: see *physicians, types of.*

ringed sideroblast: an immature red blood cell that has a ring of iron surrounding the nucleus.

rouleaux: red blood cells that appear stuck together like stacks of coins when observed on a peripheral smear.

sarcoidosis: chronic inflammatory disease of unknown origin that causes the formation of small lumps (nodules) in organs.

schistocyte: fragmented red blood cell that may be irregular in shape with pointed ends.

septicemia: bacterial infection in which the pathogens have invaded and are multiplying in the blood.

septum: partition or dividing wall in an organ; in the heart, a muscle wall separating chambers.

seronegative rheumatoid arthritis: test for rheumatoid factor is negative, common in iron-related arthritis.

serum: the watery portion of the blood left after clotting is completed.

serum glutamic-oxaloacetic transaminase (SGOT): a test used in cases of suspected coronary occlusive heart diseases or liver diseases such as hepatitis or cirrhosis.

serum glutamic-pyruvic transaminase (SGPT): an enzyme released into the bloodstream by injury or disease affecting the liver.

sex chromosomes: the pair of chromosomes responsible for sex determination. In humans and most animals, the sex chromosomes are designated X and Y; women have two X chromosomes; men have one X and one Y chromosome.

short bowel syndrome (small intestine insufficiency): a condition of malabsorption related to the surgical removal or disease of a large portion of the small intestine.

sickle-cell disease: an inherited condition characterized by red blood cells that are sickle shaped. SCD patients can experience anemia and require repeat blood transfusions, which result in iron overload. Iron chelating drugs are used to remove the excess iron.

sideroblastic anemia: a disorder in which incorporation of iron into hemoglobin and the developing red blood cells (erythroblasts) in the bone marrow is faulty. As a result, iron accumulates in the erythroblasts giving rise to ringed sideroblasts, which provide diagnosis when found on microscopic examination of bone marrow. Because ring sideroblasts develop poorly or not at all into mature red cells, anemia results (the red blood cells of the mitochondria are overloaded with iron) and hemoglobin production (heme synthesis) is defective. This presents like iron deficiency anemia (IDA) but is unlike IDA in that iron testing is normal or increased.

sideroblasts: young red blood cells that contain excess iron.

siderosis: a general term for iron leading.

sigmoid colon: the final portion of the large intestine, which empties into the rectum.

Sjogren's syndrome: an autoimmune disorder characterized by dryness of the eyes and mouth and recurrent salivary gland enlargement.

sleep apnea: the stopping of breathing during sleep for a duration of at least ten seconds.

sperm count: the measure of the number of sperm in a precise volume of fluid.

splenectomy: surgical removal of spleen.

splenomegaly: an enlargement of the spleen beyond its normal size.

steatohepatitis: fatty and inflamed liver.

steatorrhea: passage of fat in large amounts in the feces due to failure to digest and absorb it; occurs in pancreatic disease and the malabsorption syndromes; an absence of bile acids will increase steatorrhea.

stem cell: also called pluripotent, as stem cells have the potential to develop into any type of blood cell.

stool occult blood: a measure of the presence of more than minimal amounts of blood in a stool sample; may indicate abnormalities in the gastrointestinal tract.

subcutaneous: beneath the skin.

substantia nigra: a broad, thick plate of large, pigmented nerve cells in the brain; iron loading is associated with development of Parkinson's disease and iron deficit with restless legs syndrome.

sudden death: cardiac arrest caused by an irregular heartbeat.

sudden infant death syndrome (SIDS): unexpected death of normal child under six months of age; no known cause; condition may be associated with postnatal iron loading.

sugar levels: see *blood sugar, glucose.*

sugar-water hemolysis test: (also known as sucrose hemolysis test) a test to detect increased fragility of red blood cells by swelling in low ionic (low salt) solution.

synovial: pertaining to the synovia, the lubricating fluid of the joints.

synovial membrane: (also called synovium) thin lining membrane of a joint.

synovial syndrome: abnormal value or finding within the synovial (joint) fluid.

synthesis: a buildup, putting together, or composition.

systemic lupus erythematosus (SLE): a chronic, inflammatory autoimmune disorder that may affect many organ systems including the skin, joints, and internal organs.

tachycardia: rapid heartbeat.

testes: male reproductive glands (gonads) in the scrotum that produce sperm and the hormone testosterone.

testosterone: a hormone, produced primarily in the testes, that stimulates the development of secondary sexual characteristics and supports the production of sperm in males; principal male hormone.

T4: thyroxine, one of the principal hormones secreted by the thyroid gland.

thalassemia: name for a complex of hereditary anemias that occur in populations bordering the Mediterranean, in Southeast Asia, the Middle East, and in India (Cooley's anemia); a disorder in which abnormal hemoglobin is formed, and required repeated blood transfusions result in iron loading with special impairment of functions of pituitary, heart, and pancreas.

therapeutic: a healing agent or results obtained from treatment.

thiamine: one of the B vitamins, a group of water-soluble vitamins that participate in many of the chemical reactions in the body.

thrombocyte: platelet.

thrombocytopenia: a deficiency in the number of platelets.

thrombosis: abnormal blood clots.

thyroid gland: large endocrine gland located in the throat area, which produces a hormone that helps to regulate metabolism.

thyroiditis: inflammation of the thyroid gland.

thyroid profile: blood tests performed to determine thyroid function, include T3 uptake and T4 uptake, free thyroxine index (T7), thyroid-stimulating hormone (TSH), and thyrotropin.

thyrotropin-releasing factor (TRH): substance secreted by the hypothalamus that controls the release of thyroid-stimulating hormone from the anterior pituitary gland.

thyroid-stimulating hormone (TSH): substance secreted by the anterior pituitary gland that controls the release of thyroid hormone from the thyroid gland. Needed for normal thyroid growth and function. See *thyroid gland*.

thyroxine: a hormone produced by the thyroid gland.

TIA: see transient ischemic attack.

T lymphocyte: a lymphocyte that is important in the immune response but that, in aplastic anemia, suppresses the stem cells; also known as a T cell lymphocyte.

tomography: a method of producing a three-dimensional image of the internal structures of a solid object (such as the human body) by the observation and recording of the differences in the effects on the passage of waves of energy impinging on those structures.

total iron-binding capacity (TIBC): a measurement of all proteins available for binding free iron in the body; an indirect but accurate measure of transferrin (see *transferrin*). Increased TIBC levels may indicate iron-deficiency anemia; decreased TIBC may indicate cirrhosis or iron overload.

transaminases: enzymes that transfer an amino group from various amino acids to alpha-ketoglutaric acid to form glutamic acid.

transferrin (siderophilin): protein that transports iron from the intestine into the blood. It makes iron available to the bone marrow, where red blood cells are produced.

transient ischemic attack (TIA): TIAs are mini-strokes that have no lasting damage. They occur when a blood clot temporarily clogs an artery, and part of the brain doesn't get the blood it needs. The symptoms occur rapidly and last a relatively short time.

tremolite: form of asbestos consisting entirely of iron silicate; highly carcinogenic, especially when used as a whitewash covering in homes.

triglycerides (TGs): a form of fat in the bloodstream, produced in the liver.

triiodothyronine (T3): a hormone produced by the thyroid gland.

T3: triiodothyronine, one of two forms of thyroid hormone.

tumor: a spontaneous new growth of tissue that forms an abnormal mass and that does not follow normal laws of growth; may be malignant or nonmalignant.

tumor marker: a substance in blood serum whose presence may indicate a possible malignancy.

ulcer/ulceration: an open sore on the skin or on a mucous membrane.

ultrasound: the use of very high frequency sound waves to produce an image or photograph of an organ or tissue.

unbound or unsaturated iron-binding capacity (UIBC): the difference between the TIBC and the serum iron. Normal range is 70 to 390 µg/dL. Iron-binding capacity levels of TIBC and UIBC are high in anemias and low in iron overload.

upper gastrointestinal (UGI): a means of obtaining a direct look at the upper gastrointestinal tract by using a long, flexible fiber-optic scope.

urea: a substance formed in the liver and found in blood, lymph, and urine; the end product of protein metabolism in the body.

urologist: see *physicians, types of.*

vascular: pertaining to blood vessels.

ventricles: the two lower chambers of the heart. The left ventricle is the main pumping chamber in the heart.

ventricular fibrillation: rapid, irregular quivering of the heart's ventricles, with no effective heartbeat.

Vibrio vulnificus: a species of gram-negative bacteria in coastal seawater and in shellfish; requires highly saturated transferrin iron to grow in body; wounds in coastal waterways. Ingestion of raw shellfish can be fatal to iron-loaded patients.

villi: tiny, fingerlike projections that enable the small intestine to absorb nutrients from food.

viral: caused by a virus.

vitiligo: a skin condition in which there is loss of pigment from areas of skin, resulting in irregular white patches with normal skin texture.

WBCs: white blood cells.

Wilson's disease: inherited disorder of copper metabolism in which copper accumulates in the liver, red blood cells, and brain, leading to anemia, tremors, liver dysfunction, and dementia.

X chromosome: one of the two types of sex chromosomes, present twice in female cells and once in male cells.

X-ray: a name for a machine using the energy of electromagnetic waves to visualize hard tissues such as bone, or a treatment with such a machine.

Y chromosome: one of the two types of sex chromosomes; men have one X and one Y chromosome.

Yersinia: a gram-negative bacteria; some species grow in iron-loaded body fluids, and others require iron-loaded macrophages.

zinc: a metallic element, essential in the diet of all animals, including humans. Lack of zinc in the diet can cause slowed growth or slow-healing wounds among other things, and during pregnancy it may cause developmental disorders in the child. Essential for protein synthesis, insulin stability, vision, reproductive functions, and wound healing; iron supplements can interfere with normal acquisition of dietary zinc.

Glossary resources include the National Library of Medicine Medline Plus, www.marrow.org, and previous glossaries published in *The Iron Disorders Institute Guide to Anemia, The Iron Disorders Institute Guide to Hemochromatosis, First Edition,* and *Exposing the Hidden Dangers of Iron.*

Bibliography

Acton, R. T., J. C. Barton, L. V. Passmore, P. C. Adams, G. D. McLaren, C. Leiendecker-Foster, M. R. Speechley, E. L. Harris, O. Castro, J. A. Reiss, B. M. Snively, B. W. Harrison, and C. E. McLaren. 2008. "Accuracy of Family History of Hemochromatosis or Iron Overload: The Hemochromatosis and Iron Overload Screening Study." *Clinical Gastroenterology and Hepatology* 6, no. 8 (2008): 934–38.

Acton, R. T., J. C. Barton, L. V. Passmore, P. C. Adams, M. R. Speechley, F. W. Dawkins, P. Sholinsky, D. M. Reboussin, G. D. McLaren, E. L. Harris, T. C. Bent, T. M. Vogt, and O. Castro. "Relationships of Serum Ferritin, Transferrin Saturation, and HFE Mutations and Self-Reported Diabetes in the Hemochromatosis and Iron Overload Screenings (HEIRS) Study." *Diabetes Care* 29, no. 9 (2006): 2084–89.

Acton, R. T., T. Bent, C. Rivers, and M. Radojutimi-Akinsiku. "Screening for Hemochromatosis and Iron Overload: Satisfaction with Results Notification and Understanding of Mailed Results in Unaffected Participants of the HEIRS Study." *Genetic Testing* 12, no. 4 (2008): 491–500.

Adams, P. "Alcohol in Hereditary Hemochromatosis Additive Hepatoxic Effect." *Hepatology* 23 (1996): 724.

———. "Factors Affecting the Rate of Iron Mobilization During Venesection Therapy for Genetic Hemochromatosis." *American Journal of Hematology* 58 (1998): 16–19.

———. "Population Screening for Haemochromatosis." *Gut* 46 (2000): 301–3.

———. "Prevalence of Abnormal Iron Studies in Heterozygotes for Hereditary Hemochromatosis." *American Journal of Hematology* 45 (1994): 146–49.

Adams, P. C., A. E. Kertesz, C. E. McLaren, R. Barr, A. Bomford, and S. Chakrabarti. "Population Screening for Hemochromatosis: A Comparison of Unbound Iron-Binding Capacity, Transferrin Saturation, and C282Y Genotyping in 5,211 Voluntary Donors." *Hepatology* 31–5 (2000): 1160–4.

Adams, P. C., D. M. Reboussin, J. C. Barton, R. T. Acton, M. Speechley, C. Leiendecker-Foster, R. Meenan, L. Passmore, C.E. McLaren, G. D. McLaren, V. Gordeuk, F. Dawkins, and J. H. Eckfeldt. "Serial Serum Ferritin Measurements in Untreated HFE C282Y Homozygotes in the Hemochromatosis and Iron Overload Screening Study." *International Journal of Laboratory Hematology* 30, no. 4 (2008): 300–5.

Adhoute, X., J. Foucher, D. Laharie, E. Terrebonne, J. Vergniol, L. Castera, B. Lovato, E. Chanteloup, W. Merrouche, P. Couzigou, and V. de Ledinghen. "Diagnosis of Liver Fibrosis Using FibroScan and Other Noninvasive Methods in Patients with Hemochromatosis: A Prospective Study." *Gastroentérologie Clinique et Biologique* 32, no. 2 (2008): 180–87.

Aguilar-Martinez, P. A., C. Biron, F. Banc, C. Masmejean, P. Jeanjean, H. Michel, and J. F. Schved. "Compound Heterozygotes for Hemochromatosis Gene Mutations: May They Help to Understand the Pathophysiology of the Disease?" *Blood Cells, Molecules, and Disease* 23 (1997): 269–76.

Aigner, E., I. Theurl, M. Theurl, D. Lederer, H. Haufe, O. Dietze, M. Strasser, C. Datz, and G. Weiss. "Pathways Underlying Iron Accumulation in Human Nonalcoholic Fatty Liver Disease." *American Journal of Clinical Nutrition* 87, no. 5 (2008): 1374–83.

Ajioka, R. S., and J. P. Kushner. "Clinical Consequences of Iron Overload in Hemochromatosis Homozygotes." *Blood* 101 (2003): 3351–53.

Ajioka, R. S., J. E. Levy, N. C. Andrews, and J. P. Kushner. "Regulation of Iron Absorption in HFE Mutant Mice." *Blood* 100 (2002): 1465–69.

Alizadeh, B. Z., O. T. Njajou, J. M. W. Hazes, A. Hofman, P. E. Slagboom, H. A. P. Pols, and C. M. van Duijn. "The H63D Variant in the HFE Gene Predisposes to Arthralgia, Chondrocalcinosis, and Osteoarthritis." *Annals of the Rheumatic Diseases* 66 (2007): 1436–42.

Allen, K. J., A. E. Nisselle, V. R. Collins, R. Williamson, and M. B. Delatycki. "Asymptomatic Individuals at Genetic Risk of Haemochromatosis Take Appropriate Steps to Prevent Disease Related to Iron Overload." *Liver International: Official Journal of the International Association for the Study of the Liver* 28, no. 3 (2008): 363–69.

Alustiza, J. M., J. Artetxe, A. Castiella, C. Agirre, J. I. Emparanza, P. Otazua, M. Garcia-Bengoechea, J. Barrio, F. Mujica, and J. A. Recondo. "MR Quantification of Hepatic Iron Concentration."

Radiology, December 10, 2003 (published online at http://radiology.rsnajnls.org/cgi/content/abstract/2302020820v1).

Andrews, N. C., and J. E. Levy. "Iron Is Hot: An Update on the Pathophysiology of Hemochromatosis." *Blood 92* (1998): 1845–51.

Announ, N., and P. A. Guerne. "Diagnosis and Treatment of Calcium Pyrophosphate Crystal-Induced Arthropathy." [In German.] *Zeitschrift für Rheumatologie 66,* no. 7 (2007): 573–78.

———. "Treating Difficult Crystal Pyrophosphate Dihydrate Deposition Disease." *Current Rheumatology Reports* 10, no. 3 (July 2008): 228–34.

Anthone, S., C. Ambrus, R. Kohli, I. Min, R. Anthone, A. Stadler, I. Stadler, and A. Vladutiu. "Treatment of Aluminum Overload Using a Cartridge with Immobilized Desferrioxamine." *Journal of the American Society of Nephrology* 6 (1995): 1271–77.

Asberg, A., K. Hveem, K. Thorstensen, E. Ellekjter, K. Konnelonning, U. Fjosne, T. B. Halvorsen, H. B. Smethurst, E. Sagen, and K. S. Bjerve. "Screening for Hemochromatosis: High Prevalence and Low Morbidity in an Unselected Population of 65,238 Persons." *Scandinavian Journal of Gastroenterology* 36 (2001): 1108–15.

Aust, A., L. Lund, C. Chao, S. Park, and R. Fang. "Role of Iron in the Cellular Effects of Asbestos." *Inhalation Toxicology* 12 (2000): 75S–80S.

Barrett, J. F. R., P. G. Whittaker, J. G. Williams, and T. Lind. "Absorption of Non-Haem Iron from Food during Normal Pregnancy." *British Medical Journal* 309 (1994): 79–82.

Barrett-Connor, E. "Looking for the Pony in the HERS Data." *Circulation* 105 (2002): 902–3.

Bartolini, G., F. F. Italia, G. Ferraro, T. Lombardo, C. Tamburino, and S. Cordaro. "Histopathology of Thalassemie Heart Disease: An Endomyocardial Biopsy Study." *Cardiovascular Pathology* 6 (1997): 205–11.

Barton, J. C., R. T. Acton, C. Leiendecker-Foster, L. Lovato, P. C. Adams, J. H. Eckfeldt, C. E. McLaren, J. A. Reiss, G. D. McLaren, D. M. Reboussin, V. R. Gordeuk, M. R. Speechley, R. D. Press, and F. W. Dawkins. "Characteristics of Participants with Self-Reported Hemochromatosis or Iron Overload at HEIRS Study Initial Screening." *American Journal of Hematology* 83, no. 2 (2008): 126–32.

Barton, J. C., E. H. Barton, L. F. Bertoli, C. H. Gothard, and J. S. Sherrer. "Intravenous Iron Dextran Therapy in Patients with Iron Deficiency Anemia and Normal Renal Function Who Failed to Respond to or

Did Not Tolerate Oral Iron Supplementation." *American Journal of Medicine*, 109 (2000): 27–32.

Barton, J. C., and C. Q. Edwards, eds. *Genetics, Pathophysiology, Diagnosis and Treatment*. New York: Cambridge University Press, 2000.

Barton, J. C., C. Leiendecker-Foster, D. M. Reboussin, P. C. Adams, R. T. Acton, and J. H. Eckfeldt. "Hemochromatosis and Iron Overload Screening Study Research Investigators." *Thyroid* 18, no. 8 (2008): 831–38.

Barton, J. C., C. Leiendecker-Foster, D. M. Reboussin, P. C. Adams, R. T. Acton, and J. H. Eckfeldt, et al. "Thyroid-Stimulating Hormone and Free Thyroxine Levels in Persons with HFE C282Y Homozygosity, A Common Hemochromatosis Genotype: The HEIRS Study." *Thyroid* 18, no. 8 (2008): 831–38.

Barton, J. C., S. M. McDonnell, P. C. Adams, P. Brissot, L. W. Powell, C. Q. Edward, J. D. Cook, and K. V. Kowdley. "Management of Hemochromatosis." *Annals of Internal Medicine* 129 (1998): 932–39.

Barton, J. C., S. V. Rao, N. M. Pereira, T. Gelbart, E. Beutler, C. A. Rivers, and R. T. Acton. "Juvenile Hemochromatosis in the Southeastern United States: A Report of Seven Cases in Two Kinships." *Blood Cells, Molecules, and Disease* 29 (2002): 104–15.

Bartzokis, G., J. Cummings, S. Perlman, D. R. Hance, and J. Mintz. "Increased Basal Ganglia Iron Levels in Huntington Disease." *Archives of Neurology* 56 (1999): 569–74.

Bartzokis, G., D. Sultxer, J. Cummings, L. E. Hold, D. B. Hance, V. W. Henderson, and J. Mintz. "In Vivo Evaluation of Brain Iron in Alzheimer's Disease Using Magnetic Resonance Imaging." *Archives of General Psychiatry* 57 (2000): 47–53.

Bassett, M. L., S. R. Wilson, and J. A. Cavanaugh. "Penetrance of HFE Related Hemochromatosis in Perspective." *Hepatology* 36 (2002): 500–3.

Bathum, L., L. Christiansen, H. Nybo, K. A. Ramberg, D. Gaist, B. Jeune, N. E. Petersen, I. Baupel, and K. Christensen. "Association of Mutations in the Hemochromatosis Gene with Shortened Life Expectancy." *Archives of Internal Medicine* 61 (2001): 2441–44.

Beard J. L., Connor J. R. Iron status and neural functioning. *Annual Review of Nutrition* (2003) 23: 41–58.

Beaton, M., and P. C. Adams. "Assessment of Silent Liver Fibrosis in Hemochromatosis C282Y Homozygotes with Normal Transaminase Levels." *Clinical Gastroenterology and Hepatology* 6, no. 6 (2008): 713–14.

Beaton, M., D. Guyader, Y. Deugnier, R. Moirand, S. Chakrabarti, and P. Adams. "Noninvasive Prediction of Cirrhosis in C282Y-Linked Hemochromatosis." *Hepatology* 36 (2002): 673–78.

Beard, J., and B. Tobin. "Iron Status and Exercise." *American Journal of Clinical Nutrition* 72 (2001): S594–7.

Beard, J. L., "Iron Requirements in Adolescent Females." *Journal of Nutrition* 130 (2000): 440S–442S.

Bendich, A. "Calcium Supplementation and Iron Status of Females." *Nutrition* 17 (2001): 46–51.

Benyamin, B., A. F. McRae, G. Zhu, S. Gordon, A. K. Henders, A. Palotie, L. Peltonen, N. G. Martin, G. W. Montgomery, J. B. Whitfield, and P. M. Visscher. "Variant in TF and HFE Explain Approximately 40% of Genetic Variation in Serum-Transferrin Levels." *American Journal of Human Genetics* 84, no. 1 (2009): 60–65.

Beutler, E. "Targeted Disruption of the HFE Gene." *Proceedings of the National Academy of Sciences USA* 95 (1998): 2033–34.

Beutler, E., V. Felitti, T. Gelbart, and N. Ho. "The Effect of HFE Genotypes on Measurements of Iron Overload in Patients Attending a Health Appraisal Clinic." *Annals of Internal Medicine* 133 (2000): 329–37.

Beutler, E., V. Felitti, J. Koziol, J. J. Ho, and T. Gelbart. "Penetrance of 845G A (C282Y) *HFE* Hereditary Hemochromatosis Mutation in the USA." *Lancet* 359 (2002): 211–18.

Bolan, C. D., C. Conry-Cantilena, G. Mason, T. A. Rouault, and S. F. Leitman. "MCV as a Guide to Phlebotomy Therapy for Hemochromatosis." *Transfusion* 41, no. 6 (2001): 819–27.

Bonkovsky, H. L. "Iron and the Liver." *American Journal of Medical Science* 301 (1991): 32–43.

Bonkovsky, H. L., and R. W. Lambrecht. "Iron-induced Liver Injury." *Clinical Liver Disease* 4 (2000): 409–29, vi–vii.

Bonkovsky, H. L., R. W. Lambrecht, and Y. Shan. "Iron as a Co-Morbid Factor in Nonhemochromatotic Liver Disease." *Alcohol* 30, no. 2 (2003): 137–44.

Bonkovsky, H. L., and J. V. Obando. "Role of HFE Gene Mutations in Liver Diseases Other Than Hereditary Hemochromatosis." *Current Gastroenterology Reports* 1 (1999): 30–37.

Bonkovsky, H. L., R. B. Rubin, E. E. Cable, A. Davidoff, T. H. Pels Rijcken, and D. D. Stark. "Hepatic Iron Concentration: Noninvasive Estimation by Means of MR Imaging Techniques." *Radiology* 21 (1999): 227–34.

Bonkovsky, H. L., N. Troy, K. McNeal, B. F. Banner, A. Sharma, J. Obando, S. Mehta, R. S. Koff, O. Liu, and C. C. Hsieh. "Iron and HFE or TfR1 Mutations as Comorbid Factors for Development and Progression of Chronic Hepatitis C." *Journal of Hepatology* 37 (2002): 848–54.

Bothwell, T. H., R. W. Carlton, and A. G. Motulsky. "Hemochromatosis." In *The Metabolic Basis of Inherited Disease,* ed. C. R. Scriver, A. L. Beaudet, W. S. Sly, and D. Valle, 6th ed., 1411–62. New York: McGraw Information Sciences, 1989.

Bothwell, T. H., and A. P. MacPhail. "Hereditary Hemochromatosis: Etiologic, Pathologic, and Clinical Aspects." *Seminars in Hematology* 35 (1998): 55–71.

Brady, J. J., H. A. Jackson, A. G. Roberts, R. R. Morgan, S. D. Whatley, G. L. Rowlands, C. Darby, E. Shudell, R. Watson, J. Paider, M. W. Worwood, and G. H. Elder. "Co-Inheritance of Mutations in the Uroporphyrinogen Decarboxylase and Hemochromatosis Genes Accelerates the Onset of Porphyria Cutanea Tarda." *Journal of Investigative Dermatology* 115 (2000): 868–74.

Bralet, M. P., J. M. Regimbeau, P. Pineau, S. Dubois, G. Loas, F. Degos, D. Valla, J. Belghiti, C. Degott, and B. Terris. "Hepatocellular Carcinoma Occurring in Nonfibrotic Liver: Epidemiologic and Histopathologic Analysis of 80 French Cases." *Hepatology* 32 (2000): 200–4.

Brandhagen, D. J., V. F. Fairbanks, and W. Baldus. "Recognition and Management of Hereditary Hemochromatosis." *American Family Physician* 65 (2002): 853–60.

Brandhagen, D. J., V. F. Fairbanks, W. P. Baldus, C. I. Smith, K. E. Kruckeberg, D. J. Schaid, and S. N. Thibodeau. "Prevalence and Clinical Significance of HFE Gene Mutations in Patients with Iron Overload." *American Journal of Gastroenterology* 95 (2000): 2910–14.

Brissot, P., M. B. Troadec, E. Bardou-Jacquet, C. Le Lan, A. M. Jouanolle, Y. Deugnier, and O. Loreal. "Current Approach to Hemochromatosis." *Blood Reviews* 22, no. 4 (2008): 195–210.

Brittenham, G. M., A. L. Franks, and F. R. Rickles. "Research Priorities in Hereditary Hemochromatosis." *Annals of Internal Medicine* 129 (1998): 993–96.

Brittenham, G. M., G. Weiss, P. Brissot, F. Lainé, A. Guillygomarch, D. Guyader, R. Moirand, and Y. Deugnier. "Clinical Consequences of New Insights in the Pathophysiology of Disorders of Iron and Heme Metabolism." *Hematology: American Society of Hematology Education Program* (2000): 39–50.

Burdo, J. R., and J. R. Connor. "Brain Iron Uptake and Homeostatic Mechanisms: An Overview." *BioMetals* 16 (2003): 63–75.

Bureau, J. P., P. Blanc, and T. Lavabre-Bertrand. "Association of Familial Pernicious Anemia and Hereditary Haemochromatosis." *Acta Haematologica* 119, no. 1 (2008): 12–4.

Burke, M. D. "Liver Function: Test Selection and Interpretation of Results." *Clinical Laboratory Medicine* 22 (2002): 377–90.

Burke, W., G. Imperatore, S. M. McDonnell, R. C. Baron, and M. J. Khoury. "Contribution of Different *HFE* Genotypes to Iron Overload Disease: A Pooled Analysis." *Genetic Medicine* 2 (2000): 271–77.

Burke, W., E. Thomson, M. Khoury, S. McDonnell, N. Press, P. Adams, J. Barton, E. Beutler, G. Brittenham, A. Buchanan, E. Clayton–Wright, M. Cogswell, E. Meslin, A. Motulsky, L. Powell, E. Sigal, B. Wilfond, and F. Collins. "Hereditary Hemochromatosis: Gene Discovery and Its Implications for Population Based Screening." *Journal of the American Medical Association* 280 (1998): 172–78.

Camaschella, C., A. Roetto, A. Cali, M. De Gobbi, G. Garozzo, M. Carella, N. Majorano, A. Totaro, and P. Gasparini. "The Gene TFR2 Is Mutated in a New Type of Haemochromatosis Mapping to 7q22." *Nature Genetics* 25 (2000): 14–15.

Camaschella, C., A. Roetto, M. Cicilano, P. Pasquero, S. Bosio, L. Gubetta, F. Di Vito, D. Girelli, A. Totaro, M. Carella, A. Grifa, and P. Gasparini. "Juvenile and Adult Hemochromatosis Are Distinct Genetic Disorders." *European Journal of Human Genetics* 5 (1997): 371–75.

Camaschella, C., A. Roetto, and M. De Gobbi. "Genetic Haemochromatosis: Genes and Mutations Associated with Iron Loading." *Best Practices in Research Clinical Haematology* 15 (2002): 261–76.

Camaschella, C., A. Roetto, and M. De Gobbi. "Juvenile Hemochromatosis." *Seminars in Hematology* 39 (2002): 242–48.

Carroll, G. J. "Primary Osteoarthritis in the Ankle Joint Is Associated with Finger Metacarpophalangeal Osteoarthritis and the H63D Mutation in the HFE Gene: Evidence for a Hemochromatosis-Like Polyarticular Osteoarthritis Phenotype." *Journal of Clinical Rheumatology* 12, no. 3 (2006): 109–13.

Casale, G., M. Bignamini, and P. de Nicola. "Does Blood Donation Prolong Life Expectance?" *Vox Sang* 45 (1983): 398–99.

Centers for Disease Control and Prevention. "CDC Criteria for Anemia in Children and Childbearing Aged Women." *Morbidity & Mortality Weekly Report* 38 (1989): 400–4.

———. "Recommendations to Prevent and Control Iron Deficiency in the United States." *Morbidity & Mortality Weekly Report* 47 (1998): 1–28.

Charles, J., G. Miller, and C. Harrison. "Management of Haemachromatosis in General Practice." *Australian Family Physician* 36, no. 10 (2007): 792–93.

Chevrant-Breton, J., M. Simon, M. Bourel, and B. Ferrand. "Cutaneous Manifestations of Idiopathic Hemochromatosis. Study of 100 Cases." *Archives of Dermatology* 113 (1977): 161–65.

Chitturi S., and J. George. "Interaction of Iron, Insulin Resistance, and Nonalcoholic Steatohepatitis." *Current Gastroenterology Reports* 5 (2003): 18–25.

Conlon, B. J., and D. W. Smith. "Supplemental Iron Exacerbates Aminoglycoside Otoxicity in vivo." *Hearing Research* 115 (1998): 1–5.

Connor, J. R. "Iron in Central Nervous System Disorders." In *Key Topics in Brain Research*, ed. P. Riederer and M. B. H. Youdim, 1–18. Vienna: Springer-Verlag, 1993.

Connor, J. R., and S. A. Benkovic. "Iron Regulation in the Brain: Histochemical, Biochemical, and Molecular Considerations." *Annals of Neurology* 32 (1992): S51–S61.

Connor, J. R., P. J. Boyer, S. L. Menzies, B. Dellinger, R. P. Allen, W. G. Ondo, and C. J. Early. "Neuropathological Examination Suggests Impaired Brain Iron Acquisition in Restless Legs Syndrome." *Neurology* 61 (2003): 304–9.

Connor, J. R., E. A. Milward, S. Moalem, M. Sampietro, P. Boyer, M. E. Percy, C. Vergani, R. J. Scott, and M. Chorney. "Is Hemochromatosis a Risk Factor for Alzheimer's Disease?" *Journal of Alzheimer's Disease* 3 (2001): 471–77.

Conrad, M. E., J. N. Umbreit, E.G. Moore, L. N. Hainsworth, M. Porubcin, M. J. Simovich, M. T. Nakada, K. Dolan, and M. D. Garrick. "Separate Pathways for Cellular Uptake of Ferric and Ferrous Iron." *American Journal of Physiology and Gastrointestinal Liver Physiology* 279 (2000): G767–74.

Conte, D., D. Barisani, C. Mandelli, S. Fargion, A. L. Fracanzani, L. Cesarini, P. Bodini, S. Pistoso, and P. A. Bianchi. "Prevalence of Cholelithiasis in Alcoholic and Genetic Haemochromatotic Cirrhosis." *Alcohol and Alcoholism* 28 (1993): 581–84.

Cook, J. D., and C. A. Finch. "Assessing Iron Status of a Population." *American Journal of Clinical Nutrition* 32 (1979): 2115–19.

Cook, J. D., C. A. Finch, and N. J. Smith. "Evaluation of the Iron Status of a Population." *Blood* 48 (1976): 449–55.

Cook, J. D., and M. B. Reddy. "Ascorbic Acid Has a Pronounced Enhancing Effect on the Absorption of Dietary Nonheme Iron When

Assessed by Feeding Single Meals to Fasting Subjects." *American Journal of Clinical Nutrition* 73 (2001): 93–98.

Cook, J. D., B. S. Skikne, S. R. Lynch, and M. E. Reusser. "Estimates of Iron Sufficiency in the US Population." *Blood* 68 (1986): 726–31.

Crawford, D. H., T. L. Murphy, L. E. Ramm, L. M. Fletcher, A. D. Clouston, G. J. Anderson, V. N. Subramaniam, L. W. Powell, and G. A. Ramm. "Serum Hyaluronic Acid with Serum Ferritin Accurately Predicts Cirrhosis and Reduces the Need for Liver Biopsy in C282Y Hemochromatosis." *Hepatology* 49, no. 2 (2009): 418–25.

Crawford, D. H. G., E. C. Jazwinska, L. M. Cullen, and L. W. Powell. "Expression of HLA-Linked Hemochromatosis in Subjects Homozygous or Heterozygous for the C282Y Mutation." *Gastroenterology* 114 (1998): 1003–8.

Cribier, B., C. Chiaverini, N. Dali-Youcef, M. Schmitt, M. Grima, C. Hirth, J. P. Lacour, and O. Chosidow. "Porphyria Cutanea Tarda, Hepatitis C, Uroporphyrinogen Decarboxylase and Mutations of HFE Gene. A Case-Control Study." *Dermatology* 218, no. 1 (2009): 15–21.

Criswell, L. A., L. A. Merlino, J. R. Cerhan, T. R. Mikuls, A. S. Mudano, M. Burma, P. Folsom, A. R. Folsom, and K. G. Saag. "Cigarette Smoking and the Risk of Rheumatoid Arthritis among Postmenopausal Women: Results from the Iowa Women's Health Study." *American Journal of Medicine* 112 (2002): 465–71.

Crosby, W. H. "A History of Phlebotomy Therapy for Hemochromatosis." *American Journal of the Medical Sciences* 301 (1991): 28–30.

Cruickshanks, K. J., R. Klein, B. E. Klein, T. L. Wiley, D. M. Nondahl, and T. S. Tweed. "Cigarette Smoking and Hearing Loss." *Journal of the American Medical Association* 279 (1998): 1715–19.

Cutlet, P. "Iron Overload and Psychiatric Illness." *Canadian Journal of Psychiatry* 39 (1994): 8–11.

Dalhoj, J., H. Kiaer, P. Wiggers, R. W. Grady, R. L. Jones, and A. S. Knisely. "Iron Storage Disease in Parents and Sibs of Infants with Neonatal Hemochromatosis: 30-Year Follow-up." *American Journal of Medical Genetics* 37 (1990): 342–45.

Davidsen, E. S., T. Hervig, P. Omvik, and E. Gerdts. "Left Ventricular Long-Axis Function in Treated Haemochromatosis." *International Journal of Cardiovascular Imaging* 25, no. 3 (2009): 249–50.

Davidsen, E. S., P. Omvick, T. Hervig, and E. Gerdts. "Left Ventricular Diastolic Function in Patients with Treated Haemochromatosis." *Scandinavian Cardiovascular Journal* 43, no. 1 (2009): 32–38.

Davidsson, L., T. Walcyk, N. Zavaleta, and R. F. Hurrell. "Improving Iron Absorption from a Peruvian School Breakfast Meal by Adding Ascorbic Acid or Na (2) EDTA." *American Journal of Clinical Nutrition* 73 (2001): 283–87.

Davis, T. M., J. Beilby, W. A. Davis, J. K. Olynyk, G.P. Jeffrey, E. Rossi, C. Boyder, and D. G. Bruce. "Prevalence, Characteristics, and Prognostic Significance of HFE Gene Mutations in Type 2 Diabetes: The Fremantle Diabetes Study." *Diabetes Care* 31, no. 9 (2008): 1795–1801.

de Gobbi, M., F. Daraio, C. Oberkanins, A. Moritz, F. Kury, G. Fiorelli, and G. Camaschella. "Analysis of *HFE* and TFR2 Mutations in Selected Blood Donors with Biochemical Parameters of Iron Overload." *Haematologica* 4 (2003): 396–401.

de Gobbi, M. A. Roetto, A. Piperno, R. Mariani, F. Alberti, G. Papanikolaou, M. Politou, G. Lockistch, D. Girelli, S. Gargion, T. M. Cox, P. Gasparini, M. Cazzola, and C. Camaschella. "Natural History of Juvenile Haemochromatosis." *British Journal of Haematology* 117 (2002): 973–79.

Deugnier, Y., P. Brissot, and O. Loreal. "Iron and the Liver: Update 2008." *Journal of Hepatology* 48 (2008): S113–23.

Deugnier, Y., and J. Mosser. "Modifying Factors of the HFE Hemochromatosis Phenotype." *Expert Review of Gastroenterology & Hepatology* 2, no. 4 (2008): 531–40.

Deugnier, Y., and B. Turlin. "Pathology of Hepatic Iron Overload." *World Journal of Gastroenterology* 13, no. 35 (2007): 4755–60.

de Valk, B., and J. Marx. "Iron, Atherosclerosis, and Ischemic Heart Disease." *Archives of Internal Medicine* 159 (1999): 1542–48.

Dreyfus, J. "Lung Carcinoma among Siblings Who Have Inhaled Dust Containing Iron Oxides during Their Youth." *Clinical Medicine* 30 (1936): 256–60.

Drobnik, J. "Hemochromatosis." *EMedicine.com* (http://www.emedicine.com/derm/topic878.htm).

Duane, P., K. A. Raja, R. J. Simpson, and T. J. Peters. "Intestinal Iron Absorption in Chronic Alcoholics." *Alcohol and Alcoholism* 27 (1992): 539–44.

Duncan, B., R. B. Schifman, J. J. Corrigan Jr., and C. Schaefer. "Iron and the Exclusively Breast-Fed Infant from Birth to Six Months." *Journal of Pediatric Gastroenterological Nutrition* 4 (1985): 421–25.

Dunn, T., D. Blankenship, N. Beal, R. Allen, E. Schechter, W. Moore, G. Perveen, and J. Eichner. "HFE Mutations in Heart Disease." *Heart Vessels* 23, no. 5 (2008): 348–55.

Dwyer, B. E., L. R. Zacharski, D. J. Balestra, G. Perry, M. A. Smith, and X. Zhu. "Getting the Iron Out: Phlebotomy for Alzheimer's Disease?" *Medical Hypotheses* 72, no. 5 (2009): 504–9.

Ebrahim, S., and G. Davey Smith. "Mendelian Randomization: Can Genetic Epidemiology Help Redress the Failures of Observational Epidemiology?" *Human Genetics* 123, no. 1 (2008): 15–33.

Edling, C. "Lung Cancer and Smoking in a Group of Iron Ore Miners." *American Journal of Industrial Medicine* 3 (1982): 191–99.

Edwards, C. Q., T. M. Kelly, G. Ellwein, and K. P. Kushner. "Thyroid Disease in Hemochromatosis: Increased Incidence in Homozygous Men." *Archives of Internal Medicine* 143 (1983): 1890–93.

Ellervik, C., H. Birgens, A. Tybjaerg-Hansen, and B. G. Nordestgaard. "Hemochromatosis Genotypes and Risk of 31 Disease Endpoints: Meta-Analyses Including 66,000 Cases and 226,000 Controls." *Hepatology* 46, no. 4 (2007): 1071–80.

Ellervik, C., T. Mandrup-Poulsen, B. G. Nordestgaard, L. E. Larsen, M. Appleyard, M. Frandsen, P. Petersen, P. Schlichting, T. Saermark, A. Tybjaerg-Hansen, and H. Birgens. "Prevalence of Hereditary Haemochromatosis in Late-Onset Type 1 Diabetes Mellitus: A Retrospective Study." *Lancet* 358 (2001): 1405–9.

Elmberg, M., R. Hultcrantz, A. Ekbom, L. Brandt, S. Olsson, R. Olsson, S. Lindgren, L. Loof, P. Stal, S. Wallerstedt, S. Almer, H. Sandberg-Gertzen, and J. Askling. "Cancer Risk in Patients with Hereditary Hemochromatosis and in Their First-Degree Relatives." *Gastroenterology* 125–26 (2003): 1733–41.

Erdemoglu, A. K., and S. Ozbakir. "Serum Ferritin Levels and Early Prognosis of Stroke." *European Journal of Neurology* 9 (2002): 633–37.

Evert, M., and F. Dombrowski. "Hepatocellular Carcinoma in the Non-Cirrhotic Liver." [In German.] *Der Pathologe* 29, no. 1 (2008): 47–52.

Facchini, F. S., N. W. Hua, and R. A. Stoohs. "Effect of Iron Depletion in Carbohydrate-Intolerant Patients with Clinical Evidence of Non-Alcoholic Fatty Liver Disease." *Gastroenterology* 122 (2002): 931–39.

Failla, M., C. Giannattasio, A. Piperno, A. Vergani, A. Grappiolo, G. Gentile, E. Meles, and G. Mancia. "Radial Artery Wall Alterations in Genetic Hemochromatosis before and after Iron Depletion Therapy." *Hepatology* 32 (2000): 569–73.

Fallon, K.E. "The Clinical Utility of Screening of Biochemical Parameters in Elite Athletes: Analysis of 100 Cases." *British Journal of Sports Medicine* 42, no. 5 (2008): 334–37.

Feder, J. N., A. Gnirke, W. Thomas, Z. Tsuchihashi, D. A. Ruddy, A. Basava, F. Dormishian, R. Domingo Jr., M. C. Ellis, A. Fullan, L.M. Hinton, N. L. Jones, B. E. Kimmel, G. S. Kronmal, P. Lauer, V. K. Lee, D. B. Loeb, F. A. Mapa, E. McClelland, N. C. Meyer, G. A. Mintier, N. Moeller, T. Moore, E. Morikang, and R. K. Wolff, et al. "A Novel MHC Class I-Like Gene Is Mutated in Patients with Hereditary Haemochromatosis." *Nature Genetics* 13 (1996): 399–408.

Felitti, V. J. "Hemochromatosis: A Common, Rarely Diagnosed Disease." *Permanente Journal* 3 (1999): 10–22.

Fernandez-Real, J. H., G. Penarroja, A. Castro, F. Garcia-Brigado, D. Hernandez-Aguado, and W. Ricart. "Blood-Letting in High-Ferritin Type 2 Diabetes-Effects on Insulin Sensitivity and Beta-Cell Function." *Diabetes* 51 (2002): 1000–4.

Fine, D. H., D. Furgang, and F. Beydouin. "Lactoferrin Iron Levels Are Reduced in Saliva of Patients with Localized Aggressive Periodontitis." *Journal of Periodontology* 73 (2002): 624–30.

Fix, O. K., and K. V. Kowdley. "Hereditary Hemochromatosis." *Minerva Medica* 99, no. 6 (2008): 605–17.

Fleming, D. J., K. L. Tucker, P. F. Jacques, G. E. Dallal, P. W. Wilson, and R. J. Wood. "Dietary Factors Associated with the Risk of High Iron Stores in the Elderly Framingham Heart Study Cohort." *American Journal of Clinical Nutrition* 76 (2002): 1375–84.

Fleming, J., P. F. Jacques, K. L. Tucker, J. M. Massaro, R. B. D'Agostino, P. W. F. Wilson, and R. Wood. "Status of the Free-Living, Elderly Framingham Heart Study Report: An Iron-Replete Population with a High Prevalence of Elevated Iron Stores." *American Journal of Clinical Nutrition* 73 (2001): 638–46.

Fleming, R. E., K. A. Ahmad, and J. R. Ahmann, et al. "Decreased Liver Hepcidin Expression in the *HFE* Knockout Mouse." *Bioiron World Congress*, Poster No. 176, Washington, DC, May 2003.

Fleming, R. E., and W. S. Sly. "Mechanisms of Iron Accumulation in Hereditary Hemochromatosis." *Annual Reviews in Physiology* 64 (2002): 663–80.

Fletcher, L. M., K. R. Bridle, and D. H. Crawford. "Effect of Alcohol on Iron Storage Diseases of the Liver." *Best Practices in Clinical Gastroenterology* 17 (2003): 663–77.

Ford, E. S., and M. E. Cogswill. "Diabetes and Serum Ferritin Concentrations among U.S. Adults." *Diabetes Care* 22 (1999): 1978–83.

Forge, A., and J. Schacht. "Aminoclycoside Antibiotics." *Audiology and Neurotology* 5 (2000): 3–22.

Forrest, L. E., L. Curnow, M. B. Delatycki, L. Skene, and M. Aitken. "Health First, Genetics, Second: Exploring Families' Experiences of Communicating Genetic Information." *European Journal of Human Genetics* 16, no. 11 (2008): 1329–35.

Franks, A. L., and W. Burke. "Will the Real Hemochromatosis Please Stand Up?" *Annals of Internal Medicine* 130 (1999): 1018–19.

Frassinelli-Gunderson, E. P., S. Morgan, and J. R. Brown. "Iron Stores in Users of Oral Contraceptive Agents." *American Journals of Clinical Nutrition* 41 (1985): 703–12.

Frazer, D. M., K. R. Bridle, and S. J. Wilkins, et al. "Failure of Hepcidin Upregulation in Hfe-associated Haemochromatosis Implicates the Liver in the Regulation of Body Iron Homeostasis." *Bioiron World Congress*, Podium No. 25, Washington, DC, May 2003.

Fridlender, Z. G., and D. Rund. "Myocardial Infarction in a Patient with Beta-Thalassemia Major: First Report." *American Journal of Hematology* 75–1 (2004): 52–55.

Gaenzer, H., P. Marschang, W. Sturm, G. Neumayr, W. Vogel, J. Patsch, and G. Weiss. "Association between Increased Iron Stores and Impaired Endothelial Function in Patients with Hereditary Hemochromatosis." *Journal of American College of Cardiology* 40 (2002): 2189–94.

Galhenage, S. P., C. H. Viiala, and J. K. Olynyk. "Screening for Hemochromatosis: Patients with Liver Disease, Families, and Populations." *Current Gastroenterology Reports* 6 (2004): 44–51.

Ganz, T. "Hepcidin, A Key Regulator of Iron Metabolism and Mediator of Anemia of Inflammation." *Blood* 102 (2003): 783–88.

Ganz, T. "Iron Homeostasis: Fitting the Puzzle Pieces Together." *Cell Metabolism* 7, no. 4 (2008): 288–90.

Garcia, A. R., R. J. Montali, J. L. Dunn, N. L. Torres, J. A. Centeno, and Z. Goodman. "Hemochromatosis in Captive Otarids" (Proceedings AAZV and IAAAM Joint Conference, 2000), 197.

Garcia-Casal, M. N., I. Leets, and M. Layrisse. "Beta-Carotene and Inhibitors of Iron Absorption Modify Iron Uptake by Caco-2." *Cell Journal of Nutrition* 130 (2000): 5–9.

Garn, S. M., M. T. Keating, and F. Falkner. "Hematological Status and Pregnancy Outcomes." *American Journal of Clinical Nutrition* 34 (1981): 115–17.

Geleijnse, J. M., L. J. Launer, D. A. Van der Kuip, A. Hofman, and J. C. Witteman. "Inverse Association of Tea and Flavonoid Intakes with Incident Myocardial Infarction: The Rotterdam Study." *American Journal of Clinical Nutrition* 75, no. 5 (2002): 880–86.

Ghio, A. J., R. J. Pritchard, K. L. Dittrich, and J. M. Samet. "Non-heme (Fe3+) in the Lung Increases with Age in Both Humans and Rats." *Journal of Laboratory and Clinical Medicine* 129 (1997): 53–61.

Gleeson, F., E. Ryan, S. Barrett, J. Russell, and J. Crowe. "Hepatic Iron Metabolism Gene Expression Profiles in HFE Associated Hereditary Hemochromatosis." *Blood Cells, Molecules, Diseases* 38, no. 1 (2007): 37–44.

Glelijnse, J. T., L. J. Launer, A. Hofman, H. A. P. Pols, and J. C. M. Witteman. "Tea Flavonoids May Protect against Atherosclerosis." *Archive of Internal Medicine* 159 (1999): 2170–74.

Goodnough, L. T., B. Skikne, and C. Brugnara. "Erythropoietin, Iron, and Erythopoiesis." *Blood* 96 (2000): 823–33.

Gordeuk, V. R., A. Caleffi, E. Corradini, F. Ferrara, R. A. Jones, O. Castro, O. Onyekwere, R. Kittles, E. Pignatti, G. Montosi, C. Garuti, I. T. Gangaidzo, Z. A. Gomo, V. M. Moyo, T. A. Rouault, P. MacPhail, and A. Pietrangelo. "Iron Overload in Africans and African Americans and a Common Mutation in the SCL40A1 (ferroportin 1) Gene." *Blood Cells Molecules, and Diseases* 31 (2003): 299–304.

Gordeuk, V. R., C. P. McLaren, A. C. Looker, V. Hasselblad, and G. M. Brittenham. "Distribution of Transferrin Saturation in the African American Population." *Blood* 91 (1998): 2175–79.

Goswami, S. K., and D. K. Das. "Autophagy in the Myocardium: Dying for Survival?" *Experimental and Clinical Cardiology* 11, no. 3 (2006): 183–88.

Griffith, I. J., and S. A. Abrams. "Iron and Breastfeeding." *Pediatric Clinics of North America* 48 (2001): 401–13.

Guggenbuhl, P., R. Filmon, G. Mabilleau, M. F. Basle, and D. Chappard. "Iron Inhibits Hydroxyapatite Crystal Growth in vitro." *Metabolism* 57, no. 7 (2008): 903–10.

Guillen, C., I. B. McInnes, D. Vaughan, A. B. J. Speekenbrick, and J. H. Brock. "The Effects of Local Administration of Lactoferrin on Inflammation in Murine Autoimmune and Infectious Arthritis." *Arthritis and Rheumatism* 43 (2000): 2073–80.

Gum, P. A., M. Thamilarasan, J. Watanabe, E. H. Blackstone, and M. S. Lauer. "Aspirin Use and All-Cause Mortality among Patients Being Evaluated for Known or Suspected Coronary Artery Disease." *Journal of the American Medical Association* 286 (2001): 1187–94.

Guyader, D., C. Jacquelinet, R. Moirand, B. Turlin, M. H. Mendler, J. Chaperon, V. David, P. Brissot, P. Adams, and Y. Deugnier. "Noninvasive Prediction of Fibrosis in C282Y Homozygous Hemochromatosis." *Gastroenterology* 115 (1998): 929–36.

Hahn, P., A. H. Milam, and J. L. Dunaief. "Maculas Affected by Age-Related Macular Degeneration Contain Increased Chelatable Iron in the Retinal Pigment Epithelium and Bruch's Membrane." *Archives of Ophthalmology* 121 (2003): 1099–1105.

Hallberg, L., and L. Hulthen. "Prediction of Dietary Iron Absorption: An Algorithm for Calculating Absorption and Bioavailability of Dietary Iron." *American Journal of Clinical Nutrition* 71 (2000): 1147–60.

Han, O., M. L. Failla, A. D. Hill, E. R. Morris, and J. C. Smith Jr. "Inositol Phosphates Inhibit Uptake and Transport of Iron and Zinc by a Human Intestinal Cell Line." *Journal of Nutrition* 124 (1994): 580–87.

Harmatz, P., E. Butensky, K. Quirolo, R. Williams, L. Ferrell, T. Moyer, D. Golden, L. Neumayr, and E. Vichinsky. "Severity of Iron Overload in Patients with Sickle Cell Disease Receiving Chronic Red Blood Cell Transfusion Therapy." *Blood* 96 (2000): 76–79.

Harris, Z. L., A. Durley, T. Man, and J. Gitlin. "Targeted Gene Disruption Reveals an Essential Role for Ceruloplasmin in Cellular Iron Efflux." *Proceedings of the National Academy of Sciences USA* 96 (1999): 10812–7.

Harris, Z. L., Y. Takahashi, H. Miyajima, M. Serizawa, R. MacGillivray, and J. Gitlin. "Aceruloplasminemia: Molecular Characterization of this Disorder of Iron Metabolism." *Proceedings of the National Academy of Sciences USA* 92 (1995): 2539–43.

Harrison, S. A., and B. R. Bacon. "Hereditary Hemochromatosis: Update for 2003." *Journal of Hepatology* 38 (2003): S14–S23.

Hellman, N. E., and J. D. Gitlin. "Ceruloplasmin Metabolism and Function." *Annual Review of Nutrition* 22 (2002): 439–58.

Hemminki, E., K. Nemet, M. Horvath, M. Malin, D. Schuler, and S. Hollan. "Impact of Iron Fortification of Milk Formulas on Infants' Growth and Health." *Nutrition Research* 15 (1995): 491–503.

Hemminki, E., and U. Rimpela. "A Randomized Comparison of Routine versus Selective Iron Supplementation during Pregnancy." *Journal of the American College of Nutrition* 10 (1997): 344–51.

Hernell, O., and B. Lonnerdal. "Iron Status of Infant Fed Low-Iron Formula: No Effect of Added Bovine Lactoferrin or Nucleotides." *American Journal of Clinical Nutrition* 76 (2002): 858–64.

Hsiao, T. J., J. C. Chen, and J. D. Wang. "Insulin Resistance and Ferritin as Major Determinants of Nonalcoholic Fatty Liver Disease in Apparently Healthy Obese Patients." *International Journal of Obesity and Related Metabolic Disorders* 28, no. 1 (2004): 167–72.

Ikeda, M. "Iron Overload without C282Y Mutation in Patients with Epilepsy." *Journal of Neurology & Neurosurgical Psychiatry* 70 (2001): 551–53.

Imperatore, G., L. E. Pinsky, A. Motulsky, M. Reyes, L. A. Bradley, and W. Burke. "Hereditary Hemochromatosis: Perspectives of Public Health, Medical Genetics, and Primary Care." *Genetic Medicine* 5 (2003): 1–8.

Imaizumi, M., C. S. Matsumoto, K. Yamada, Y. Nanba, Y. Takaki, and K. Nakatsuka. "Electroretinographic assessment of early changes in ocular siderosis." *Ophthalmologica.* (Sept.–Oct. 2000) 214 (5): 354–59.

Jacobs, E. M., J. C. Hendriks, J. J. Marx, C. T. van Deursen, H.G. Kreeftenberg, R. A. de Vries, A. F. Stalenhoef, A. L. Verbeek, and D. W. Swinkels. "Morbidity and Mortality in First-Degree Relatives of C282Y Homozygous Probands with Clinically Detected Haemochromatosis Compared with the General Population: The Hemochromatosis Family Study (HEFAS)." *Netherlands Journal of Medicine* 65, no. 11 (2007): 425–33.

Jacobs, E. M., J. C. Hendriks, C. T. van Deursen, H. G. Kreeftenberg, R.A. de Vries, J. J. Marx, A. F. Stalenhoef, A. L. Verbeek, and D. W. Swinkels. "Severity of Iron Overload of Proband Determines Serum Ferritin Levels in Families with HFE-Related Hemochromatosis: The Hemochromatosis Family Study." *Journal of Hepatology* 50, no. 1 (2009): 174–83.

Jacobs, E. M., A. L. Verbeek, H. G. Kreeftenberg, C. T. van Deursen, J. J. Marx, A. F. Stalenhoef, D. W. Swinkels, and R. A. de Vries. "Changing Aspects of HFE-Related Hereditary Haemochromatosis and Endeavors to Early Diagnosis." *Netherlands Journal of Medicine* 65, no. 11 (2007): 419–24.

Jiang, R., J. Ma, A. Ascherio, M. J. Stampfer, W. C. Willett, and F. B. Hu. "Dietary Iron Intake and Blood Donations in Relations to Risk of Type II Diabetes in Men: A Prospective Cohort Study." *American Journal of Clinical Nutrition* 79 (2004): 70–75.

Jordan, J. M. "Arthritis in Hemochromatosis or Iron Storage Disease." *Current Opinion in Rheumatology* 16 (2004): 62–66.

Kaltwasser, J. P., R. Gottschalk, and C. H. Seidl. "Severe Juvenile Hemochromatosis (JH) Missing HFE Gene Variants: Implications for a Second Gene Locus Leading to Iron Overload." *British Journal of Haematology* 102 (1998): 1111–12.

Kaltwasser, J. P., E. Werner, K. Schalk, C. Hansen, R. Gottschalk, and C. Seidl. "Clinical Trial on the Effect of Regular Tea Drinking on

Iron Accumulation in Genetic Haemochromatosis." *Gut* 43 (1998): 699–704.

Kamp, D. W., M. J. Greenberger, J. S. Sbalchierro, S. E. Preusen, and S. A. Weitzman. "Cigarette Smoke Augments Asbestos-Induced Alveolar Epithelial Cell Injury: Role of Free Radicals." *Free Radical Biology and Medicine* 25 (1998): 728–39.

Kamp, D. W., V. A. Israbian, A. V. Yeldand, R. J. Panos, P. Graceffa, and S. A. Weitzman. "Phytic Acid, an Iron Chelator, Attenuates Pulmonary Inflammation and Fibrosis in Rats after Intratracheal Instillation of Asbestos." *Toxicologic Pathology* 23 (1995): 689–95.

Kew, M. D. "Pathogenesis of Hepatocellular Carcinoma in Hereditary Hemochromatosis Occurrence in Noncirrhotic Patients." *Hepatology* 11 (1990): 1086–87.

Kiechl, S., J. Willeit, G. Egger, W. Poewe, and F. Oberhollenzer. "Body Iron Stores and the Risk of Carotid Atherosclerosis." *Circulation* 96 (1997): 3300–7.

Kirk, L., J. Bird, S. Ramadan, A. Samad, G. Adebayo, W. Lourens, and J. Williams. "Haemochromatosis Gene Frequency in a Control and Diabetic Irish Population." *Irish Journal of Medical Service* 178, no. 1 (2009): 39–42.

Klaassen, C. H., Y. A. van Aarssen, and J. W. van der Stappen. "Improved Real-Time Detection of the H63D and S65C Mutations Associated with Hereditary Hemochromatosis Using a Simple Probe Assay Format." *Clinical Chemistry and Laboratory Medicine* 46, no. 7 (2008): 985–86.

Klipstein-Grobusch, K., J. F. Koster, D. E. Grobbee, J. Lindermans, H. Boeing, A. Hofman, and C. M. Witterman. "Serum Ferritin and Risk of Myocardial Infarction in the Elderly: The Rotterdam Study." *American Journal of Clinical Nutrition* 69 (1999): 1231–36.

Knisely, A. S. "Neonatal Hemochromatosis." *Advances in Pediatrics* 39 (1992): 383–403.

Ko, C., N. Siddaiah, J. Berger, R. Gish, D. Brandhagen, R. K. Sterling, S. J. Cotler, R. J. Fontana, T. M. McCashland, S. H. Han, F. D. Gordon, M. L. Schilsky, and K. V. Kowdley. "Prevalence of Hepatic Iron Overload and Association with Hepatocellular Cancer in End-Stage Liver Disease: Results from the National Hemochromatosis Transplant Registry." *Liver International: Official Journal of the International Association for the Study of the Liver* 27, no. 10 (2007): 1394–1401.

Kudva, G. C., and B. R. Bacon. "Iron Deficiency Anemia in Hereditary Hemochromatosis after Gastric Bypass Surgery." *Annals of Hematology* 88, no. 3 (2009): 291–92.

Kuryshev, Y. A., G. M. Brittenham, H. Fujioka, P. Kannan, C. C. Shieh, S. A. Cohen, and A. M. Brown. "Decreased Sodium and Increased Transient Outward Potassium Currents in Iron-Loaded Cardiac Myocytes." *Circulation* 100 (1999): 675–83.

Lachili, B., I. Hininger, H. Faure, J. Arnaud, M. J. Richard, A. Favier, and A. M. Roussel. "Increased Lipid Peroxidation in Pregnant Women after Iron and Vitamin C Supplementation." *Biological Trace Element Research* 83 (2001): 103–10.

Laird, A. R., N. Ramchandani, E. M. deGoma, B. Avula, I. A. Khan, and N. Gesundheit. "Acute Hepatitis Associated with the Use of an Herbal Supplement (Polygonum Multiflorum) Mimicking Iron-Overload Syndrome." *Journal of Clinical Gastroenterology* 42, no. 7 (2008): 861–62.

Lamarche, J. B., M. Cote, and B. Lemieux. "The Cardiomyopathy of Friedreich's Ataxia Morphological Observations in Three Cases." *Canadian Journal of Neurological Sciences* 7 (1980): 389–96.

Lambrecht, R. W., and H. L. Bonkovsky. "Hemochromatosis and Porphyria." *Seminars in Gastrointestinal Disease* 13 (2002): 109–19.

Lamoril, J., C. Andant, L. Gouya, E. Malonova, B. Grandchamp, P. Martasek, J. C. Deybach, and H. Puy. "Hemochromatosis (HFE) and Transferrin Receptor-1 (TfR-1) Genes in Sporadic Porphyria Cutanea Tarda (PCT)." *Cell Molecular Biology* 48 (2002): 33–41.

Lapenna, D., S. De Gioia, A. Mezzett, G. Ciofani, A. Consoli, L. Marzio, and F. Cuccurullo. "Cigarette Smoke, Ferritin, and Lipid Peroxidation." *American Journal of Respiratory and Critical Care Medicine* 151 (1995): 431–35.

Lauffer, R. *Iron and Your Heart*. New York: St. Martin's Press, 1991.

Lauret, E., M. Rodriguez, S. Gonzalez, A. Linares, A. Lopez-Vasquez, J. Martinez-Borra, L. Rodrigo, and C. Lopez-Larrea. "HFE Gene Mutations in Alcoholic and Virus-Related Cirrhotic Patients with Hepatocellular Carcinoma." *American Journal of Gastroenterology* 97 (2002): 1016–21.

Lawless, M. W., M. White, A. K. Mankan, M. J. O'Dwyer, and S. Norris. "Elevated MCP-1 Serum Levels Are Associated with the H63D Mutation and Not the C282Y Mutation in Hereditary Hemochromatosis." *Tissue Antigens* 70, no. 4 (2007): 294–300.

Layrisse, M., M. Garcia-Casal, L. Solano, M. Baron, F. Arguello, D. Llovera, J. Ramirez, I. Leets, and E. Tropper. "Iron Bioavailability in Humans from Breakfasts Enriched with Iron Bis-Glycine Chelate, Phytates and Polyphenols." *Human Nutrition and Metabolism* 9 (2000): 2195–99.

Layrisse, M., C. Martinez-Torres, M. Renzi, F. Velez, and M. Gonzalez. "Sugar as a Vehicle for Iron Fortification." *American Journal of Clinical Nutrition* 29 (1976): 8–18.

Lee, P. L., T. Gelbart, C. West, C. Halloran, V. Felitti, and E. Beutler. "A Study of Genes That May Modulate the Expression of Hereditary Hemochromatosis: Transferrin Receptor-1, Ferroportin, Ceruloplasmin, Ferritin Light and Heavy Chains, Iron Regulatory Proteins (IRP)-1 and 2, and Hepcidin." *Blood Cells, Molecules, and Disease* 27 (2001): 783–802.

Lefkowitch, J. H. "Hepatobiliary Pathology." *Current Opinion in Gastroenterology* 24, no. 3 (2008): 269–77.

Leigh, M. J., and D. D. Miller. "Effects of pH and Chelating Agents on Iron Binding by Dietary Fiber: Implications for Iron Availability." *American Journal of Clinical Nutrition* 38 (1983): 202–13.

Leong, W. I., and B. Lonnerdal. "Hepcidin, the Recently Identified Peptide That Appears to Regulate Iron Absorption." *Journal of Nutrition* 134 (2004): 1–4.

Lewis, A. S., C. H. Courtney, and A. B. Atkinson. "All Patients with 'Idiopathic' Hypopituitarism Should Be Screened for Hemochromatosis." *Pituitary* 12 (2009): 273–5.

Lieber, C. S. "Biochemical and Molecular Basis of Alcohol-Induced Injury to Liver and Other Tissues." *New England Journal of Medicine* 319 (1988): 1639–50.

Lonnerdal, B. "Effects of Milk and Milk Components on Calcium, Magnesium, and Trace Element Absorption during Infancy." *Physiological Reviews* 77 (1997): 643–69.

Lonnerdal, B., and O. Hernell. "Iron, Zinc, Copper, and Selenium Status of Breast-Fed Infants and Infants Fed Trace Element Fortified Milk-Based Infant Formula." *Acta Pediatrica* 83 (1994): 367–73.

Looker, A. C., M. Loyevsky, and V. R. Gordeuk. "Increased Serum Transferrin Saturation Is Associated with Lower Serum Transferrin Receptor Concentration." *Clinical Chemistry* 45 (1999): 2191–99.

Lubitz, S. A., S. H. Goldbarg, and D. Mehta. "Sudden Cardiac Death in Infiltrative Cardiomyopathies: Sarcoidosis, Scleroderma, Amyloidosis, Hemochromatosis." *Progress in Cardiovascular Diseases* 51, no. 1 (2008): 58–73.

Mainous III, A., Diaz, V. "Cardiovascular Fitness Among Young Men." *The American Journal of Cardiology* 103 (2009): 1, 115–118.

Mallory, M. A., C. Sthapanachai, and K. V. Kowdley. "Iron Overload Related to Excessive Vitamin C Intake." *Annals of Internal Medicine* 139, no. 6 (2003): 532–33.

Martin, E. D., P. Bedossa, and P. Oudinot. "Lesions of the Area of Oddi's Sphincter: Incidence and Association with Biliary and Pancreatic Lesions in a Series of 109 Autopsies." *Gastroenterology Clinical Biology* 11 (1987): 574–80.

Mateos, F., J. Brock, and J. L. Perez-Arellano. "Iron Metabolism in the Lower Respiratory Tract." *Thorax* 53 (1998): 594–600.

McCord, J. M. "Effects of Positive Iron Status at a Cellular Level." *Nutritional Reviews* 54 (1996): 85–88.

———. "Iron, Free Radicals and Oxidative Injury." *Seminars in Hematology* 35 (1998): 5–12.

McCullen, M. A., L. M. Fletcher, G. Dimeski, A. Pink, L.W. Powell, D. H. Crawford, and P. E. Hickman. "Patient-Focused Outcomes Following Detection in a Hospital-Based Screening Programme for C282Y Haemochromatosis." *Internal Medical Journal* 38, no. 8 (2008): 651–56.

McDonnell, S. M., P. D. Phatak, V. Felitti, A. Hover, and G. D. McLaren. "Screenings for Hemochromatosis in Primary Care Settings." *Annals of Internal Medicine* 129 (1998): 962–70.

McDonnell, S. M., B. L. Preston, S. A. Jewell, J. C. Barton, C. Q. Edwards, P. Adams, and R. Yip. "A Survey of 2,851 Patients with Hemochromatosis: Symptoms and Response to Treatment." *American Journal of Medicine* 106 (1999): 619–24.

McDonnell, S. M., D. L. Witte, M. E. Cogswell, and R. McIntyre. "Strategies to Increase Detection of Hemochromatosis." *Annals of Internal Medicine* 129 (1998): 987–92.

McLaren, G. D., C. E. McLaren, P. C. Adams, J. C. Barton, D. M. Reboussin, V. R. Gordeuk, R. T. Acton, E. L. Harris, M. R. Speechley, P. Sholinsky, F. W. Dawkins, B. M. Snively, T. M. Vogt, and J. H. Eckfeldt. "Hemochromatosis and Iron Overload Screen (HEIRS) Study Research Investigators." *Canadian Journal of Gastroenterology* 22, no. 11 (2008): 923–30.

Melis, M. A., M. Cau, F. Deidda, S. Barella, A. Cao, and R. Galanello. "H63D Mutation in the *HFE* Gene Increases Iron Overload in Beta-thalassemia Carriers." *Haematologica* 87 (2002): 242–45.

Mennella, G., S. Valverde, S. Forzan, M. Fezzi, G. Munaretto, and G. Gessoni. "High Prevalence of HFE Gene Mutations in Hemodialysis Patients." *Minerva Urologica e Nefrologica = The Italian Journal of Urology and Nephrology* 60, no. 2 (2008): 81–84.

Merryweather-Clarke, A. T., E. Cadet, A. Bomford, D. Capron, V. Viprakasit, A. Miller, P. J. McHugh, R. W. Chapman, J. J. Pointon, V. L. Wimhurst, K. J. Livesey, V. Tanphaichitr, J. Rochette, and

K. J. Robson. "Digenic Inheritance of Mutations in HAMP and HFE Results in Different Types of Haemochromatosis." *Human Molecular Genetics* 12 (2003): 2241–47.

Merryweather-Clarke, A. T. et al. "Heterozygosity for Novel Hepcidin Mutations May Modify the C282Y Heterozygotes." *Bioiron World Congress*, Poster No. 80, Bethesda, MD, 2003.

Merryweather-Clarke, A. T., M. G. Zaahl, and E. Cadet, et al. "Heterozygosity for Novel Hepcidin Mutations May Modify the Phenotype of HFE C282Y Heterozygotes." *Bioiron World Congress*, Poster No. 50, Washington, D.C., May 2003.

Meyers, D. G., D. McCall, T. D. Sears, T. S. Olson, and G. L. Felix. "Duplex Pulsed Doppler Echocardiography in Mitral Regurgitation." *Journal of Clinical Ultrasound* 14 (1986): 117–21.

Meyers, D. G., D. Strickland, P.A. Maloley, J. K. Seburg, J. E. Wilson, and B. F. McManus. "Possible Association of a Reduction in Cardiovascular Event with Blood Donation." *Heart* 78 (1997): 188–93.

Milward, E. A., S. K. Baines, M. W. Knuiman, H. C. Bartholomew, M. L. Divitini, D. G. Ravine, D. G. Bruce, and J. K. Olynyk. "Noncitrus Fruits as Novel Dietary Environmental Modifiers of Iron Stores in People with or without HFE Gene Mutations." *Mayo Clinic Proceedings* 83, no. 5 (2008): 543–49.

Moirand R., P. C. Adams, V. Bicheler, P. Brissot, and Y. Deugnier. "Clinical Features of Genetic Hemochromatosis in Women Compared with Men." *Annals of Internal Medicine* 127 (1997): 105–10.

Montosi, G., P. Paglia, C. Garuti, C. A. Guzman, J. M. Bastin, M. P. Colombo, and A. Pietrangelo. "Wild-Type HFE Protein Normalizes Transferrin Iron Accumulation in Macrophages from Subjects with Hereditary Hemochromatosis." *Blood* 96 (2000): 1125–29.

Morck, T. A., S. R. Lynch, and J. D. Cook. "Inhibition of Food Iron Absorption by Coffee." *American Journal of Clinical Nutrition* 37 (1983): 416–20.

Morrison, E. D., D. J. Brandhagen, P. D. Phatak, J. C. Baron, E. L. Krawitt, H. B. El-Serag, S. C. Gordon, M. V. Galan, B. Y. Tung, G. N. Ioannou, and K. V. Kowdley. "Serum Ferritin Level Predicts Advanced Hepatic Fibrosis Among U.S. Patients with Phenotypic Hemochromatosis." *Annals of Internal Medicine* 138 (2003): 627–33.

Muckenthaler, M., C. N. Roy, A. O. Custodio, B. Minana, J. deGraaf, L. K. Montross, N. C. Andrews, and M. W. Hentze. "Regulatory Defects in Liver and Intestine Implicate Abnormal Hepcidin and Cybrd1 Expression in Mouse Hemochromatosis." *Nature Genetics* 34 (2003): 102–7.

Muckenthaler, M. U. "Fine Tuning of Hepcidin Expression by Positive and Negative Regulators." *Cell Metabolism* 8, no. 1 (2008): 1–3.

Muller-Berghaus, J., A. S. Knisely, R. Zaum, A. Vierzig, E. Kirn, D. V. Michalk, and B. Roth. "Neonatal Haemochromatosis: Report of a Patient with Favorable Outcome." *European Journal of Pediatrics* 156 (1997): 296–98.

Murray, K. F., and K. V. Kowdley. "Neonatal Hemochromatosis." *Pediatrics* 108 (2001): 960–4.

Murugan, R. C., P. L. Lee, M. R. Kalavar, and J. C. Barton. "Early Age of Onset Iron Overload and Homozygosity for the Novel Hemojuvelin Mutation HJV R54X (exon 3; c.160A→T) in an African American Male of West Indies Descent." *Clinical Genetics* 74, no. 1 (2008): 88–92.

Nelson, R. L. "Iron and Colorectal Cancer Risk: Human Studies." *Nutrition Reviews* 59 (2001): 140–8.

Niederau, C. "Hereditary Hemochromatosis." *Der Internist* 44 (2003): 191–205.

Niederau, C. "Iron Overload and Atherosclerosis." *Hepatology* 32 (2000): 672–74.

Niederau, C., R. Fischer, A. Sonnenberg, W. Stremmel, H. J. Trampisch, and G. Strohmeyer. "Survival and Causes of Death in Cirrhotic and in Noncirrhotic Patients with Primary Hemochromatosis." *New England Journal of Medicine* 313 (1985): 1256–62.

Niederau, C., G. Strohmeyer, and W. Stremmel. "Epidemiology, Clinical Spectrum and Prognosis of Hemochromatosis." *Advances in Experimental Medicine and Biology* 356 (1994): 293–302.

Nittis, T., and J. D. Gitlin. "The Copper-Iron Connection: Hereditary Aceruloplasminemia." *Seminars in Hematology* 39 (2002): 282–89.

Obejero-Paz, C., T. Yang, W. Q. Dong, M. N. Levy, G. M. Brittenham, Y. A. Kuryshev, and A. M. Brown. "Deferoxamine Promotes Survival and Prevents Electocardiographic Abnormalities in the Gerbil Model of Iron-Overload Cardiomyopathy." *Journal of Laboratory Clinical Medicine* 141 (2003): 121–30.

O'Brien, K. O., N. Zavaleta, L. E. Caulfield, J. Wen, and S. A. Abrams. "Prenatal Iron Supplements Impair Zinc Absorption in Pregnant Peruvian Women." *Journal of Nutrition* 130 (2000): 2251–55.

O'Brien-Ladner, A. R., S. R. Nelson, W. J. Murphy, B. M. Blumer, and L. J. Wesselius. "Iron Is a Regulatory Component of Human Il-1B Production." *American Journal of Respiration and Cell Molecular Biology* 23 (2000): 112–19.

Oken, E., and C. Duggan. "Update on Micronutrients: Iron and Zinc." *Current Opinion in Pediatrics* 14 (2002): 350–53.

Oldenburg, B., J. C. Koningsberger, G. P. Van Berge Henegouwen, B. S. Van Asbeck, and J. J. Rarx. "Iron and Inflammatory Bowel Disease." *Alimentary Pharmacological Therapy* 15 (2001): 429–38.

Olivieri, N. F. "The Thalassemias." *New England Journal of Medicine* 341 (1999): 99–109.

Olivieri, N. F., G. M. Brittenham, C. E. McLaren, D. M. Templeton, R. G. Cameron, R. A. McClelland, A. D. Burt, and K. A. Fleming. "Long-Term Safety and Effectiveness of Iron-Chelation Therapy with Deferiprone for Thalassemia Major." *New England Journal of Medicine* 339 (1998): 417–23.

Olynyk, J., D. Cullen, S. Aquilia, E. Rossi, L. Summerville, and L. Powell. "A Population-Based Study of the Clinical Expression of the Hemochromatosis Gene." *New England Journal of Medicine* 341 (1999): 718–24.

Olynyk, J. K., E. Gan, and T. Tan. "Predicting Iron Overload in Hyperferritinemia." *Clinical Gastroenterology and Hepatology* 7 (2009): 359–62.

Olynyk, J. K., D. Trinder, G. A. Ramm, R. S. Britton, and B. R. Bacon. "Hereditary Hemochromatosis in the Post-HFE Era." *Hepatology* 48, no. 3 (2008): 991–1001.

O'Sullivan, E. P., J. H. McDermott, M. S. Murphy, S. Sen, and C. H. Walsh. "Declining Prevalence of Diabetes Mellitus in Hereditary Haemochromatosis—The Result of Earlier Diagnosis." *Diabetes Research and Clinical Practice* 81, no. 3 (2008): 316–20.

Pankow, J. S., E. Boerwinkle, P. C. Adams, E. Guallar, C. Leiendecker-Foster, J. Rogowski, and J. H. Eckfeldt. "HFE C282Y Homozygotes Have Reduced Low-Density Lipoprotein Cholesterol: The Atherosclerosis Risk in Communities (ARIC) Study." *Translational Research: The Journal of Laboratory and Clinical Medicine* 152, no. 1 (2008): 3–10.

Pantopoulos, K. "Function of the Hemochromatosis Protein HFE: Lessons from Animal Models." *World Journal of Gastroenterology* 14, no. 45 (2008): 6893–6901.

Papakonstantinu, O., A. V. R. Mohana-Borges, L. Campell, D. Trudell, P. Haghighi, and D. Resnick. "Hip Arthropathy in a Patient with Primary Hemochromatosis: MR Imaging Findings with Pathologic Correlation." *Skeletal Radiology* 34 (2005): 180–84.

Papanikolaou, G., M. E. Samuels, E. H. Ludwig, M. L. MacDonald, P. L. Franchini, M. P. Dube, L. Andres, J. MacFarlane, N. Sakellaropoulos, M. Politou, E. Nemeth, J. Thompson, J. K. Risler, C. Zaborowska, R. Babakaiff, C. C. Radomski, T. D. Pape, O. Davidas, J. Christakis, P. Brissot, G. Lockitch, T. Ganz, M. R. Hayden, and Y. P. Goldberg. "Mutations in HFE2 Cause Iron Overload in Chromosome 1q-Linked Juvenile Hemochromatosis." *Nature Genetics* 34 (2004): 77–82.

Park, S. K., H. Hu, R. O. Wright, J. Schwartz, Y. Cheng, D. Sparrow, P. S. Vokonas, and M. G. Weisskopf. "Iron Metabolism Genes, Low-Level Lead Exposure, and QT Interval." *Environmental Health Perspectives* 117, no. 1 (2009): 80–85.

Patel, R. R., E. S. Yi, and J. H. Ryu. "Systemic Iron Overload Associated with Welder's Siderosis." *American Journal of Medical Science* 337, no. 1 (2009): 57–59.

Pawlotsky, Y., P. LeDarter, R. Moirand, P. Guggenbuhl, A. M. Juanolle, E. Catheline, J. Meadeb, P. Brissot, Y. Deugnier, and G. Chales. "Elevated Parathyroid Hormone 44–68 and Osteoarticular Changes in Patients with Genetic Hemochromatosis." *Arthritis and Rheumatism* 42 (1999): 799–806.

Pedersen, P., and N. Milman. "Genetic Screening for HFE Hemochromatosis in 6,020 Danish Men: Penetrance of C282Y, H63D, and S65C Variants." *Annals of Hematology* 88 (2009): 775–84.

Pennell, D. J. "Cardiovascular Magnetic Resonance: Twenty-First Century Solutions in Cardiology." *Clinical Medicine* 3, no. 3 (2003): 273–78.

Percy, M., S. Moalem, A. Garcia, M. J. Somerville, M. Hicks, D. Andrews, A. Azad, P. Schwarz, R. B. Zavareh, R. Birkan, C. Choo, V. Chow, S. Dhaliwal, V. Duda, A. L. Kupferschmidt, K. Lam, D. Lightman, K. Machalek, W. Mar, F. Nguyen, P. J. Rytwinski, E. Svara, M. Tran, K. Wheeler, L. Yeung, K. Zanibbi, R. Zener, M. Ziraldo, and M. Freedman. "Involvement of ApoE E4 and H63D in Sporadic Alzheimer's Disease in a Folate-Supplemented Ontario Population." *Journal of Alzheimer's Disease* 14, no. 1 (2008): 69–84.

Petrovich, I. U. A., R. P. Podorozhnaia, T. I. Genesina, and G. F. Beloklitskaia. "Iron in Oral Cavity Fluid in Gingival Inflammation." [In Russian.] *Patologicheskaia Fiziologiia Eksperimentalnaia Terapiia* 3 (1996): 22–24.

———. "Haemochromatosis." *Gut* 52 (2003, suppl.): ii23–30.

———. "Iron in NASH, Chronic Liver Diseases and HCC: How Much Iron Is Too Much?" *Journal of Hepatology* 50, no. 2 (2008): 249–51.

Phatak, P. D., and J. C. Barton. "Phlebotomy-Mobilized Iron as a Surrogate for Liver Iron Content in Hemochromatosis Patients." *Hematology* 8 (2003): 429–32.

Phatak, P. D., H. L. Bonkovsky, and K. V. Kowdley. "Hereditary Hemochromatosis: Time for Targeted Screening." *Annals of Internal Medicine* 149, no. 4 (2008): 270–72.

Phatak, P. D., D. H. Ryan, J. Cappuccio, D. Oakes, C. Braggins, K. Provenzano, S. Eberly, and R. L. Sham. "Prevalence and Penetrance of HFE Mutations in 4,865 Unselected Primary Care Patients." *Blood Cells, Molecules, and Disease* 29 (2002): 41–47.

Phatak, P. D., R. L. Sham, R. F. Raubertas, K. Dunnigan, M. T. O'Leary, C. Braggins, and J. D. Cappuccio. "Prevalence of Hereditary Hemochromatosis in 16,031 Primary Care Patients." *Annals of Internal Medicine* 129 (1998): 954–61.

Philpott, C. C. "Molecular Aspects of Iron Absorption: Insight into the Role of *HFE* in Hemochromatosis." *Hepatology* 35 (2002): 993–1001.

Pietrangelo, A. "EASL International Consensus, Conference on Haemochromatosis." *Journal of Hepatology* 33 (2000): 485–504.

Pollitz, K., B. N. Peshkin, E. Bangit, and K. Lucia. "Genetic Discrimination in Health Insurance: Current Legal Protections and Industry Practices." *Inquiry* 44, no. 3 (2007): 350–68.

Porto, B., R. Vieira, and G. Porto. "Increased Capacity of Lymphocytes from Hereditary Hemochromatosis Patients in Homozygous for the C282Y HFE Mutation to Respond to the Genotoxic Effect of Diepoxybutane." *Mutation Research* 673, no. 1 (2009): 37–42.

Pruchnicki, M. C., J. D. Coyle, S. Hoshaw-Woodard, and W. H. Bay. "Effect of Phosphate Binders on Supplemental Iron Absorption in Healthy Subjects." *Journal of Clinical Pharmacology* 42, no. 10 (2002): 1171–76.

Qian, M., and J. Eaton. "Glycochelates and the Etiology of Diabetic Peripheral Neuropathy." *Free Radical Biology and Medicine* 28 (2000): 652–56.

Reyes, M., D. O. Dunet, K. B. Isenberg, M. Trisolini, and D. K. Wagener. "Family-Based Detection for Hereditary Hemochromatosis." *Journal of Genetic Counseling* 17, no. 1 (2008): 92–100.

Roest, M., Y. T. von der Schouw, B. de Valk, J. J. Marx, M. I. Tempelman, P. G. de Groot, J. J. Sixma, and J. D. Banga. "Heterozygosity for a Hereditary Hemochromatosis Gene Is Associated with Cardiovascular Death." *Circulation* 100 (1999): 1268–73.

Roetto, A., F. Alberti, F. Daraio, A. Cali, M. Cazzola, A. Totaro, P. Gasparini, and C. Camaschella. "The Juvenile Hemochromatosis Locus Maps to Chromosome 1q." *American Journal of Human Genetics* 64 (1999): 1388–93.

Roetto, A., F. Daraio, F. Alberti, P. Porporato, A. Cali, M. De Gobbi, and C. Camaschella. "Hemochromatosis Due to Mutations in Transferrin Receptor 2." *Blood Cells, Molecules, and Disease* 29 (2002): 465–70.

Roetto, A., G. Papanikolaou, M. Politou, F. Alberti, D. Girelli, J. Christakis, D. Loukopoulos, and C. Camaschella. "Mutant Antimicrobial Peptide Hepcidin Is Associated with Severe Juvenile Hemochromatosis." *Nature Genetics* 33 (2003): 21–22.

Rohlfs, E. M., N. J. Shaheen, and L. M. Silverman. "Is the Hemochromatosis Gene a Modifier Locus for Cystic Fibrosis?" *Genetic Testing* 2 (1998): 85–88.

Rolfs, A., H. L. Bonkovsky, J. G. Kohlroser, K. McNeal, A. Sharma, U. V. Berger, and M. A. Hediger. "Intestinal Expression of Genes Involved in Iron Absorption in Humans." *American Journal of Physiology & Gastrointestinal Liver Physiology* 282 (2002): G598–G607.

Ross, J. M., R. M. Kowalchuk, J. Shaulinsky, L. Ross, D. Ryan, and P. D. Phatak. "Association of Heterozygous Hemochromatosis C282Y Gene Mutation with Hand Osteoarthritis." *Journal of Rheumatology* 30 (2003): 121–25.

Rosmorduc, O., R. Poupon, I. Nion, D. Wendum, J. Feder, G. Bereziat, and B. Hermelin. "Differential HFE Allele Expression in Hemochromatosis Heterozygotes." *Gastroenterology* 119 (2000): 1075–86.

Roughead, Z. K., C. A. Zito, and J. R. Hunt. "Initial Uptake and Absorption of Non-heme Iron and Absorption of Heme Iron in Humans Are Unaffected by the Addition of Calcium as Cheese to a Meal with High Iron Bioavailability." *American Journal of Clinical Nutrition* 76, no. 2 (2002): 419–25.

Roughead, Z. K., and J. R. Hunt. "Adaptation in Iron Absorption: Iron Supplementation Reduces Nonheme-Iron but Not Heme-Iron Absorption from Food." *American Journal of Clinical Nutrition* 72 (2000): 982–89.

Rubio-Tapia, A., and J. A. Murray. "The Liver in Celiac Disease." *Hepatology* 46, no. 5 (2007): 1650–58.

Ryan, E., V. Byrnes, B. Coughlan, A. M. Flanagan, S. Barrett, J. C. O'Keane, and J. Crowe. "Underdiagnosis of Hereditary Haemochromatosis: Lack of Presentation or Penetration?" *Gut* 51 (2002): 108–12.

Saarinen, U. M., and M. A. Siimes. "Developmental Changes in Serum Iron, Total Iron-Binding Capacity, and Transferrin Saturation in Infancy." *Journal of Pediatrics* 91 (1977): 875–77.

Salonen, J. T., K. Nyyssonen, H. Korpela, J. Tuomilehto, R. Seppanen, and R. Salonen. "High Stored Iron Levels Are Associated with Excess Risk of Myocardial Infarction in Eastern Finnish Men." *Circulation* 86 (1992): 802–11.

Salonen, J. T., T. P. Tuomainen, R. Salonen, T. A. Lakka, and K. Nyyssonen. "Donation of Blood Is Associated with Reduced Risk of Myocardial Infarction." *American Journal of Epidemiology* 148 (1998): 445–61.

Sampietro, M., L. Caputo, A. Casatta, M. Meregalli, A. Pellagatti, J. Tagliabue, G. Annoni, and C. Vergani. "The Hemachromatosis Gene Affects the Age of Onset Sporadic Alzheimer's Disease." *Neurobiology & Aging* 22 (2001): 563–68.

Sandberg, A. S., M. Brune, N. G. Carlsson, L. Hallberg, E. Skoglund, and L. Rossander-Hulthen. "Inositol Phosphates with Different Numbers of Phosphate Groups Influence Iron Absorption in Humans." *American Journal of Clinical Nutrition* 70 (1999): 240–46.

Sattar, N., D. C. Scott, D. McMillan, D. Talwar, S. J. O'Reilly, and G. S. Fell. "Acute Phase Reactants and Plasma Trace Element Concentrations in Non-Small Cell Lung Cancer Patients and Controls." *Nutrition & Cancer* 28 (1997): 308–12.

Schatzkin, A., C. C. Abnet, A. J. Cross, M. Gunter, R. Pfeiffer, M. Gail, U. Lim, and G. Davey-Smith. "Mendelian Randomization: How It Can—and Cannot—Help Confirm Casual Relations between Nutrition and Cancer." *Cancer Prevention Research (Philadelphia, PA)* 2, no. 2 (2009): 104–13.

Schumacher, H. R. "Hemochromatosis and Arthritis." *Arthritis and Rheumatology* 7 (1964): 41–50.

Schumacher, H. R., P. C. Straka, M. A. Krikker, and A. T. Dudley. "The Arthropathy of Hemochromatosis." *Annals of the New York Academy of Sciences* 526 (1988): 224–33.

Scotet, V., M. C. Merour, A. Y. Mercier, B. Chanu, T. Le Faou, O. Raguenes, G. Le Gac, C. Mura, J. B. Nousbaum, and F. Ferec. "Hereditary Hemochromatosis: Effect of Excessive Alcohol Consumption on Disease Expression in Patients Homozygous for the C282Y Mutation." *American Journal of Epidemiology* 158, no. 2 (2003): 129–34.

Serrao, R., M. Zirwas, and J. C. English. "Palmar Erythema." *American Journal of Clinical Dermatology* 8, no. 6 (2007): 347–56.

Shaheen, N. J., L. B. Lawrence, B. R. Bacon, J. C. Barton, N. H. Barton, J. Galanko, C. F. Martin, C. K. Burnett, and R. S. Sandler. "Insurance, Employment, and Psychosocial Consequences of a Diagnosis of Hereditary Hemochromatosis in Subjects without End Organ Damage." *American Journal of Gastroenterology* 98 (2003): 1175–80.

Sheth, S., and G. M. Brittenham. "Genetic Disorders Affecting Proteins of Iron Metabolism: Clinical Implications." *Annual Review of Medicine* 51 (2000): 443–64.

Siemens, L. J., and C. H. Mahler. "Hypogonadotrophic Hypogonadism in Human Hemochromatosis: Recovery of Reproductive Function after Iron Depletion." *Clinical Endocrinology and Metabolism* 65 (1987): 585–87.

Siimes, M. A. "Hematopoeisis and Storage of Iron in Infants." In *Iron Metabolism in Infants*, ed. B. Lonnerdal, 34–62. Boca Raton, FL: CRC Press, 1990.

Silber, M. H., and J. W. Richardson. "Multiple Blood Donation Associated with Iron Deficiency in Patients with Restless Legs Syndrome." *Mayo Clinic Procedures* 78, no. 1 (2003): 52–54.

Simsek, S., P. W. B. Nanayakkara, J. M. F. Keek, L. M. Fber, K. F. Bruin, and G. Pals. "Two Dutch Families with Hereditary Hyperferritinaemia-Cataract Syndrome and Heterozygosity for an HFE Related Haemochromatosis Gene Mutation." *Netherlands Journal of Medicine* 61 (2003): 291–95.

Steenland, K., and W. Saderson. "Lung Cancer among Industrial Sand Workers Exposed to Crystalline Silica." *American Journal of Epidemiology* 153 (2001): 695–703.

Steiber, Z., N. Ehlers, S. Heegaard, J. Hjortdal, A. Berta, and J.U. Prause. "Brown Cornea." *Graefe's Archive for Clinical and Experimental Ophthalmology* 246, no. 4 (2008): 537–41.

Stephansson, O., P. Dickman, A. Johansson, and S. Cnattingius. "Maternal Hemoglobin Concentration during Pregnancy and Risk of Stillbirth." *Journal of the American Medical Association* 284 (2000): 2611–17.

Strachan, A. S. "Haemosiderosis and Haemochromatosis in South Africans with a Comment on Etiology of Haemochromatosis." Master's thesis, University of Glasgow, 1929.

Stremmel, W., H. D. Riedel, C. Niederau, and G. Strohmeyer. "Pathogenesis of Genetic Haemochromatosis." *European Journal of Clinical Investigation* 23 (1993): 321–29.

Stuart, K. A., G. J. Anderson, D. M. Frazer, L. W. Powell, M. McCullen, L. M. Fletcher, and D. H. Crawford. "Duodenal Expression of Iron

Transport Molecules in Untreated Haemochromatosis Subjects." *Gut* 52 (2003): 953–59.

Sullivan, J. L. "Blood Donation May Be Good for the Donor." *Vox Sang* 61 (1991): 161–64.

———. "Iron in Arterial Plaque: A Modifiable Risk Factor for Atherosclerosis." *Biochimica et Biophysica Acta* (published online June 19, 2008).

———. "Iron, Plasma Antioxidants, and the Oxygen Radical Disease of Prematurity." *American Journal of Diseases in Children* 12 (1998): 1341–44.

———. "Iron Therapy and Cardiovascular Disease." *Kidney International* 55 (1999): S135–37.

Surber, R., H. H. Sigusch, H. Huehnert, and H. R. Figulla. "Haemochromatosis (HFE) Gene C282Y Mutation and the Risk of Coronary Artery Disease and Myocardial Infarction: A Study in 1279 Patients Undergoing Coronary Angiography." *Journal of Medical Genetics* 40 (2003): e58.

Tamagno, G., E. De Carlo, G. Murialdo, and C. Scandellari. "A Possible Link between Genetic Hemochromatosis and Autoimmune Thyroiditis." *Minerva Medica* 98, no. 6 (2007): 769–72.

Tamura, T., R. L. Goldenberg, J. Hou, K. E. Johnston, S. P. Cliver, S. L. Ramey, and K. G. Nelson. "Cord Serum Ferritin Concentrations and Mental and Psychomotor Dab Development of Children at Five Years of Age." *Journal of Pediatrics* 140 (2002): 165–70.

Tandon, N., V. Thakur, R. Kumar, C. Gupton, and S. K. Sarin. "Beneficial Influence of an Indigenous Low-Iron Diet on Serum Idicators of Iron Status in Patients with Chronic Liver Disease." *British Journal of Nutrition* 83 (2000): 235–39.

Tao, M., and D. L. Pelletier. "The Effect of Dietary Iron Intake on the Development of Iron Overload among Homozygotes for Haemochromatosis." *Public Health Nutrition*, 6 (2009): 1–7.

Thorburn, D., G. Curry, R. Spooner, E. Spence, K. Oien, D. Halls, R. Foxe, E. A. B. McCruden, R. N. M. MacSween, and P. R. Mills. "The Role of Iron and Haemochromatosis Gene Mutations in the Progression of Liver Disease in Chronic Hepatitis C." *Gut* 50 (2002): 248–52.

Toumainen, T. P., K. Kontula, K. Nyssonen, T. A. Lakka, T. Helio, and J. T. Salonen. "Increased Risk of Acute Myocardial Infarction in Carriers of the Hemochromatosis Gene Cys282Tyr Mutation." *Circulation* 100 (1999): 1274–79.

Tsuji, T. "Experimental Hemosiderosis: Relationship between Skin Pigmentation and Hemosiderin." *Acta Derma Venerology* 60 (1980): 109–14.

Tweed, M. J., and J. M. Roland. "Hemochromatosis as an Endocrine Cause of Subfertility." *British Medical Journal* 316 (1998): 915–16.

Umbreit, J. N., M. E. Conrad, E. G. Moore, and L. F. Latour. "Iron Absorption and Cellular Transport: The Mobilferrin/Paraferritin Paradigm. *Seminars in Hematology* 35 (1998): 13–26.

Vaiopoulos, G., G. Papanikolaou, M. Politou, I. Jebreel, N. Sakellaropoulos, and D. Loukopoulos. "Arthropathy in Juvenile Hemochromatosis." *Arthritis and Rheumatology* 48 (2003): 227–30.

Valenti, L., A. L. Fracanzani, V. Rossi, C. Rampini, E. Pulixi, M. Varenna, S. Fargion, and L. Sinigaglia. "The Hand Arthropathy of Hereditary Hemochromatosis Is Strongly Associated with Iron Overload." *Journal of Rheumatology* 35, no. 1 (2008): 153–58.

Varkonyi, J., J. P. Kaltwasser, C. Seidl, G. Kollai, H. Andrikovics, and A. Tordai. "A Case of Non-HFE Juvenile Hemochromatosis Presenting with Adrenocortical Insufficiency." *British Journal of Haematology* 109 (2000): 248–53.

Von Herbay, A., H. de Groot, U. Hegi, W. Stremmel, G. Strohmeyer, and H. Sies. "Low Vitamin E Content in Plasma of Patients with Alcoholic Liver Disease, Hemochromatosis and Wilson's Disease." *Journal of Hepatology* 20 (1994): 41–46.

Vujic Spasic, M., J. Kiss, T. Herrmann, B. Galy, S. Martinache, J. Stolte, H. J. Grone, W. Stremmel, M. W. Hentze, and M. U. Muckenthaler. "HFE Acts in Hepatocytes to Prevent Hemochromatosis." *Cell Metabolism* 7, no. 2 (2008): 173–78.

Waalen, J., V. Felitti, and E. Beutler. "Haemoglobin and Ferritin Concentration in Men and Women: Cross Sectional Study." *British Medical Journal* 325 (2002): 137.

Wang, X., C. Leiendecker-Fost, R. T. Acton, J. C. Barton, C. E. McLaren, G. D. McLaren, V. R. Gordeuk, and J. J. Eckfeldt. "Beme Carrier Protein 1 (HCP1) Genetic Variants in the Hemochromatosis and Iron Overload Screening (HEIRS) Study Participants." *Blood Cells, Molecules, and Diseases* 42, no. 2 (2009): 150–54.

Watkins, S., D. Thorburn, N. Joshi, M. Neilson, T. Joyce, R. Spooner, A. Cooke, P. R. Mills, A. J. Morris, and A. J. Stanley. "The Biochemical and Clinical Penetrance of Individuals Diagnosed with Genetic Haemochromatosis by Predictive Genetic Testing." *European Journal of Gastroenterology and Hepatology* 20, no. 5 (2008): 379–83.

Weinberg, Gene. "Development of Clinical Methods of Iron Deprivation for Suppression of Neoplastic and Infectious Diseases." *Cancer Investigations* 17 (1999): 507–13.

Weinberg, Gene. Bacteriol Rev. *Roles of metallic ions in host-parasite interactions*. Mar. 1966. 30 (1): 136–51.

———. "The Development of Awareness of the Carcinogenic Hazard of Inhaled Iron." *Oncology Research* 11 (1999): 109–13.

———. "Do Some Carriers of Hemochromatosis Gene Mutations Have Higher Than Normal Rates of Disease and Death?" *BioMetals* 15 (2002): 347–50.

———. "Iron and Susceptibility to Infectious Disease." *Science* 184 (1974): 952–56.

———. "Iron Therapy and Cancer." *Kidney International* 55 (1999, Suppl.): S131–34.

———. "Iron Withholding: A Defense against Viral Infections." *Biometals* 9 (1996): 393–99.

———. "The Role of Iron in Cancer." *European Journal of Cancer Prevention* 5 (1996): 19–36.

———. "The Role of Iron in Protozoan and Fungal Infectious Diseases." *Journal of Eukaryotic Microbiology* 46 (1999): 231–36.

———. "Survival Advantage of the Hemochromatosis C282Y Mutation." *Perspectives in Biology and Medicine* 51, no. 1 (2008): 98–102.

———. "The Therapeutic Potential of Human Lactoferrin." *Expert Opinion on Investigational Drugs* 12 (2003): 841–51.

———. "Therapeutic Potential of Human Transferrin and Lactoferrin." *American Society of Microbiology News* 68 (2002): 65–69.

Weinberg, G. A. "Iron Chelators as Therapeutic Agents against Pneumocystis." *Antimicrobial Agents and Chemotherapy* 38 (1994): 997–1003.

Weinberg, R. Ell, Sr., and E. D. Weinberg. "Blood-letting, Iron Homeostasis, and Human Health." *Medical Hypotheses* 21 (1986): 441–43.

Weiss, K. H., D. Gotthardt, J. Schmidt, P. Schemmer, J. Encke, C. Riediger, W. Stremmel, P. Sauer, and U. Merle. "Liver Transplantation for Metabolic Diseases in Adults: Indications and Outcome." *Nephrology, Dialysis, Transplantation: Official Publication of the European Dialysis and Transplant Association—European Renal Association* 22 (2007, Suppl.): viii9–viii12.

Wenzel, L. B., R. Anderson, D. C. Tucker, S. Palla, E. Thomson, M. Speechley, H. Harrison, O. Lewis-Jack, M. Fadojutimi-Akinsiku, J.

H. Eckfeldt, J. A. Reiss, C. A. Rivers, E. Bookman, B. M. Snively, and C. E. McLaren. "Health-Related Quality of Life in a Racially Diverse Population Screened for Hemochromatosis: Results from the Hemochromatosis and Iron Overload Screening (HEIRS) Study." *Genetics in Medicine* 9, no. 10 (2007): 705–12.

Wesselius, L. J., M. E. Nelson, and B. S. Skikne. "Increased Release of Ferritin and Iron by Iron-Loaded Alveolar Macrophages in Cigarette Smokers." *American Journal of Respiratory Critical Care Medicine* 150 (1994): 690–95.

Wesselius, L. J., I. M. Smirnov, M. E. Nelson, A. R. O'Brien-Ladner, C. H. Flowers, and B. S. Skikne. "Alveolar Macrophages Accumulate Iron and Ferritin after in vivo Exposure to Iron or Tungsten Dusts." *Journal of Laboratory and Clinical Medicine* 127 (1996): 401–9.

Westwood, M. A., L. J. Anderson, D. N. Firmin, P. D. Gatehouse, C. H. Lorenz, B. Wonke, and D. J. Pennell. "Interscanner Reproducibility of Cardiovascular Magnetic Resonance T2* Measurements of Tissue Iron in Thalassemia." *Journal of Magnetic Resonance Imaging* 18, no. 5 (2003): 616–20.

Whitington, P. F., and S. Kelly. "Outcome of Pregnancies at Risk for Neonatal Hemochromatosis Is Improved by Treatment with High-dose Intravenous Immunoglobulin." *Pediatrics* 121, no. 6 (2008): e1615–21.

Wigg, A. J., H. Harley, and G. Casey. "Heterozygous Recipient and Donor HFE Mutations Associated with a Hereditary Haemochromatosis Phenotype after Liver Transplantation." *Gut* 52 (2003): 433–35.

Wilson, J. G., J. H. Lindquist, S. C. Grambow, E. D. Crook, and J. F. Maher. "Potential Role of Increased Iron Stores in Diabetes." *American Journal of Medical Science* 325 (2003): 332–39.

Witte, D., W. Crosby, C. Edwards, V. Fairbanks, and F. Mitros. "Hereditary Hemochromatosis." *Clinica Chimica Acta* 245 (1996): 139–200.

Wolff, B., Völzke, H., Lüdemann, J., Robinson, D., Vogelgesang, D., Staudt, A., Kessler, C., Dahm, J. B., John, U., Felix, S. B. "Association between high serum ferritin levels and carotid atherosclerosis in the study of health in Pomerania (SHIP)." *Stroke.* 2004 35 (2): 453–57.

Wrighting, D. M., and N. C. Andrews. "Iron Homeostasis and Erythropoieses." *Current Topics in Developmental Biology* 82 (2008): 141–67.

Wu, C. H., Y. C. Yang, W. J. Yan, F. H. Lu, J. S. Wu, and C. J. Chang. "Epidemiological Evidence of Increased Bone Mineral Density in

Habitual Tea Drinkers." *Archives of Internal Medicine* 162 (2002): 1001–6.

Ye, Z., and J. Connor. "Screening of Transcriptionally Regulated Genes Following Iron Chelation in Human Astrocytoma Cells." *Biochemical and Biophysical Research Communications* 264 (1999): 709–13.

Young, L.C. "Porphyria Cutanea Tarda Associated with Cys282Tyr Mutation in HFE Gene in Hereditary Hemochromatosis: A Case Report and Review of the Literature." *Cutis* 80, no. 5 (2007): 415–18.

Zacharski, L. R., B. K. Chow, P. S. Howes, G. Shamayeva, J. A. Baron, R. L. Dalman, D. J. Malenka, C. K. Ozaki, and P. W. Lavori. "Reduction of Iron Stores and Cardiovascular Outcomes in Patients with Peripheral Arterial Disease: A Randomized Controlled Trial." *Journal of the American Medical Association* 297, no. 6 (2007): 603–10.

Zacharski, L. R., D. L. Ornstein, S. Woloshin, and L. M. Schwartz. "Association of Age, Sex, and Race with Body Iron Stores in Adults: Analysis of NHANES III Data." *American Heart Journal* 140 (2000): 98–104.

Zandman-Goddard, G., and Y. Shoenfeld. "Hyperferritinemia in Autoimmunity." *Israel Medical Association Journal* 10, no. 1 (2008): 83–84.

Zijp, I. M., O. Korver, and L. B. Tijburg. "Effect of Tea and Other Dietary Factors on Iron Absorption." *Critical Reviews in Food Science and Nutrition* 40, no. 5 (2000): 371–98.

Index

A

abdominal pain, 65, 66
acetaminophen, 71, 81
Aclasta, 84
acquired iron overload, 208. See also iron
    overload
Actonel, 84
adrenal function, 101
AFP, 73
African siderosis, 6, 110
age-related macular degeneration (AMD),
    107
AHS, 254–255
alanine transaminase (ALT), 71, 73
albumin, 71
alcohol use, alcoholism
    accusations of, 151–154
    detecting, 72
    dietary guidelines for, 233
    iron accumulation and, 8, 225–226
    in liver disease, 66, 67, 68–69
alendronate (Fosamax), 84
alkaline phosphatase (ALP), 72
alpha-antitrypsin-1 deficiency, 71
alpha-fetoprotein (AFP), 73
ALT, 71, 73
alveolar macrophages, 110
AMD, 107
amenorrhea, 130–132, 168–169
American Hemochromatosis Society
    (AHS), 254–255
amikacin, 106
aminoglycosides, 106
Andrews, Nancy, 249
anemia
    blood test indicators, 37–38
    as diagnosis, 145–146

Geritol for, 16–17
    from phlebotomy, 132, 216
anterior pituitary gland, 101
antibiotics, 106
antidepressants, 71
antioxidants, 11
antiseizure medications, 71
anxiety, during phlebotomy, 210
apheresis, 209, 212–214
arrhythmia, 85, 88, 216
arthralgia. See joint pain or disease
arthritis, 77–79, 130–132
Arthritis Foundation, 252
arthropathy. See joint pain or disease
asbestos exposure, 108
ascorbic acid, 225
aspartate aminotransferase (AST), 71–72,
    73
aspirin, 80, 210
AST, 71–72, 73
atherosclerosis, 89–90
at-risk populations, 5
Aust, Ann, 245
awareness, of hemochromatosis, 189. See
    also Iron Disorders Institute, outreach
    and advocacy

B

Bacon, Bruce R., 245
Bartzokis, George, 245
basophil cells, 40
Beard, John, 249
beta-carotene, 226–227, 235
beta cells, 98
bilirubin, 70
biopsy, liver, 41–43, 67
bisphosphonates, 84

blood bags, 205
blood centers, 199–201
blood clots, during phlebotomy, 210, 215
blood donation
    versus phlebotomy, 203
    as treatment, 12, 99
    use of blood from, 199–201
blood sugar levels, 97, 99
blood tests
    CBC, 34–40
    iron panels, 29–34, 146
    LFTs, 70–71
    phlebotomy and, 208
    procedural changes in, 47–48,
        191–192
    records of, 33–34
    role in diagnosis, 27, 155
bone health, 82–84
Boniva, 84
Bonkovsky, Herbert L., 245
brain iron balance, 92–95
Brandhagen, David, 249
breast milk, 218, 223–224
Brick, Mardi, 253
bronze diabetes, 5, 103
The Bronze Killer (Warder), 257
Buchanan, Alan, 249
butterfly needles, 205, 206, 216

C
C282S mutation, 52, 53
C282Y mutation
    carriers, 178
    explained, 51–54
    heterozygote, 140
    lung disease and, 108, 110
    PCT and, 104
calcium, 222, 232
Canadian Hemochromatosis Society,
    256–257
Caplan, Arthur, 245–246
Capnocytophaga canimorsus, 116
cardiomyopathy, 86–88
cast-iron cookware, 234
CBC, 34–40
CBC differentials, 38–39
CDC, 260
celiac sprue, 71
Centers for Disease Control and
    Prevention (CDC), 260
ceruloplasmin, 9–10
chelation therapy. See iron-chelation
    therapy
chest port, 176–177, 214–216
children, 143–144, 218, 223

cholesterol levels, 67, 70–71
cholesterol-lowering drugs, 71
chondrocalcinosis, 77, 79
chromosomes, 51
chronic fatigue, 22
chronic hemolysis, 75
chronic hepatic porphyria, 67
cirrhosis, 64, 69–70, 73
colchicine, 81
complete blood count (CBC), 34–40
compound heterozygote, 52–53, 140
Connor, James, 246
Cook, James, 246
copper, 10, 235
copper overload (Wilson's disease), 66, 71
coronary artery disease, 86, 89–90
Cottingham, Charm, 257
Crawford, Roberta, 255–256
cyberchondria, 142–144

D
DDN, 261
deferasirox (Exjade), 217
deferiprone/DMHP/L1 (Ferriprox), 176,
    217
deferoxamine (Desferal), 176, 217
de-ironing (induction) phase, 207, 208
DEM, 261
depression, 92–95, 148–149
Desferal, 176, 217
de Sterke, Irene, 174–178
de Sterke, Philip, 177–178
diabetes mellitus
    liver disease and, 66
    risk, 98, 99
    as symptom, 120–124, 151–152
    symptoms of, 98
    types, 96–98
diagnosis, of hemochromatosis
    cyberchondria and, 142–144
    delayed, in men, 3–4, 120–125
    delayed, in women, 125–139
    elevated serum iron in, 155–160
    genetic testing for, 58
    incidence rates, 119
    multiple symptoms and, 148–152
    wrong diagnosis and, 145–146
diagnostic algorithm, 34, 35
diagnostic tests and tools. See also specific
    tests or tools
    biopsies, 41–43
    blood tests, 27, 29–40
    genetic testing, 27
    lab tests, 27–29
    liver function tests, 70–71

quantitative phlebotomy, 43–44
  scans, 44–46
dietary guidelines
foods to avoid, 209, 221
for iron avidity, 211
iron bioavailability and, 221–232
phlebotomy and, 220–221
recommendations, 232–236
divalent metal transport ions (DMT1), 10
Division of Diabetes, Endocrinology, and
  Metabolic Diseases (DEM), 261
Division of Digestive Diseases and
  Nutrition (DDN), 261
Division of Kidney, Urologic, and
  Hematologic Diseases (KUH), 261–262
DMHP (Ferriprox), 176, 217
DMT1, 10
DNA, 51
doctors. See physicians
double red-blood-cell apheresis (DRCA),
  209, 212–214
drug side effects, 66, 71, 106

E
E. coli, 114
EDTA, 216
egg factor, 232
electrocardiogram (EKG), 90–91
ELSI, 56–57
emergency preparedness, 237–240
Emla cream, 210
emotions, 142–144, 148–149. See also
  depression
endocrine system, 96–102
environmental hazards, 108–112
eosonophils, 40
erythrocytes. See red blood cells (RBCs)
esophageal varices, 69
Ethical, Legal, and Social Implications
  (ELSI) Research Program, 56–57
ethnicity, 53–54, 110
ethylenediaminetetraacetic acid (EDTA), 216
executive panels (blood tests), 47–48, 155
exercise, 81
Exjade, 217
exocrine system, 100

F
family medical history
  data collection tool, 21
  diabetes risk and, 98
  heart disease in, 85
  hemochromatosis and, 125–127, 130–
    139, 161–165 (See also genetics;
    genetic testing)

family planning, 59
fatigue, 16–17, 22
fats, in diet, 66, 221, 232, 233
Feder, John, 250
feEDTA, 227
Ferriprox, 176, 217
FerriScan, 45
ferritin. See serum ferritin
Ferritometer, 45–46
Ferrochel, 227
ferrous iron, 223
ferrous sulfate, 227
fibromyalgia, 83
first documented cases, 181–187
Forman, Rhonda, 168–169
Fosamax, 84
free-radical activity
  antibiotics and, 106
  diabetes, 98, 99
  dietary fats and, 232
  heart disease or failure, 88, 89–90
  hyperpigmentation, 103
  joint pain, 82
  unbound ("free") iron and, 9, 11–12
fruits, 233
funding for research, outreach, 191, 194

G
G6PD, 210
gallbladder, 75–76
gamma glutamyl transferase (GGT), 72
Garrison, Cheryl, 188
gender bias, 128–139
genetic counselors, 55
Genetic Information Nondiscrimination
  Act (GINA), 55–56, 61
genetics, 17, 51–54, 98
genetic testing
  benefits and risks, 55–57, 61
  candidates for, 58–60
  as diagnostic tool, 27, 58, 140–141
  as screening tool, 49, 161–165
  setbacks in, 190
gentamicin, 106
Geritol, 16–17
GGT, 72
GINA, 55–56, 61
gingivitis, 105
glucosamine chondroitin, 81–82
glucose-6-phosphate dehydrogenase deficiency (G6PD), 210
gonadotrophic hormones, 101–102
government health agencies, 258–265
grans (GRs), 39
grapefruit juice, 225

gravity bags, 205
green tea, 229
GRs, 39
gum disease, 105

H

H63D mutation
    explained, 52
    heterozygote, homozygote, 54,
        140–141
    joint disease and, 82
HA, 81
hair loss, 105, 149–151
HCl, 223, 227–228
Hct, 37
health care costs, 49
hearing loss, 106
heart disease or failure
    atherosclerosis, 89–90
    cardiomyopathy, 86–88
    gerbil heart study, 90–91
    HCC and, 85
    heart attack signs, 86
    liver enzymes and, 71, 72
    minimal extraction and, 216
    as symptom, 151–152
Heberden's nodes, 77
HEIRS project (hemochromatosis iron
    overload study), 190
hematocrit (Hct), 37
heme iron, 222–223
hemochromatosis, term and definition, 4
Hemochromatosis Adventures (Brick), 253
Hemochromatosis Cookbook, 119, 209,
    221, 232–233
hemochromatosis iron overload study
    (HEIRS project), 190
Hemochromatosis Research Foundation,
    255–256
hemoglobin (Hgb), 37, 130
hemosiderin, 10, 31
heparin, 215
hepatic iron index (HII), 42–43
hepatitis, 66, 67–68, 69
hepatomegaly (enlarged liver), 22, 66
hepcidin, 65
herbal remedies, 81, 219, 221
hereditary hemochromatosis (HHC), 4–6,
    51–54
Herr, Charlie, 169–174
heterozygote, 52–53, 140
HFE gene, 51–54, 188. See also specific
    mutations
Hgb, 37, 130
HHC, 4–6, 51–54

HII, 42–43
historical perspectives
    chelation therapy, 174–178
    disease recognition, 5–6, 187–188
    first documented cases, 181–187
    premature deaths, 168–174, 178–181
HIV, 116
homozygote, 52–53, 140–141
hormone replacement therapy, 102
hormones, 100–102
H. pylori, 9, 114
Human Genome Project, 56–57
human immunodeficiency virus (HIV), 116
Hume, C. R., 242–243
hyaluronic acid (HA), 81
hydration, 234
hydrochloric acid (HCl), 223, 227–228
hyperpigmentation, 5, 103
hypochondria, 3–4
hypoglycemia, 97–98
hypogonadism, 101
hypothalamus, 100
hypothyroidism
    reference ranges, 194–195
    as symptom, 120–124, 129–130
    symptoms of, 101

I

ibandronate (Bonvia), 84
IDI. See Iron Disorders Institute (IDI)
imipramine, 94
immune system, 94–95, 113–116
impotence, 149–151
incidence rates, of hemochromatosis, 21,
    119
induction phase, 207, 208
infants and children, 143–144, 218,
    223–225
infections, 71, 113–116
infertility, 136–139
inflammation, 94, 116, 145–146
informed consent, 55, 61
insulin, 97, 99
interferon, 67–68
iron. See also iron supplements
    absorption and transport, 8–10,
        14–15, 99
    airborne, 108–112
    bioavailability, 221–232
    body distribution and requirements,
        12–14, 30
    defined, 8
    removing excess, 12 (See also specific
        methods)
    sources, 8, 108

types, 222–223
unabsorbed, 12
unbound ("free"), 9, 11–12
iron avidity, 137–138, 211
iron-chelation therapy
   ineffective, 176
   side effects, 218–219
   as treatment, 12, 99–100, 209, 216–219
Iron Disorders Centers of Excellence, 191
Iron Disorders Institute (IDI)
   advisory board members, 245–250
   infrastructure, 244–245
   logo, 242
   mascot, 242–243
   outreach and advocacy, 119, 187–
      190, 194–195, 244, 251–252
   products and services, 243
Iron Disorders Institute Network of
   Charitable Health Alliances, 251–253
iron fist, 22, 77
iron-fortified foods, 17, 227
iron overload
   blood tests for, 29
   versus hemochromatosis, 4, 208
   hemoglobin levels and, 37
   liver and, 66, 71
   quantitative phlebotomy and, 43–44
   screening for, 48–49
   undiagnosed, 75
Iron Overload Diseases (organization), 256
iron panels, 29–34, 146
iron supplements
   for anemia, 146
   excessive, 8
   Geritol, 16–17
   iron absorption and, 14–15
   for iron avidity, 211
iron-withholding defense system (IWDS),
   94–95, 110, 113–114

J

joint pain or disease
   phlebotomy and, 79–80
   as symptom, 22, 124–125, 130–132,
      149–151
   treatment of, 80–82
   types, 77–79
Jordan, Joanne M., 246

K

kanamycin, 106
koilonychia, 103–104
Kowdley, Kris, 246
Krikker, Margit, 255–256
KUH, 261–262

L

L1 (Ferriprox), 176, 217
lab tests, 27–28
lactoferrin (Lf), 9, 105
leukocytes. See white blood cells (WBCs)
Lf, 9, 105
LFTs, 70–71
liver biopsy, 41–43, 67
liver cancer, 64, 66–67
liver disease or damage. See also alcohol
   use, alcoholism; cirrhosis
   as cause of death, 22
   cirrhosis, 64, 69–70, 73
   hepatitis, 66, 67–68, 69
   from herbal remedies, 81, 219
   as symptom, 133–136, 151–152
   symptoms and diagnosis, 65–67,
      72–73
   tannins and, 229–230
   topical anesthetics and, 210
   vitamin A and, 235
liver enzymes, 22, 71–72
liver function, 65
liver function tests (LFTs), 70–71
liver transplant, 73–74
Longshore, John, 246
lungs, lung diseases, 108–112, 115
luteinizing hormone (LH), 101–102
Lyme disease, 114
lymphocytes, 39–40

M

MacPhail, Patrick, 247
macrophages. See white blood cells
magnesium carbonate, 81
magnetic resonance imaging (MRI),
   44–45, 90
Main, Christopher, 169–174
Main, Laura, 169–174, 188
Mainous, Arch III, 247
maintenance phase, 207, 208
Martin, Sam, 178–181
MCH, 38
McLaren, Gordon, 247
mean cell (corpuscular) volume (MCV),
   37–38, 209
mean corpuscular hemoglobin (MCH), 38
mean platelet volume (MPV), 38
Means, Robert T. Jr., 247
meat, in diet
   iron absorption and, 228
   iron avidity and, 211
   limiting, 209, 221
medical ID bracelets, 240
Medicare, 47, 258

medication side effects, 66, 71, 106
menstruation, 60. See also amenorrhea
metabolic disorders, 20
Meyers, David, 247
minimal extraction, 216
monocytes, 40
mononuclear phagocytes, 40
mood swings, 148–149
MPV, 38
MRI, 44–45, 90
multivitamins, 234–235
muscle-wasting disease, 71

N

NASH. See nonalcoholic steatohepatitis
National Heart, Lung, and Blood Institute
    (NHLBI), 263–264
National Human Genome Research
    Institute, 56–57, 264
National Institute of Neurological
    Disorders and Stroke (NINDS),
    264–265
National Institutes of Diabetes and
    Digestive and Kidney Diseases
    (NIDDK), 260–262
National Institutes of Health (NIH),
    260–265
needles, 205, 206, 216
neomycin, 106
neonatal hemochromatosis, 143–144
Netherlands Hemochromatosis Society, 178
netilmicin, 106
neutrophils, 39
NHLBI, 263–264
NIDDK, 260–262
NIH, 260–265
NINDS, 264–265
nonalcoholic steatohepatitis (NASH)
    liver damage and, 66, 69, 154
    liver enzymes and, 71
nonheme iron, 222–223
nonsteroidal anti-inflammatory drugs
    (NSAIDs), 80

O

oatmeal, 230
oldest survivors, 163–165
Olivieri, Nancy, 250
osteoarthritis, 77–79
osteomalacia, 82–84
osteoporosis, 82–84
overbleeding, 137–138, 160
oxalates, 231
oxidative stress. See free-radical activity

P

PAD, 89
Paget's disease, 84
pancreas, 96–97, 99–100
pathogens, 71, 113–116
patient apathy, 192–193
patient checklist, 269
PCT, 104–105
Penn State College of Medicine, 262
peripheral arterial disease (PAD), 89
phagocytes, 39, 40
Phatak, P. D., 247–248
phenolic compounds, 229
phlebotomy
    alternatives to, 209, 212–219 (See also
        specific treatments)
    compliance, 234
    as diagnostic tool, 43–44
    dietary changes and, 220–221
    excessive, 137–138, 160
    FAQ, 203–211
    joint pain and, 79–80, 82
    misguided, 142–143, 146–147
    in PAD study, 89
    records of, 209–210
    side effects, 202
    as treatment, 12, 99, 202–203
    vein appearance and, 240
phosphates, 231
phosvitin, 232
physicians
    checklist for, 267
    educating, 119, 187–190, 194–195,
        199, 244
    finding, 198–199
    ignoring advice from, 158–160
phytate, 230–231
pituitary gland, 100–101
platelets, 38
PMNs, 39
Polymorphonuclear Neutrophils (PMNs),
    39
polyphenols, 226, 229
porphyria cutanea tarda (PCT), 104–105
portal hypertension, 69
portal-systemic shunts, 69–70
preexisting diseases, 21–22
premature deaths, 168–174, 178–181
Princell, Mark, 248
prothrombin time, 70
Prozac, 94
pseudogout (chondrocalcinosis), 77, 79
publications, from IDI, 243

Q

quantitative phlebotomy, 43–44. See also
  phlebotomy

R

RBCs, 36–37
RDAs, 13–14
RDW, 38
Reclast, 84
recommended dietary allowances (RDAs),
  13–14
record-keeping
  blood tests, 33–34
  phlebotomies, 209–210
red-blood-cell distribution width (RDW),
  38
red blood cells (RBCs), 36–37, 213
red wine, 226
reference ranges
  defined, 28
  hemoglobin, 37
  hypothyroidism, 194–195
  serum ferritin, 34
  standardizing, 194–195
  TS percentage, 32, 115
research
  future funding for, 194
  gerbil heart study, 90–91
  NHLBI funded, 264
  NIDDK funded, 262–263
  setbacks in, 190–191
restrictive cardiomyopathy, 87–88
rheumatoid arthritis, 77–78
risedronate (Actonel), 84
Ritter, Jack, 181–187

S

S65C mutation, 52
Salonen, Jukka, 250
Satcher, David, 259
scans, 44–46
screening, 47–50
Scripps Research Institute, 190, 262–263
secondhand smoke. See tobacco smoke
  or use
segs, 39
septicemia, 115–116
serotonin, 94–95
serum ferritin (SF)
  defined, 10, 30–31
  in heart, 90
  in hepatitis patients, 67–68
  in liver, 65
  in misguided treatment, 142–143
  phlebotomy and, 208

reference range, 34
removal from blood panel, 191–192
role in diagnosis, 155–160
serum glutamate pyruvate transaminase
  (SGPT), 71
serum glutamic oxaloacetic transaminase
  (SGOT), 72
serum iron (SI), 31–32, 47
SF. See serum ferritin
SGOT, 72
SGPT, 71
shellfish, raw, 115–116, 221, 233
SI, 31–32, 47
siderophilin, 9
Skikne, Barry, 248
skin color, 5, 103
social implications, of hemochromatosis,
  26
sphincter of Oddi, 75
spinach, 222, 231
spleen, 75, 114
spoon nail, 103–104
SQUID, 45–46
steroids, 81
stomach acid, 223, 227–228
streptomycin, 106
strontium renelate, 84
subways, 109
superconducting quantum interference
  device (SQUID), 45–46
supplements, 221, 234–235. See also iron
  supplements
support groups, 253–254
survivors, oldest, 163–165
symptoms of hemochromatosis. See also
  specific symptoms
  multiple, in diagnosis, 148–152
  preexisting diseases as, 21–22
  reported by patients, 22–25

T

tannins, 229–230
testosterone, 102
tests. See diagnostic tests and tools
thrombocytopenia, 38
thyroid function, 101–102. See also hypothyroidism
thyroid-stimulating hormone (TSH),
  194–195
TIBC, 32, 47, 50
TIPS, 69–70
tobacco smoke or use, 8, 106, 108, 110,
  234
tobramycin, 106
tooth loss, 105

topical antiseptic, 210
total iron-binding capacity (TIBC), 32,
47, 50
total protein test, 71
tourniquets, 204
toxin exposure, 66, 108–112
transferrin, 9, 30
transferrin saturation (TS) percentage. See
TS percentage
transjugular intrahepatic portal-systemic
shunts (TIPS), 69–70
travel, 168–174, 239–240
treatment. See phlebotomy
triglycerides, 70–71
TSH, 194–195
TS percentage
calculating, 32, 33
defined, 32
as diagnostic tool, 142–143
infections and, 115
phlebotomy and, 208
reference range, 32, 115
as screening tool, 49–50
tuberculosis, 108, 110, 115

U
UIBC, 33, 50
UL, 13–14
unsaturated iron-binding capacity (UIBC),
33, 50
upper intake level (UL), 13–14
U.S. Department of Health and Human
Services, 259
U.S. surgeon general, 259

V
vacuum bags or bottles, 205, 206,
214–215
vegetables, 233
veins, appearance of, 240
vision problems, 106–107
vitamin A, 235
vitamin C, 225, 233
vitamin D, 83
V. vulnificus, 115, 233

W
Warder, Marie, 255–257
WBCs, 36, 38–40
weakness, 22
weight loss, 66
Weinberg, Gene, 248
well water, 226
Wesselius, Lewis, 248

white blood cells (WBCs)
airborne iron and, 109, 110
in immune function, 114
types and purposes, 36, 39–40
Wilson's disease (copper overload), 66, 71
women, 60, 125–139
workplace hazards, 108
Wurster, Mark, 248

Z
Zacharski, Leo R., 248–249
zinc, 235
zoledronic acid (Reclast, Aclasta), 84

Contacts

The Iron Disorders Institute provides resources on its websites such as treatment centers, healthcare providers, disease specific organizations, Web links, reading materials, educational literature, calendar of events for workshops, conferences, clinical trials, and services. Visit www.irondisorders.org or www. hemochromatosis.org for the most current information about these resources.